Radiology Fundamentals

Jennifer Kissane • Janet A. Neutze
Harjit Singh
Editors

Shalin Patel
Illustrator and Graphics Editor

Radiology Fundamentals

Introduction to Imaging & Technology

Sixth Edition

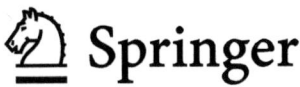 Springer

Editors
Jennifer Kissane, MD
Penn State Health Heart
and Vascular Institute
Department of Radiology
Penn State Hershey Medical Center
Hershey, PA
USA

Janet A. Neutze, MD, FACR
Department of Radiology
Penn State Hershey Medical Center
Hershey, PA
USA

Harjit Singh, MD, FSIR
Department of Radiology and
Radiological Science
Johns Hopkins Medical Institutions
Baltimore, MD
USA

Illustrator and Graphics Editor
Shalin Patel, MD
Department of Radiology
Penn State Health
Hershey, PA
USA

ISBN 978-3-030-22172-0   ISBN 978-3-030-22173-7   (eBook)
https://doi.org/10.1007/978-3-030-22173-7

This Springer imprint is published by the registered company Springer Nature Switzerland AG
The registered company address is: Gewerbestrasse 11, 6330 Cham, Switzerland

*Thank you to the sixth edition team.
I couldn't have done it without you. I am in
awe of the energy and effort put into this
project by so many, past and present—it is
what makes this such a remarkable textbook.*

*To my family, thank you for the love, support,
and encouragement.
To my Dad, thanks for watching over me.*
— Harjit Singh

*Thank you learners for giving us the
opportunity to share our passions. Thank you
family for your patience; now it's your turn.*
— Janet A. Neutze

*JN and HS, thank you for the guidance.
Contributors, thank you for the hard work.
SP, thanks for making it pretty!*

*To my husband, thank you for being
awesome; to my parents, thank you for my
work ethic; to my crazy kids, keep reading!
Remember, "N" is for the knowledge cause
I'm very, very smart.*
— Jennifer Kissane

*Thank you to my family and to the entire
RadFun team, specifically JK for the
opportunity.*
— Shalin Patel

PREFACE

The sixth edition of the *Radiology Fundamentals: Introduction to Imaging & Technology* is directed toward medical students, non-radiology house staff, physician assistants, nurse practitioners, radiologist assistants, and other allied health professionals as a curriculum guide to supplement their radiology education. This book serves only as an introduction to the dynamic field of radiology. The goal of this text is to provide the reader with examples and brief discussions of the basic radiographic principles that should serve as the foundation for further learning. We hope that it will foster and further stimulate the process at the heart of medical education: self-directed learning.

Each edition continues to expand upon the first edition of the photocopied pages and films, written and organized by the original authors, Dr. William Hendrick and Dr. Carlton "Tad" Phelps. As mentors, Dr. Hendrick and Dr. Phelps of Albany Medical Center wanted a curriculum guide to reinforce the teaching concepts of their radiology elective. Dr. Harjit Singh, editor and author of much of the text of the first print edition, formalized the material in 1988. Our third edition, updated by the faculty and students at Penn State Hershey, was a first effort at organizing and digitizing the information for publication. The fourth edition expanded and reinforced the original authors' work. The fifth edition expanded on the positive aspects of the fourth edition, including a pediatrics imaging section. The fifth edition wouldn't have been possible without the hard work of Jonathan Enterline, MD.

Our sixth edition introduces SAFE radiology, an exciting new way to approach the application of imaging to patient care. Easy to learn and easy to remember, SAFE reminds us all that safety and appropriateness should precede any imaging testing and that all results should be applied expeditiously and thoughtfully. Dr. Jennifer Kissane joins us as a new editor and brings both her diagnostic and interventional radiology expertise to those chapters.

Radiology continues to expand in breadth and depth. As consultants to our clinician colleagues and from both cost and safety standpoints, radiologists are poised to be the navigators for clinical imaging well into the future. We hope this book, used in conjunction with lectures, electives, and discussions, is a start.

Hershey, Pennsylvania

Jennifer Kissane, MD
Janet A. Neutze, MD, FACR
Harjit Singh, MD, FSIR

January 2019

CONTENTS

CONTRIBUTORS

Original Authors

William J. Hendrick Jr., MD
Albany Medical Center
Albany, NY, USA

Carlton (Tad) Phelps, MD
Albany Medical Center
Albany, NY, USA

Harjit Singh, MD, FSIR
Johns Hopkins University
Baltimore, MD, USA

Editors of the Sixth Edition

Jennifer Kissane, MD
Penn State Heart and Vascular Institute
Penn State Health
Hershey, PA, USA

Janet A. Neutze, MD, FACR
Penn State Health
Hershey, PA, USA

Harjit Singh, MD, FSIR
Johns Hopkins University
Baltimore, MD, USA

Illustrator and Graphics Editor of the Sixth Edition

Shalin Patel, MD
Penn State Health
Hershey, PA, USA

Contributors to the Sixth Edition

Amit K. Agarwal, MD
Peter O'Donnell Jr. Brain Institute
UT Southwestern Medical Center
Dallas, TX, USA
Chapters 51, 52, 53

Anita Ankola, MD
University of Florida
Jacksonville, FL, USA
Chapters 25, 27, 29, 31, 33, 35

Barry Amos, DO
Penn State Health
Hershey, PA, USA
Chapters 44, 46

James Birkholz, MD
Penn State Health
Hershey, PA, USA
Chapters 26, 28, 30, 32, 34

James M. Brian, MD
Penn State Health
Hershey, PA, USA
Chapter 56

Karen L. Brown, MS
Penn State Health
Hershey, PA, USA
Chapter 2

Rekha A. Cherian, DMRD, DNB, FRCR
Penn State Health
Hershey, PA, USA
Chapters 10, 12, 13, 14, 15, 16, 17, 18, 19, 20, 22

Christopher Enwonwu, MD
Penn State Health
Hershey, PA, USA
Chapters 9, 41

Joseph S. Fotos, MD
Penn State Health
Hershey, PA, USA
Chapters 36, 37, 38, 39, 40

Jason Gold, DO
Penn State Health
Hershey, PA, USA
Chapters 42, 45

Michael Goldenberg
Medical Student, Class of 2020
Penn State College of Medicine
Hershey, PA, USA
Chapters 36, 37, 38, 39, 40

Cristy N. Gustas-French, MD
Penn State Health
Hershey, PA, USA
Chapters 47, 48, 49, 50

Jennifer Kissane, MD
Penn State Heart and Vascular Institute
Penn State Health
Hershey, PA, USA
Chapters 9, 24, 41, 42, 45

Steven H. King, MA
Penn State Health
Hershey, PA, USA
Chapter 2

Bryce Lowrey, MD
Penn State Health
Hershey, PA, USA
Chapters 10, 12, 13, 14, 15, 16

Frank C. Lynch, MD, FSIR
Penn State Heart and Vascular Institute
Penn State Health
Hershey, PA, USA
Chapters 42, 45

Tyler McKinnon, DO
Penn State Health
Hershey, PA, USA
Chapters 17, 18, 19, 20, 22

Janet A. Neutze, MD, FACR
Penn State Health
Hershey, PA, USA
Chapters 1, 2, 3, 4, 5, 6, 7, 8

Tao Ouyang, MD
Penn State Health
Hershey, PA, USA
Chapters 54, 55

Shalin Patel, MD
Department of Radiology
Penn State Health
Hershey, PA, USA
Chapter 23

Shyamsunder Sabat, MD
Penn State Health
Hershey, PA, USA
Chapters 51, 52, 53, 54, 55

Harjit Singh, MD, FSIR
Johns Hopkins University
Baltimore, MD, USA
Chapters 11, 21

Lindsay Stratchko, DO
Penn State Health
Hershey, PA, USA
Chapter 43

Jonelle Thomas, MD, MPH
Penn State Health
Hershey, PA, USA
Chapters 47, 48, 49, 50

Mark Tulchinsky, MD
Penn State Health
Hershey, PA, USA
Chapters 36, 37, 38, 39, 40

PART I
INTRODUCTION

1 PRACTICING SAFE RADIOLOGY

It is no longer good enough to just know how to interpret imaging studies. All imaging modalities have bioeffects on tissue. Many imaging examinations ordered today are unnecessary or inappropriate, inflating healthcare costs. Imaging reports reflect the complexity of the image information and may be difficult to interpret by the ordering providers. Patients are now able to access their imaging information via electronic portals and are holding clinicians and radiologists accountable for the information in those reports.

In response to these new requirements, medical student educators in the Department of Radiology at Penn State College of Medicine created an educational program to improve patient care and increase value, utilizing a new scaffold curriculum for medical students and learners of all levels.

We created the acronym **SAFE** – **S**afety-**A**ppropriateness-(interpreting) **F**ilms-**E**xpedite and **E**xecute – as a way to remember the order in which safely, timely and appropriately ordered, interpreted, and implemented imaging should be provided. Without safety and appropriateness practiced *first*, even the best imaging interpretation may not provide the desired imaging results a patient deserves. We designed this program to align with the American College of Radiology's (ACR) Imaging 3.0 goals of providing safe, appropriate, timely, and value-based imaging to all patients and clinicians. It will also give students some insight into Centers for Medicare and Medicaid Services' (CMS) Qualified Provider Led Entity (QPLE)/Appropriate Use Criteria (AUC) programs, due to be fully implemented by 2021.

The description that follows elaborates on the concepts in each part of the SAFE program. In addition, in each of the chapters which follow, we have noted key SAFE points that relate to the modality and/or the image interpretation.

© Springer Nature Switzerland AG 2020
J. Kissane et al. (eds.), *Radiology Fundamentals: Introduction to Imaging
& Technology*, https://doi.org/10.1007/978-3-030-22173-7_1

We hope you will find the SAFE radiology concept valuable to your learning, your teaching, and your practice of applying the best imaging to the care of all patients.

S: Safety: Discuss patient and physician safety considerations in the use of ionizing radiation, magnetic resonance imaging, ultrasound, and radiology contrast materials. Describe radiology safety applicable to the pediatric, pregnant, and elderly patient. List resources available to accomplish these goals including the role of Health Physics personnel available at your practice.

A: Appropriateness: Utilize resources such as radiologists, ACR Appropriateness Criteria™, Image Gently™, Image Wisely™, and Choosing Wisely™ to order appropriate studies while managing resources and maximizing safety. Observe the role that radiology studies and radiologists play in the overall care and management of the patient.

F: Films: Use a systemic approach when evaluating chest and abdominal radiographs. Discuss core concepts in advanced imaging such as Hounsfield units (CT), T1 and T2 weighting on MRI, and fluid on ultrasound exams. Describe patient preparation for radiology studies. Observe how imaging studies are obtained.

E: Expedite and Execute: Expedite patient management by recognizing common emergent findings. Execute the knowledge you have learned about safety, appropriateness, and image interpretation to provide safe and effective patient-centered care.

2 PATIENT RADIATION SAFETY AND RISK

Objectives:
1. Understand the difference between nonionizing and ionizing radiation.
2. Understand the difference between stochastic and non-stochastic effects.
3. Be able to discuss the concept of ALARA.

Everyone is concerned about patient radiation dose. From 1993 through 2008, radiation dose attributed to medical radiation rose from 0.54 to 3 mSv per capita. The largest component of the medical patient radiation dose was CT scanning (49%). This is despite the fact that CT scanning makes up only 17% of the total medical procedures that contributes to a patient's radiation dose.

The radiation dose for all diagnostic exams should be minimized to the lowest amount of radiation needed to produce a diagnostic quality exam [1].

What Is Radiation?

Radiation is emitted from unstable atoms. Unstable atoms are said to be "radioactive" because they release energy (radiation). The radiation emitted may be electromagnetic energy (x-rays and gamma rays) or particles such as alpha or beta particles. Radiation can also be produced by high-voltage devices, such as x-ray machines. X-rays are a form of electromagnetic energy with a wavelength that places it into an ionizing radiation category. In a diagnostic exam, these photons can penetrate the body and are recorded on digital or film medium to produce an image of various densities that show details inside the body.

Light, radio, and microwaves are nonionizing types of electromagnetic radiation. Radio waves are used to generate MR images. X-rays and gamma rays are *ionizing*

© Springer Nature Switzerland AG 2020

J. Kissane et al. (eds.), *Radiology Fundamentals: Introduction to Imaging & Technology*, https://doi.org/10.1007/978-3-030-22173-7_2

forms of electromagnetic radiation and can produce charged particles (ions) in matter. When ionizations occur in tissue, they can lead to cellular damage. Most damage is repaired by natural processes. In some cases, the damage cannot be repaired or is not repaired correctly which can lead to biological effects.

There are two categories of biological effects related to radiation exposure:

Non-stochastic (also called deterministic)
Stochastic (also called probabilistic)

- *Non-stochastic* effects can occur when the amount of radiation energy imparted to tissue (dose) exceeds a threshold value. Below the threshold, no effect is observed. Above the threshold, the effect is certain.

Examples:

- Skin injury
- Cataracts

- Stochastic effects can manifest at any dose, meaning there is no threshold below which the effect cannot occur. In reality, the probability of a stochastic effect increases as radiation dose imparted to the tissue increases.

Examples:

- Cancer
- Leukemia

Where Do We Use Radiation in a Hospital?

- Radiography:

  - Fluoroscopy
  - Mammography
  - Cardiac catheterization
  - Computed tomography
  - Radiation therapy (linear accelerator)

- Radioactive material:

  - Nuclear medicine
  - Radiation therapy

Listed below are three tables – they provide an estimate of effective radiation dose from common diagnostic exams and interventional procedures (Tables 2.1, 2.2, and 2.3). As a reference standard, the average annual background radiation we all receive from the sun and soil is 3 mSv.

Table 2.1 Typical effective radiation dose from diagnostic x-ray-single exposure

Exam [1]	Effective dose mSv (mrem)
Chest	0.1 (10)
Cervical spine	0.2 (20)
Thoracic spine	1.0 (100)
Lumbar spine	1.5 (150)
Pelvis	0.7 (70)
Abdomen or hip	0.6 (60)
Mammogram (2 views)	0.36 (36)
Dental bitewing	0.005 (0.5)
Dental (panoramic)	0.01 (1)
DEXA (whole body)	0.001 (0.1)
Skull	0.1 (10)
Hand or foot	0.005 (0.5)

Adapted with permission from Mettler et al. [2]

Table 2.2 The dose a patient could receive if undergoing an entire procedure that may be diagnostic or interventional. For example, a lumbar spine series usually consists of five x-ray exams

Examinations and procedures	Effective dose mSv (mrem)
Intravenous pyelogram	3.0 (300)
Upper GI	6.0 (600)
Barium enema	7.0 (700)
Abdomen, kidney, ureter, bladder (KUB)	0.7 (70)
CT head	2.0 (200)
CT chest	7.0 (700)
CT abdomen/pelvis	10.0 (1000)
Whole-body CT screening	10.0 (1000)
CT biopsy	1.0 (100)
Calcium scoring	2.0 (200)
Coronary angiography	20.0 (2000)
Cardiac diagnostic and intervention	30.0 (3000)
Pacemaker placement	1.0 (100)
Peripheral vascular angioplasties	5.0 (500)
Noncardiac embolization	55.0 (5500)
Vertebroplasty	16.0 (1600)

Adapted with permission from Mettler et al. [2]

Table 2.3 Typical effective radiation dose from nuclear medicine examinations

Nuclear medicine scan radiopharmaceutical (common trade name)	Effective dose mSv (mrem)
Brain (PET) 18F FDG	14.1 (1410)
Brain (perfusion) 99mTc HMPAO	6.9 (690)
Hepatobiliary (liver flow) 99mTc sulfur colloid	2.1 (210)
Bone 99mTc MDP	6.3 (630)
Lung perfusion/ventilation 99mTc MAA & 133Xe	2.5 (250)
Kidney (filtration rate) 99mTc DTPA	1.8 (180)
Kidney (tubular function) 99mTc MAG3	2.2 (220)
Tumor/infection 67Ga	2.5 (250)
Heart (stress-rest) 99mTc sestamibi (Cardiolite)	9.4 (940)
Heart (stress-rest) 201Tl chloride	41.0 (4100)
Heart (stress-rest) 99mTc tetrofosmin (Myoview)	11.0 (1100)
Various PET studies 18F FDG	14.0 (1400)

Adapted with permission from Mettler et al. [2]

What Are the Risks?

There is no threshold for stochastic effects so any imaging procedure or therapy that involves the use of radiation involves some risk. When performed properly, the risk is usually very small and is far outweighed by the medical benefit of having the procedure. Regardless, the concept of ALARA (keeping the radiation dose **as low as reasonably achievable**) should always be employed to minimize the risk.

A small percentage of imaging and therapy studies performed in the hospital can potentially exceed threshold values for non-stochastic effects.

Radiation therapy and interventional fluoroscopy procedures may result in radiation doses that exceed the threshold dose for skin injuries, and less frequently for cataract induction. The procedures performed in these areas are often lifesaving, and every effort to minimize the magnitude of these effects is taken.

Resources

As you continue your career in medicine, you will specialize. Part of medicine, in virtually all areas of specialization, involves ordering x-rays or nuclear medicine based procedures for your patients.

In the news media, great attention has been paid to the increase in medical radiation dose to members of the public. Currently, there are discussions and debates over the appropriateness of ordering certain exams without need. This will become a health system financial restraint (CMS' QPLE/AUC program) as well as a public health question.

Some Resources to Look into:

- ACR Appropriateness Criteria
  http://www.acr.org/secondarymainmenucategories/quality_safety/app_criteria.
    aspx
- Image Wisely Campaign (adult)
  http://www.rsna.org/Media/rsna/upload/Wisely_525.pdf
- Image Gently Campaign (pediatrics)
  http://www.pedrad.org/associations/5364/ig/
- Health Physics Society
  http://hps.org/physicians/blog/
  http://hps.org/publicinformation/asktheexperts.cfm

S: Ionizing radiation is the first thing we think about when we think about safety in imaging. In addition to radiologists, cardiologists, orthopedic surgeons, emergency physicians, podiatrists as well as medical professionals with office "x-ray" machines need radiation safety education and support. Know about and use these resources such as your health physicists.

A: Resources such as health physicists, radiologists, ACR Appropriateness Criteria™, Image Gently™, Image Wisely™, and Choosing Wisely™ will help you to order appropriate studies while managing resources and maximizing safety.

F: Be aware that your imaging specialists are using techniques such as collimation of the examined area, reducing fluoroscopy time, and selecting appropriate number of images to answer the clinical question asked.

E: Resources such as health physicists and radiologists can help to advise and manage inappropriate or excessive radiation exposure to patients such as pediatric and pregnant patients. The ALARA principle is key to the SAFE use of ionizing radiation and, as we shall see, other imaging modalities such as MRI and ultrasound.

References

1. Schauer DA, Linton OW. National Council on Radiation Protection and Measurements Report No. 160. Ionizing Radiation Exposure of the Population of the United States, medical exposure--are we doing less with more, and is there a role for health physics? Health Phys 2009 Jul;97(1):1–5.
2. Mettler Jr FA, Huda W, Yoshizumi TT, Mahesh M. Effective doses in radiology and diagnostic nuclear medicine: a catalog. Radiology. 2008;248(1):254–63.

3 INTRODUCTION TO RADIOLOGY CONCEPTS

Objectives:
1. Identify the four (4) naturally occurring densities visible on a conventional radiograph in order from the highest to lowest density.
2. Define and give two examples of the silhouette sign on a frontal chest radiograph.

Radiographic Densities

Let us disregard the anatomy seen on the radiograph for now and concentrate on basic radiographic principles. In Fig. 3.1, you can see examples of the four basic densities, bone, soft tissue, fat, and air, which are visible on a conventional radiograph.

Main Radiographic Densities

1. *Bone* – this is the densest of the four basic densities and appears white or "radiodense" as radiologists prefer to say.
2. *Soft Tissue* – all fluids and soft tissues have the same density on a conventional radiograph. This density is slightly less than the bone but slightly greater than fat. One advantage of CT scanning is that various soft tissues and fluids can be discriminated as different radiographic densities to a much greater degree than conventional radiographs.

© Springer Nature Switzerland AG 2020
J. Kissane et al. (eds.), *Radiology Fundamentals: Introduction to Imaging & Technology*, https://doi.org/10.1007/978-3-030-22173-7_3

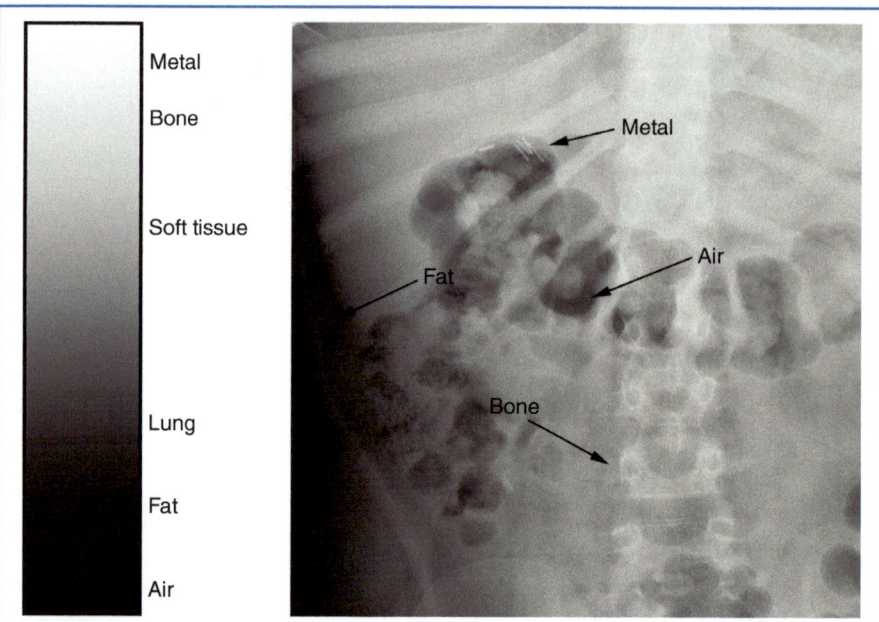

FIGURE 3.1 - RADIOGRAPHIC DENSITIES
Note how the four basic densities are visible on an abdominal radiograph

3. *Fat* – this density may seem the least obvious to you. Fat can be seen interposed between various soft tissue and fluid densities. Abdominal fat allows us to see the edges of various soft tissue structures since the fat is slightly less dense than the organs themselves.
4. *Air* – the lungs, "bowel gas," and the air surrounding the patient are examples of air densities. Air densities are generally quite dark, almost black, on the radiograph. Thus, the lungs are not radiodense but are instead said to be "radiolucent." Why does the air in the lungs appear less black (more radiodense) than the air around the patient? This is because the air density in the lungs is added to the densities of the superimposed chest wall structures.

There is an additional density on some radiographs which may be denser than bone: metal density. This is not included in the above classification because it is not a naturally occurring density. Examples of metallic density on the radiograph include orthopedic hardware, wire sutures in the sternum in patients who have undergone cardiac surgery, and wire leads seen in a pacemaker.

Radiographic densities are normally additive in an arithmetic way. This means that a soft tissue density which is twice as thick as an adjacent soft tissue structure will be twice as white. Conversely, a structure which is half as dense as an adjacent structure but twice as thick will demonstrate an identical radiographic density.

The Silhouette Sign

What is the effect of juxtaposition of structures of varying density upon each other? When two structures of *different densities* are adjacent (i.e., abutting each other), the interface between them will be clearly delineated on the radiograph. For example, the soft tissue density of the heart is clearly delineated from the air density of the lung along the cardiac border. However, when two structures of the *same density* are adjacent or overlapping, their margins cannot be distinguished. For example, when pneumonia fills the alveoli of the right lung with fluid, the lung becomes fluid density, and the normal interface between the right heart border (soft tissue density) and the lung (air) may become invisible; the right heart border can no longer be seen (Fig. 3.2).

This is called the silhouette sign and is one of the most useful principles in radiology.

Other examples of the silhouette sign include the following:

1. The heart cannot be distinguished separately from the blood within the cardiac chambers because both have soft tissue/fluid density.
2. The dome of the liver and the inferior aspect of the right hemidiaphragm cannot be distinguished radiographically since both have soft tissue density. You would

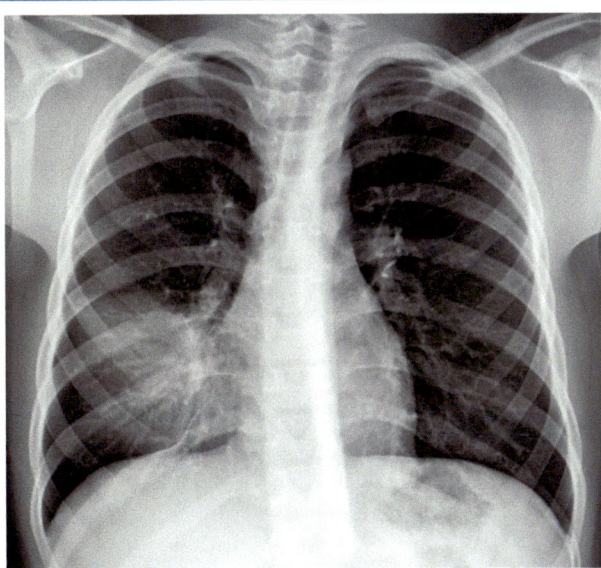

FIGURE 3.2 - THE SILHOUETTE SIGN
Right middle lobe pneumonia illustrates silhouetting of the right heart border by the area of consolidation. Compare to the crisp left heart border

only see the dome of the liver and the right hemidiaphragm separately when free intraperitoneal air is present. This is because the air density is interposed between the two soft tissue densities.

The silhouette sign will be used repeatedly in many sections of this course and in interpreting radiographs clinically. It is very important that you have a clear understanding of this principle.

S: Recognizing densities on conventional imaging may result in cancelling advanced imaging that could cause harm. For example, recognizing metal within the eye on an x-ray would result in cancellation of a brain MRI as the strong magnetic field of the MRI can cause the metal to heat up or migrate, causing blindness.

A: Conventional imaging, such as x-rays of chest, abdomen, and bones, is often the first-line modality to decide if further imaging is needed. ACR Appropriateness Criteria is a good place to start learning about the appropriate order of imaging or if imaging is even necessary.

F: Conventional radiography is dependent on experts such as radiology technologists to acquire images with techniques that allow different densities to be displayed. Improper techniques, large and small patients, or uncooperative patients may contribute to images that are difficult to interpret.

E: Identifying unexpected densities such as air outside of an expected location (pneumothorax or pneumoperitoneum) or metal density such as bullet fragments or foreign bodies will result in appropriate identification and management.

4 CONVENTIONAL RADIOLOGY

Objectives:
1. State the convention for describing standard radiographic projections.
2. Explain why cardiac size differs on AP versus PA radiographs.
3. Define the "lordotic projection" view and two indications for its use.
4. Discuss how the following variables and techniques may alter the appearance of a conventional chest radiograph: underexposure, rotation, inspiration, and expiration.

Many technical factors impact the appearance of conventional radiographs. This chapter will introduce the main factors you should be aware of when interpreting radiographs.

The Radiographic Projection

The radiographic projection is named according to the direction in which the x-ray beam passes through the body of the patient when the radiograph is taken (Fig. 4.1).

In other words, if the x-ray detector was placed behind the patient and the x-ray tube was placed in front of the patient, the x-rays would pass from the front of the patient through the back of the patient onto the x-ray detector in an anteroposterior (AP) radiograph. In a posterior-anterior (PA) radiograph, the detector is located along the anterior aspect of the patient's body with the x-ray tube posterior to the patient. In this situation, the x-ray beam passes through the patient from posterior to anterior.

Note the difference in the size of the heart shadow between the AP and PA radiograph in Fig. 4.1. Because x-rays diverge from a point source, objects that are situ-

© Springer Nature Switzerland AG 2020
J. Kissane et al. (eds.), *Radiology Fundamentals: Introduction to Imaging & Technology*, https://doi.org/10.1007/978-3-030-22173-7_4

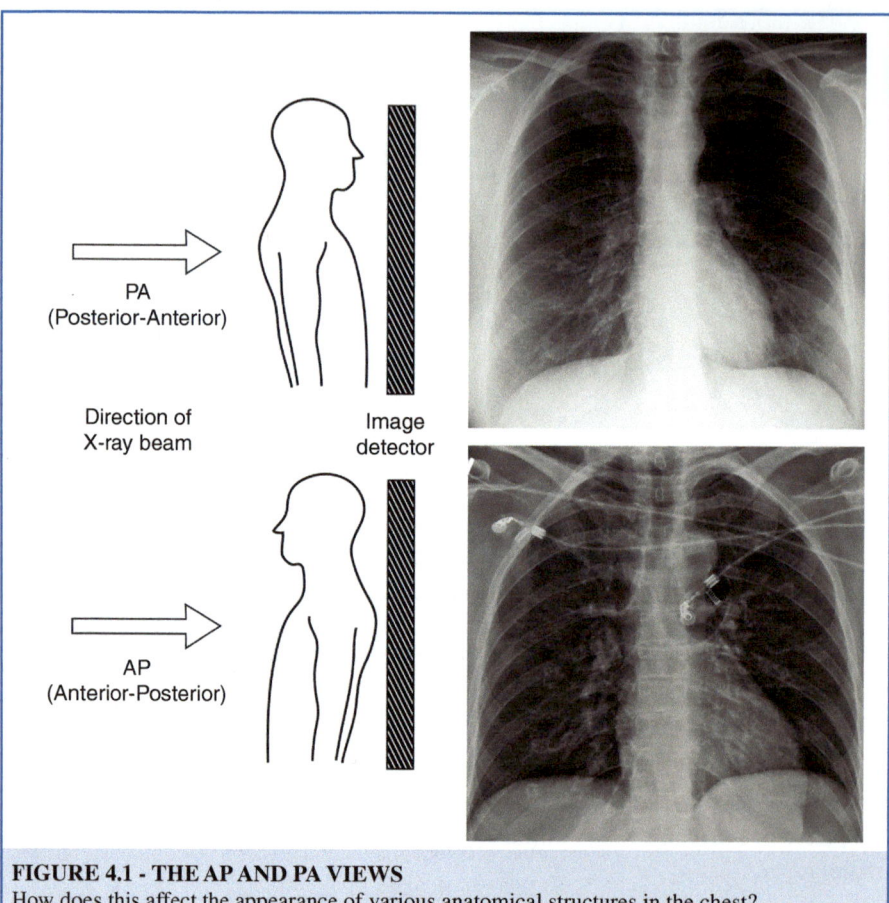

FIGURE 4.1 - THE AP AND PA VIEWS
How does this affect the appearance of various anatomical structures in the chest?

PA
(Posterior-Anterior)

Direction of
X-ray beam

Image
detector

AP
(Anterior-Posterior)

ated farther from the detector will cast a larger shadow. Since the heart is an anterior structure, it is magnified more on the AP radiograph because the anterior structures are farther from the radiographic detector. Demonstrate this principle for yourself by shining a flashlight on your hand so that it casts a shadow on the wall. The farther your hand is from the wall (which in this case acts like the x-ray detector), the more magnified and fuzzy the shadow becomes. Portable radiographs are most commonly performed AP, because the patient can be imaged in a semi-upright or supine position. The radiographic trade-off is that image quality may not be as good, as the supine patient's chest x-ray is often underinflated.

Next, look at Fig. 4.2. This is the "lordotic projection." With this projection, the x-ray source is angled toward the head, and the clavicles project superior to the lung apex on the radiograph. This view is used to detect possible apical abnormalities such as tuberculosis or a lung tumor in the apex, called a Pancoast tumor. CT scans are now more commonly used because of increased sensitivity and specificity relative to the apical lordotic chest x-ray.

Look at Fig. 4.3. The heads of the clavicles and the spinous processes have been drawn on the diagram on the left. Since the clavicular heads are anterior structures

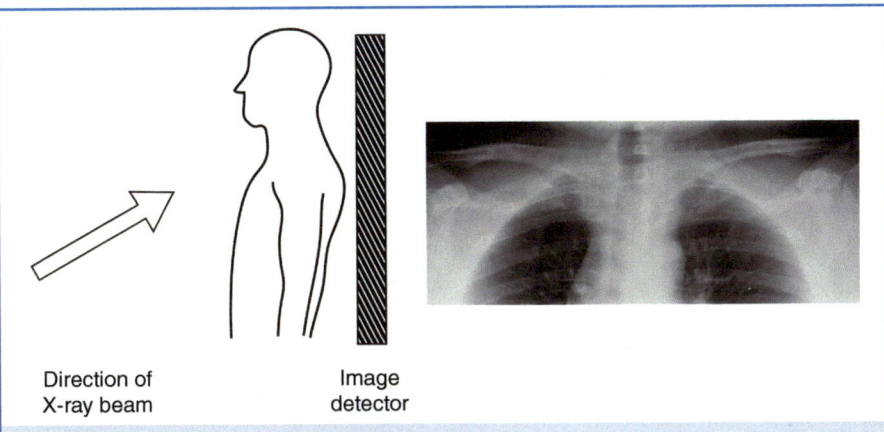

FIGURE 4.2 - THE LORDOTIC PROJECTION
The lordotic view is especially useful for visualizing the lung apices. The clavicles are projected cephalad, allowing a clear view of the lung apices

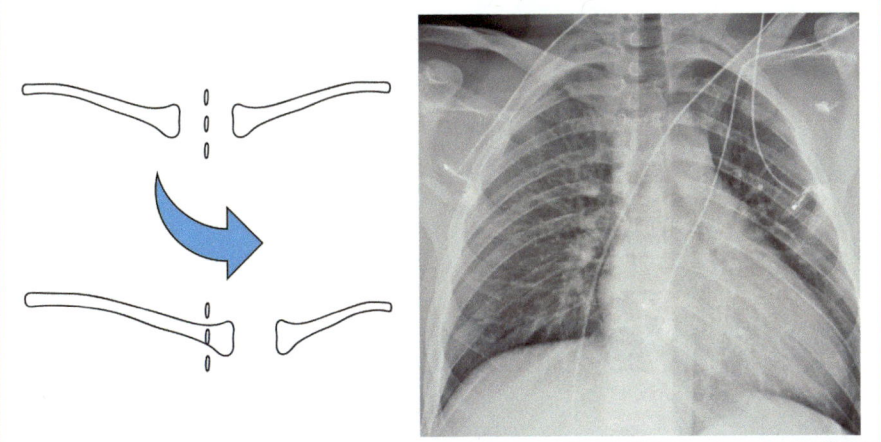

FIGURE 4.3 - ROTATION OF THE CHEST
In this illustration, note how the clavicular heads and spinous processes of the vertebral bodies appear in the AP position and with the rotation of the chest to the left. On the chest x-ray, the right clavicular head has rotated past the spinous processes, indicating that the patient is rotated to the left

and the spinous processes are quite posterior, they will move in opposite directions on the radiographs relative to a central axis of rotation. Using this principle of rotation, acquiring two radiographs, one in straight PA and one in slight rotation, may help to determine the position of an abnormality in the lung.

Finally, note Fig. 4.4. The two radiographs were obtained within minutes of each other. Although this is an extreme example, it is important to realize that radiographs exposed at less than full inspiration produce artifactual crowding of the pulmonary vasculature which can simulate pulmonary edema.

In some situations, expiratory radiographs are intentionally obtained. The most common situation is when looking for a small pneumothorax. In this situation, the pneumothorax will become slightly larger relative to the lung as air is expired.

Next, examine Fig. 4.5. Can you find examples of the four basic densities? Can you find examples of summation of radiographic densities due to superimposition of structures? Superimposed kidneys and stool-filled colon will be denser than each structure by itself. Examples of the silhouette sign? Kidneys adjacent to the liver or spleen will silhouette and obscure each other's margins.

And last, but certainly not the least, Fig. 4.6 is an image from a normal air contrast barium enema. This demonstrates how certain substances such as barium can be used to make certain anatomic structures more visible on the radiograph (in this case, white barium and dark air in the large bowel).

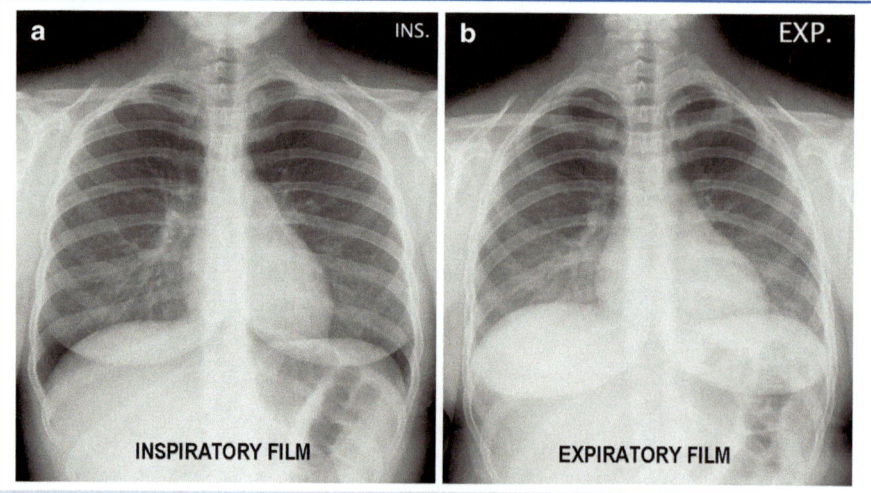

FIGURE 4.4 - INSPIRATORY AND EXPIRATORY FILMS
The radiographs here are those of inspiration (**a**) and expiration (**b**). Note the difference in the size of the lungs and their apparent difference in densities

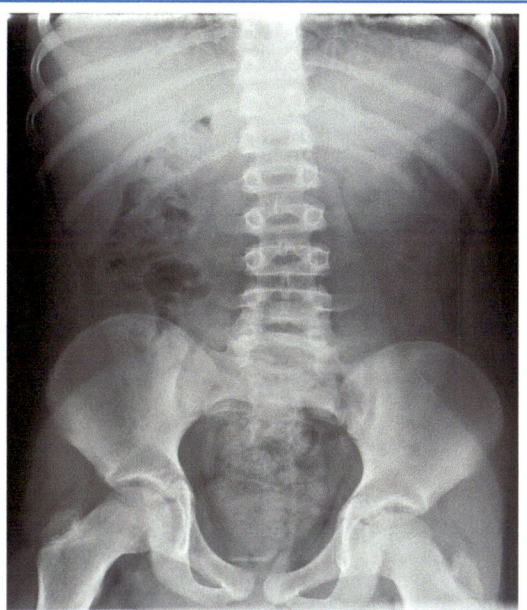

FIGURE 4.5 - NORMAL ABDOMINAL RADIOGRAPH

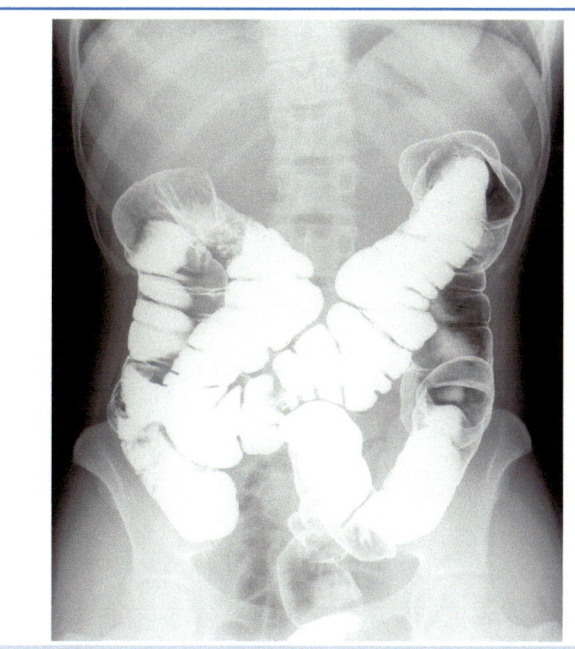

FIGURE 4.6 - NORMAL BARIUM ENEMA

S: Portable radiographs are commonly performed from an AP projection, which allows for seated or supine position, good for an unstable patient.

A: Whenever possible, minimize technical factors such as a portable chest x-ray (often seated, hypoinflated, and rotated) when a standard standing, well-inflated chest x-ray can be performed and is more likely to give information to answer the clinical question.

F: Technical factors such as expiration are used to answer specific questions such a presence of pneumothorax. Unintentional factors such as rotation may reduce the image quality of a conventional radiograph.

E: Act on the information you receive. Understand why a radiologist suggests repeating a poor quality radiograph because of technical factors, but also let them know if the information you have answers your clinical question without repeat imaging.

5 ULTRASOUND

Objectives:
1. State the function of the transducer used in ultrasonography.
2. Define the term "sonolucent."
3. Give examples of structures that transmit sound well and that transmit sound poorly.

Ultrasound

Ultrasound uses no ionizing radiation and it can image directly in any body plane. In practice, an ultrasonographer (either an ultrasound technologist called a sonographer or a physician) places gel on the patient's skin and moves a transducer across the surface of the patient's body. The gel forms an acoustic seal between the transducer and the skin for better transmission of sound, which results in better images.

The transducer can both send out and receive high-frequency sound waves, which transmit through, or reflect off, structures in the body. The returning sound waves are categorized by their intensity (referred to as echogenicity) and duration of time that it takes for them to return. It is the time that it takes for the echo to return from its encounter with an acoustic interface (a structure within the body which reflects sound) that allows its location within the image to be assigned (Fig. 5.1).

The intensity of the returning echo (echogenicity) of tissues varies greatly. Some tissues, like abdominal fat, are higher in echogenicity than other soft tissues. On the ultrasound image, such structures will appear whiter and are described as being increased in echotexture or "hypERechoic." Tissues/interfaces that return echoes of lower intensity are displayed as darker on ultrasound images and are described as decreased in echotexture or "hypOechoic." By evaluating the echotexture of tissues, we can distinguish one organ from another and look for pathologic processes.

© Springer Nature Switzerland AG 2020
J. Kissane et al. (eds.), *Radiology Fundamentals: Introduction to Imaging & Technology*, https://doi.org/10.1007/978-3-030-22173-7_5

Fluid-filled structures (such as the gallbladder or urinary bladder) have few or no internal acoustic interfaces and hence appear clear black or sonolucent on ultrasound. Look at the simple cyst found when scanning the breast of a patient in Fig. 5.2. Note that the cyst depicted in this image is "anechoic," having no detect-

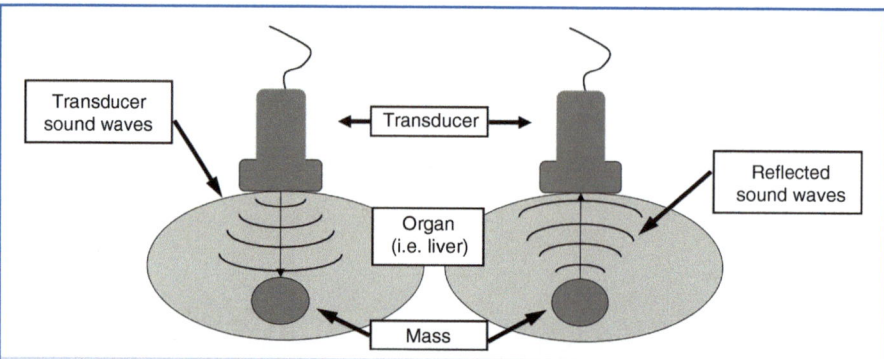

FIGURE 5.1 - ULTRASOUND
The ultrasound transducer acts similar to the sonar on a submarine. The transducer sends a short burst of high-frequency sound into the tissue. Some part of the sound is reflected back by the tissues, the reflected signal is "read" by the transducer, and an image is created

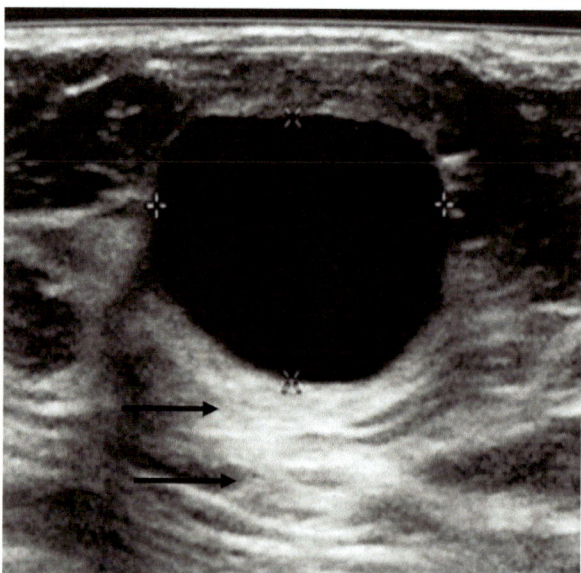

FIGURE 5.2 - SIMPLE BREAST CYST
"Anechoic" cyst having no internal echoes. Note the increased echodensity behind the cyst (*arrows*)

able internal echoes. Sound waves traveling through the fluid-filled cyst retain their energy (since they encounter fewer acoustic interfaces). For this reason, they can pass through with more intensity when they reach the far wall of the cyst. This phenomenon is referred to as "acoustic enhancement" (arrows).

Some structures that are very dense, such as calcified structures or bone, will prevent sound waves from passing beyond them. As a result, there is no imaging information that can be obtained deep to those structures. A dark band-like "shadow" is produced beyond the echodense structure. This dark shadow can be quite prominent, helping identify even very small calcifications, such as kidney stones. This is known as the headlight sign as is seen in Fig. 5.3.

The orientation of the plane of the section on an ultrasound image is indicated by the sonographer, who annotates the plane of the section on images, either with text or with an indicator image.

Scans are normally viewed in "real time." This means that structures can be seen to move in the image (e.g., cardiac valves) and structures can pass into and out of the field of view. The images that the ultrasonographer records are only selected "frozen" images from an extensive examination. In some situations, it may be advantageous to record the examination in real time, known as a video or cine clip.

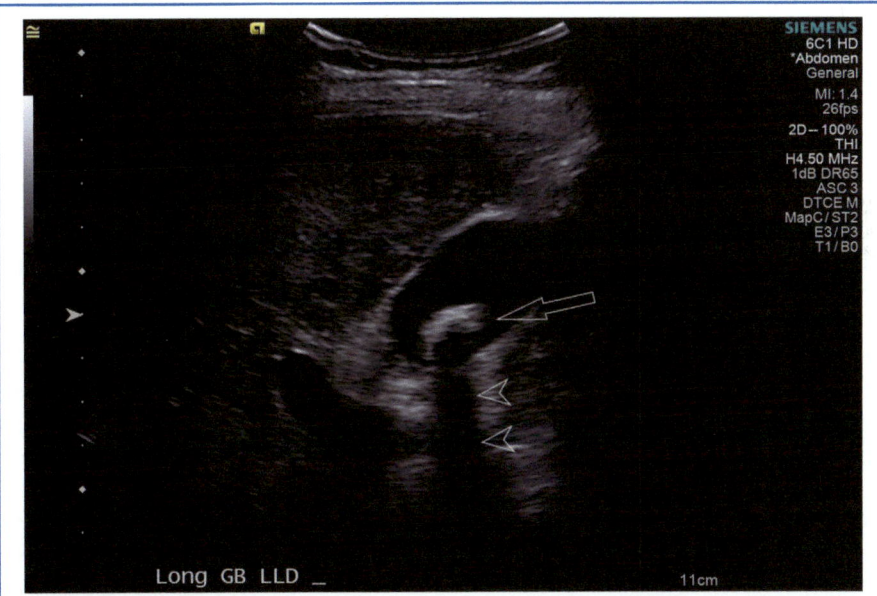

FIGURE 5.3 - HEADLIGHT SIGN
Note the band-like "shadow" (*white lined arrowheads*) beyond the bright echogenic gallstone (*white lined arrow*) due to inability of the sound waves to travel through the dense stone

$$X \propto \left(\frac{1}{D}\right)^2$$

FIGURE 5.4 - INVERSE SQUARE LAW
This is the inverse square law, as it applies to radiography, where X is the exposure at a given distance, D, from a radiation source. If, for example, the distance is doubled, the exposure would be one-fourth of its original strength. The same law applies to the strength of the ultrasound beam

Ultrasound weakens or attenuates rapidly by the inverse square law with distance from the transducer; therefore, structures closer to the transducer are better visualized. Many transducers have been adapted to get them close to the imaged structures. Transducers are included on endoscopes, allowing assessment of the duodenum, common bile duct, and pancreas. An endovaginal transducer provides very detailed imaging of the uterus and ovaries. Endorectal transducers allow high-resolution imaging of the prostate and rectum. By placing the transducer closer to the imaged object, you can also use higher wavelengths of ultrasound, improving detail (Fig. 5.4).

Color and Power Doppler Imaging in Ultrasound

When an ultrasound beam encounters a moving structure a change in the pitch or frequency of the returning echo, compared to the echo sent out by the transducer, occurs. This is called the Doppler shift and it is encountered in real life when you hear a siren from a police car as it drives past you; the pitch or frequency of the sound you hear changes as the vehicle passes.

By using the information generated by this Doppler shift, images can be generated, giving information about the speed and direction of the moving structure. This is most commonly used in evaluating blood vessels and blood flow. In conventional color Doppler, the displayed color identifies the direction of flow as well as the speed of flow. Power Doppler, which measures the concentration of moving structures, is more sensitive to low-flow states, but does not allow an evaluation of direction or speed.

Calculating the velocity of moving red blood cells numerically can allow an estimation of the diameter of the vessel in which the cells are flowing. This is the basis of a vascular spectral (duplex) assessment of vessels such as the carotid arteries. A spectral Doppler study will display grayscale images, color images, and waveform images of the vessel being evaluated. As the vessel lumen narrows, generally the velocity of red cells moving through it increases. By using multiple calculations along the path of the vessel, multiple velocity measurements and ratios of velocities can be calculated, allowing one to diagnose, quantify, and monitor focal areas of vascular narrowing.

Color/power Doppler and spectral imaging are used to assess for possible clot in veins, to evaluate areas of arterial narrowing/stenosis, and to determine if masses and organs have increased blood flow. You might see increased blood flow in a malignant tumor or reduced blood flow in a torsed testicle or ovary. Doppler imaging is also used to diagnose vascular malformations and assess for the presence of varicose veins.

Indications for Ultrasound Use

Ultrasound is most efficient in thinner individuals or when evaluating structures closer to the transducer. It does not require the use of ionizing radiation, but still should be used cautiously. Studies have shown that prolonged exposure to ultrasound can increase the temperature of tissue and that cavitation can occur when sound waves pass through a structure containing a gas bubble or air pocket (such as bowel and lung). Like any other imaging modality, ultrasound should be used judiciously, only when necessary, and by someone appropriately trained in the modality.

Ultrasound is most commonly used to image specific organs such as the liver, gallbladder, kidneys, spleen, uterus/adnexa, and scrotum. Despite knowing the limitations of ultrasound when evaluating air- and fecal-filled bowel loops (and structures around them), ultrasound is being used increasingly to evaluate diseased bowel (which tends to be thicker and often fluid-filled). With appropriate training, point-of-care ultrasound can aid in the detection of pneumothorax, pleural effusions, and peritoneal fluid and in guiding the placement of central lines.

S: Unlike conventional radiography, CT scanning and angiography, ultrasound does not use ionizing radiation to generate images. However, ultrasound does deposit energy into tissue and so must be used safely. Think about therapeutic uses of ultrasound such as lithotripsy and ultrasound for physical therapy. Anyone using ultrasound for diagnostic and therapeutic purposes should have proper ultrasound safety training.

A: Ultrasound is best used to answer specific questions, in appropriate organs and locations, and in proper patients. Ultrasound is not a good modality to use to just "look around" for pathology. Ultrasound may provide limited diagnostic images in the obese patient, the uncooperative patient and the patient with thick bandages or large scars.

F: Obtaining ultrasound images is aided by knowledge of anatomy and experience to conceptualize what you are seeing. Tissue display is unique to ultrasound such as adipose tissue which is dark on CT and bright on ultrasound.

E: Ultrasound can provide quick real-time assessment and information to answer a clinical question and direct treatment. For example, ultrasound can be used to identify large amounts of free fluid in the abdomen after trauma, directing the next steps in patient care.

6

COMPUTED TOMOGRAPHY

Objectives:
1. State how the densities on a CT scan are assigned.
2. Define the terms "pixel" and "voxel."
3. Compare and contrast the spatial and density resolution achieved with a CT scan with that of conventional radiographs.
4. State how to determine if contrast material is used when viewing a CT.

CT Imaging Orientation

Computed tomography (CT) uses ionizing radiation to create an image. This allows visualization of a greater variety of tissue structures beyond the four basic densities (air, bone, soft tissue, and fat) that are seen on a conventional radiograph. Unlike conventional x-rays, which utilize one projection to form an image, CT uses multiple small projections across the body and combines the information to form the image. It is this combination of the images that allows greater soft tissue detail to be displayed (Fig. 6.1).

Each individual picture of a computed tomography (CT) study is referred to as a section or an axial "slice." This is because the picture must be interpreted as if the patient has been completely sectioned in an axial plane, like a loaf of bread, with the viewer looking at the section from the feet toward the head.

J. Kissane et al. (eds.), *Radiology Fundamentals: Introduction to Imaging & Technology*, https://doi.org/10.1007/978-3-030-22173-7_6

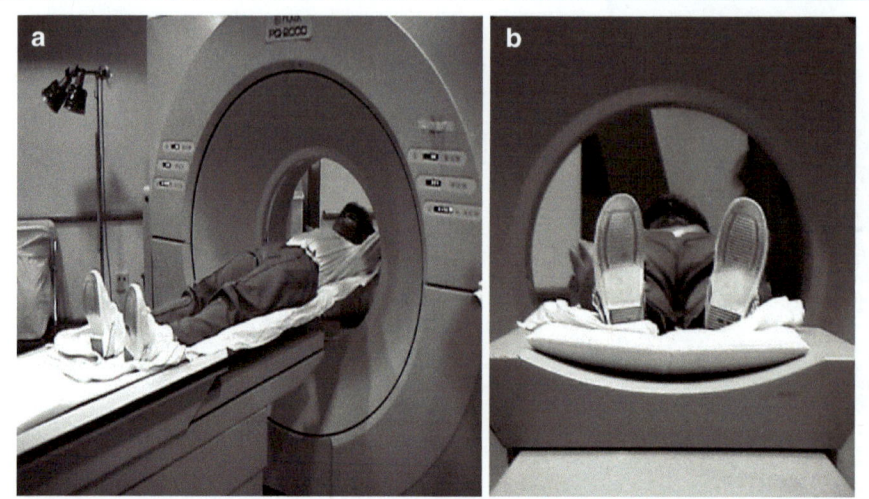

FIGURE 6.1 - COMPUTED TOMOGRAPHY (CT)
(**a**) The patient is placed in the CT gantry and images are obtained in axial sections called "slices." (**b**) When reviewing the axial images, the radiologist interprets each image as if he/she were at the patient's feet, looking toward the patient's head

Pixels and Voxels

If you look closely at the CT scan, you will realize that the picture is actually made up of thousands of little squares called "pixels" (picture elements) (Fig. 6.2). Each pixel represents tissue that is about 1 mm or less on each of two sides and is assigned a grayscale value from 0 (black) to 255 (white). The grayscale value reflects how much of the x-ray beam that small piece of tissue (represented by the pixel) attenuated or blocked as it was passing through the patient. Darker shades (closer to black) represent structures that attenuate very little of the beam (like gas), while whiter shades represent structures that strongly attenuate the beam (like bone or calcification).

The thickness of the slice of a CT study is typically 1 mm or less, creating a three-dimensional volume element or "voxel" which is shaped like a cube. The word voxel is short for "volume pixel," the smallest distinguishable box-shaped part of a three-dimensional image. Pixel intensity represents an average from tissue within the "voxel." Although the spatial resolution of the CT scan is less than that of a conventional radiograph, the density resolution is much greater. Earlier models of CT scanners used the "step and shoot" method to acquire images. While lying on a motorized table, the patient was slowly moved into the scanning gantry, and a single slice was obtained while the patient was asked to hold his or her breath. These scanners, though remarkable for their generation, sometimes caused small pathology to be missed as patients would not hold their breath in the same fashion each time. These studies had long acquisition times.

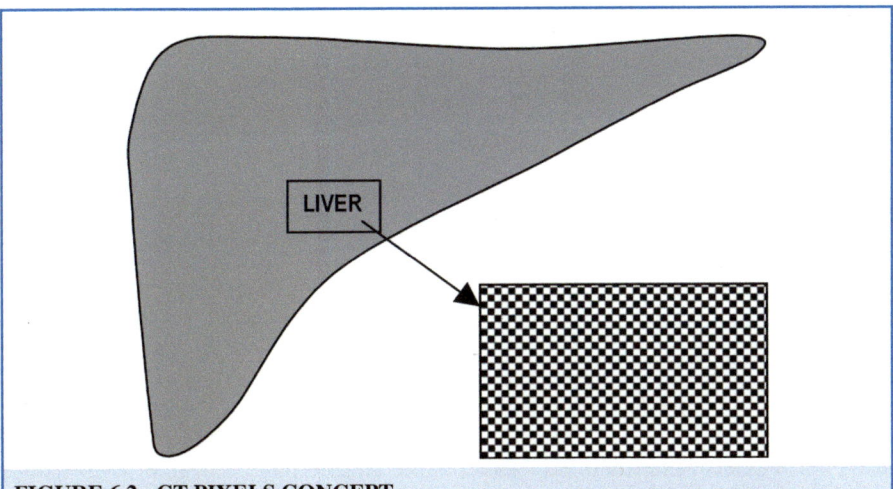

FIGURE 6.2 - CT PIXELS CONCEPT
As you look at the CT slice, it is important to keep in mind that each image is really made up of thousands of pixels (picture elements), each representing tissue about 1 mm^2

Current generation scanners move the patient continuously through the scanning gantry during a single breath-hold. The patient is advanced while the x-ray tube continuously rotates, acquiring a data set that is much like a spiral in configuration (thus the name "spiral CT"). Current scans are performed much more rapidly than with the old "step and shoot" method. The data can then be reformatted into coronal, sagittal, and oblique planes. Current scanners have the capability of obtaining voxels of data so small that the reformatted images in other planes offer nearly identical resolution.

CT Values or Hounsfield Units (HU)

The amount of the x-ray beam that a particular voxel of tissue attenuates can be represented by a number called the Hounsfield unit, named after Sir Godfrey N. Hounsfield, an electrical engineer who won the Nobel Prize in 1979 for his pioneering work in the development of CT in the 1960s. By looking at the Hounsfield unit value of a structure one can get an idea of what types of tissue may be present (bone, calcification, water, blood, etc.). Also, by looking at changes in the Hounsfield unit value of tissue on images obtained before intravenous contrast compared to after intravenous contrast, one can determine how vascular a structure is. Listed below is a basic guide to HU values prior to contrast (Table 6.1).

Table 6.1 Typical HU for different tissues

Substance	Hounsfield units (HU)
Air	−1000
Fat	−100
Water	0
Muscle/soft tissue	+40
Contrast	+130
Bone	+1000

Contrast Studies

Intravenous contrast as well as oral and sometimes rectal contrast agents may be used in CT scans. The small "+C" label in the alphanumeric image of each section indicates that intravenous contrast was used. Also, if the aorta, kidneys, or ureter is radiopaque or white, it is a good indication that IV contrast was used. If the stomach or small or large bowel is radiopaque, oral contrast has been given.

Optimizing the Visualization of Specific Structures

Since CT scans are created from digital data, the grayscale display can be manipulated in such a way as to display the same information in various formats. These different formats are called window settings and amount to changing the total number of grayscales displayed and the value at which the grayscale is centered. Such changes determine which type of tissue is best displayed. Commonly used window settings include the soft tissue (mediastinal and abdomen), bone, and lung (pulmonary). In Fig. 6.3, the same image is displayed using different windows. In the mediastinal window, soft tissue structures are discernible from each other. In the pulmonary window, the lung parenchyma is well seen, but the soft tissue structures all look the same. Additional electronic manipulation with filters and subtraction will provide more information and perhaps answer the clinical question that the raw images can only infer.

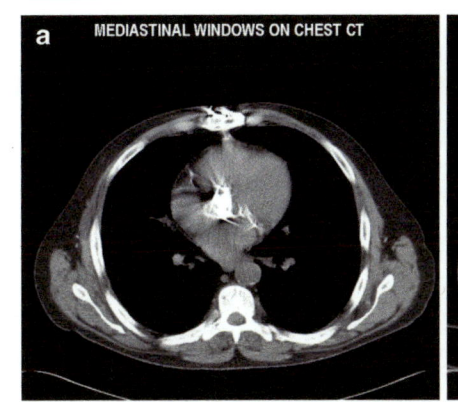 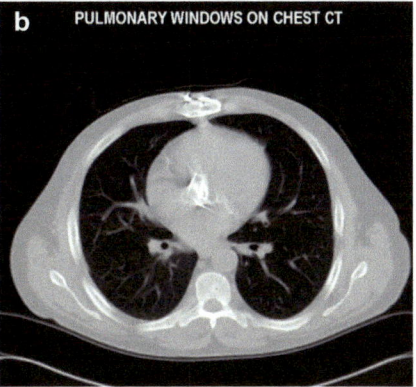

FIGURE 6.3 - CT SCAN OF THE CHEST
Note how the mediastinal window (**a**) allows for optimal visualization of the mediastinal and soft tissue structures and the pulmonary window (**b**) for lung parenchyma

S: A significant amount of ionizing radiation is used to perform a CT scan. Attention to appropriate ordering, judicious scanning of just the body part of concern, and use of contrast only when needed are very important.

A: It is so easy to just "get a CT" of almost everyone for almost any indication that it is paramount to utilize resources such as radiologists, ACR Appropriateness Criteria™, Image Gently™, Image Wisely™, and Choosing Wisely™ to order appropriate studies while managing resources and maximizing safety. Using other modalities such as ultrasound and MRI, delaying imaging if a patient is responding to treatment, and reviewing recent imaging are some of the many ways to use CT scanning appropriately.

F: CT scanning has become the workhorse of diagnostic imaging. Images can be acquired at sub-centimeter thickness and in single breath hold. The data can be reconstructed in various planes to best answer clinical questions, plan surgery and direct patient management.

E: CT scans are readily available, and scan results can be quickly acted upon with precision, such as following trauma or surgery.

7

MRI

Objectives:
1. Identify and characterize the tissue appearance of normal and common abnormal findings on CT and MRI.
2. State one advantage and three disadvantages that MRI has over CT.

Magnetic resonance imaging (MRI) has its greatest application in the fields of neuroradiology and musculoskeletal radiology.

To form a magnetic resonance image, the patient is placed in a strong uniform magnetic field. The magnetic field aligns hydrogen nuclei within the patient in the direction of the field. The nuclei are "disturbed" from this orientation by application of an external radiofrequency (RF) pulse. After the RF pulse is stopped, the hydrogen nuclei return to their alignment within the externally imposed magnetic field, giving off RF signals as they lose energy (Fig. 7.1).

The frequency of the RF signal emitted from the hydrogen nucleus as it returns to its orientation within the field is determined by the strength of that field. Therefore, the location of the RF signal given off by each hydrogen nucleus can be calculated. Each RF signal is analyzed by the computer for its intensity and other criteria. The signals are then assigned grayscale values (white to black) on the detector by the computer. Since this process of creating an image based on tissue characteristics is completely different from the absorption of x-rays by different tissues, MR images can show different types of pathologies and hence its utility. For example, MRI can discriminate soft tissue differences better than CT scans and is often used to define soft tissue abnormalities like herniated discs, ligament tears, and soft tissue tumors in the spine.

There are two basic sequences in MRI that are important to understand and recognize. These sequences are known as the T1-weighted and T2-weighted sequences.

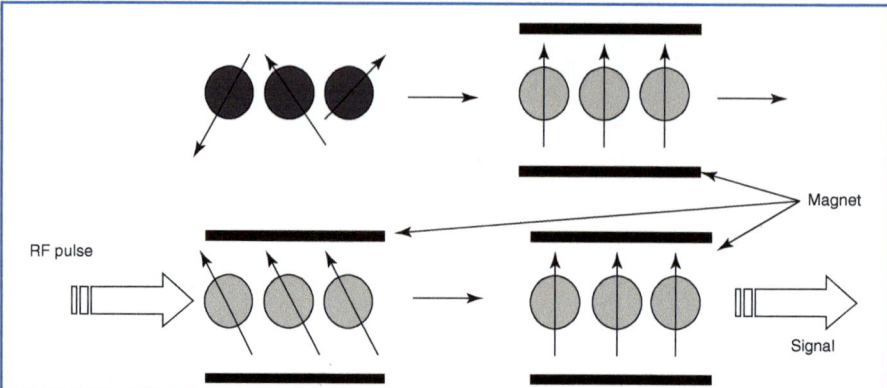

FIGURE 7.1 - MAGNETIC RESONANCE IMAGING: HYDROGEN NUCLEI
In their natural state, hydrogen atoms are spinning with their axes of rotation randomly oriented. When placed in a magnetic field, they align in a uniform direction. An RF pulse is applied, knocking the H-atoms out of their magnetic field orientation. Once the RF pulse is stopped, the atoms return to their previous alignment, giving off a signal which is then used to form the image

The "weighting" represents the exploitation of specific properties of hydrogen atoms that are exposed to a magnetic field. T1-weighted images classically demonstrate water as hypointense (dark) and fat as hyperintense (bright), with different soft tissues expressed as a gradient in between. In T2-weighted images, water is represented as hyperintense and fat as hypointense (again with soft tissues in the middle). Many of the more complicated sequences (gradient echo, FLAIR, etc.) are based on these two sequences.

Advantages and Disadvantages of MRI

With the advent of multi-slice CT scanners, CT scans can be acquired or reformatted in many planes. Therefore, a prior advantage that MRI had, exclusive multiplane capacity, is nearly gone. However, MRI's clear advantage is that it uses no ionizing radiation. Disadvantages of MRI are that it is generally more costly than CT, is less available, and takes longer to perform. Another disadvantage is the inability to scan patients who have ferromagnetic material such as some shrapnel in them. These metallic fragments can actually move with the magnetic field and cause the patient significant discomfort or damage. Although MRI-compatible pacemakers are in development, generally speaking pacemakers are contraindicated because of their ferromagnetic properties: the MRI can heat the leads and inappropriately trigger the pacemaker. But some metal, based on location, type, or duration in place, may not be a contraindication to an MRI. Check with a radiologist if you are not sure if a device is MR compatible. Additionally, there are web resources that can ascertain the MR safety of different medical devices.

S: One of MRI's unique safety advantages is its ability to generate images without the use of ionizing radiation. Two unique disadvantages are (1) that the MRI magnet may move or disrupt metals such as metal foreign bodies and metal devices such as pacemakers and cochlear implants and (2) the contrast used can cause nephrogenic systemic fibrosis (NSF), an irreversible complication in a small minority of patients with baseline renal insufficiency who receive gadolinium-based contrast. Knowledge of patient medical devices and foreign bodies as well as renal function will minimize harm.

A: One of MRI's many strengths is the ability to display soft tissue anatomy, making MRI particularly useful in evaluating neuroradiology (brain and spine) and musculoskeletal (joints, tendons and ligaments, bone and soft tissue tumors) pathology.

F: Different magnetic field sequences result in different displays of tissue in the same field of view, resulting in incredible amounts of information.

E: MR imaging acquisition is lengthy and is not usually the modality of choice in emergent situations.

8 INTRODUCTION TO NUCLEAR MEDICINE

Objectives:
1. Define the nuclear medicine (NM) specialty.
2. Be able to define key terms – isotope, radiopharmaceutical, gamma rays, gamma probe, gamma camera, planar imaging, etc.
3. Define how the component parts of a radiopharmaceutical and the route of its administration contribute to diagnostic and therapeutic nuclear medicine.
4. Define the unique characteristics of different imaging methods in nuclear medicine.

Introduction

The terms specific to the nuclear medicine (NM) section will be displayed in *italics* when first mentioned, and the same abbreviations will be used from its first appearance to subsequent NM chapters.

Basic Definitions

Nuclear medicine (NM) is a medical specialty where practitioners are skilled in using radioactive isotopes for the diagnosis and therapy of disease. Isotopes are variants of stable elements that have an identical number of *protons* (p), which determines the atomic number and element's chemical characteristics, but differ in the number of *neutrons* (n). The sum of p and n equals the atomic mass. Some isotopes are radioactive, which means that they emit energy from the nucleus in the

© Springer Nature Switzerland AG 2020
J. Kissane et al. (eds.), *Radiology Fundamentals: Introduction to Imaging & Technology*, https://doi.org/10.1007/978-3-030-22173-7_8

process of transformation to a more stable form – a process called *radioactive decay*. Every radioactive isotope decays exponentially with a specific rate that can be expressed as its *half-life* ($T_{1/2}$), which is the time required for an isotope to decay to half of its starting activity.

An example of iodine (I) may be helpful to illustrate the isotope concept. The stable element is ^{127}I, which contains 53 p and 74 n in its nucleus, thus having an atomic mass of 127. The common radioactive isotopes of iodine used in nuclear medicine are ^{123}I (p53, n70) and ^{131}I (p53, n78). These isotopes can be administered to patients in the simplest of chemical forms, such as *sodium iodide salt* (also called *radioactive iodine, radioiodide,* or *radioiodine*). *Radiopharmaceutical* (RF) is another term for a chemical combination containing an isotope, where it is combined with (or *labeled* to) more complex molecules (pharmaceuticals), such as antibodies, hormones, or peptides, just to name a few. The pharmaceutical component of the RF would determine its biological distribution in the body, as well as its utility for diagnostic and/or therapeutic applications.

Radioisotopes and Radiopharmaceuticals

The most commonly used isotope in nuclear medicine is *metastable technetium-99* (^{99m}Tc). Its popularity is chiefly based on physical qualities, including the gamma ray emitted in the decay process that carries the energy of 140 *kiloelectron volts* (KeV), which is ideally suited for efficient detection by NM imaging equipment. Another useful quality is its $T_{1/2}$ of 6 h, which is ideal for the majority of diagnostic applications. It also has advantageous chemical qualities which allow for convenient labeling to different pharmaceuticals, resulting in a wide array of RFs. Some of them are listed in Table 8.1. The biodistribution of RFs varies according to the route of administration. One of the oldest RFs is ^{99m}Tc-labeled sulfur colloid, which demonstrates how different routes of administration influence biodistribution and diagnostic utilization (Table 8.1). In general, the routes of RF administration include oral, intravenous, subcutaneous, intradermal, inhaled, and instilled into a body cavity or an organ through a catheter or a needle.

The use of different isotopes is also based on the type of rays (*photons*) they emit. These include *gamma, beta,* and *alpha* photons. Gamma photons have the physical quality of a longer emission range (meters), and thus they are well suited for imaging. In contrast, alpha and beta photons travel very short distances (millimeters) before their energy is absorbed into tissues, which makes them ideal for *unsealed (internal) radiotherapy or radioisotope therapy* applications.

Table 8.1 Commonly used ^{99m}Tc-labeled radiopharmaceuticals in nuclear medicine

Radiopharmaceutical	Administration via	Test name	Main organ(s)/ system(s) tested	Physiologic function(s) tested
Tc-99 m-diethylenetriaminepenta-acetic acid (DTPA)	Intravenous	Renal scan (scintigraphy)	Kidneys	Glomerular function, drainage
Tc-99 m-diethylenetriaminepenta-acetic acid (DTPA)	Inhaled	Lung ventilation scan	Lung	Ventilation, ciliary clearance
Tc-99 m-hydroxymethylene diphosphonate (HDP)	Intravenous	Bone scan (scintigraphy)	Bone	Osteoblast activity
Tc-99 m-macroaggregated albumin (MAA)	Intravenous	Lung perfusion scan	Lung	Perfusion
Tc-99 m-mebrofenin	Intravenous	Hepatobiliary ("HIDA") scan	Liver, biliary ducts, gallbladder	Bile production, gallbladder
Tc-99 m-mercaptoacetyl triglycine (MAG3)	Intravenous	Renal scan (scintigraphy)	Kidneys	Tubular function, drainage
Tc-99 m-methylene diphosphonate (MDP)	Intravenous	Bone scan (scintigraphy)	Bone	Osteoblast activity
Tc-99 m-pertechnetate	Intravenous	Thyroid scan (scintigraphy)	Thyroid	Sodium iodide symporter
Tc-99 m-pertechnetate	Intravenous	Salivary scan (scintigraphy)	Salivary glands	Saliva production, drainage
Tc-99 m-pertechnetate	Intravenous	Meckel's scan	Stomach and bowel	Gastric mucosa
Tc-99 m-red blood cells	Intravenous	Radionuclide ventriculography	Heart chambers	Wall motion, ejection fraction
Tc-99 m-red blood cells	Intravenous	Gastrointestinal bleeding scan	Intestinal extravasation	Hemostasis
Tc-99 m-sulfur colloid	Intravenous	Liver-spleen scan	Liver, spleen, bone marrow	Mononuclear phagocyte system
Tc-99 m-sulfur colloid	Intradermal	Lymphangiography	Lymph vasculature and nodes	Lymphatic drainage
Tc-99 m-sulfur colloid	Bladder catheter	Voiding cystourethrogram (VCUG)	Bladder, ureters, kidney	Vesicoureteral valve
Tc-99 m-sulfur colloid (cooked with eggs)	Orally	Gastric emptying test	Stomach	Gastric motility (emptying)

Detection, Imaging, and Quantification

The principle of gamma photon detection is based on its interaction with certain materials that produce a spark of light (or *scintillation* – Latin origin), which is converted into an electric pulse. This pulse is recorded as one *count*. The simplest method for clinical detection and quantification of gamma ray emissions is a *gamma probe* (Fig. 8.1a). A smaller version of this instrument is available for the detection of radioactivity intraoperatively by a surgeon (Fig. 8.1b). This is useful in a number of circumstances when a focus targeted by a RF needs to be surgically excised, but cannot be

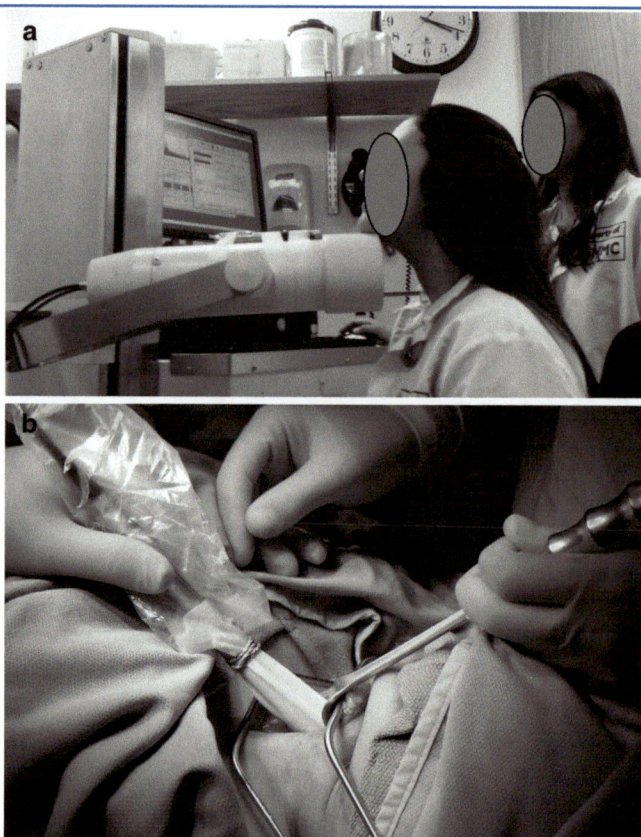

FIGURE 8.1 - GAMMA PROBES
The stationary thyroid gamma probe is shown measuring thyroid activity (**a**). This equipment is often used to calculate iodine-131 uptake. The handheld miniaturized gamma probe is used in the operating room to find radioactive thyroid tissue that was labeled before surgery (**b**)

readily distinguished from surrounding anatomy on visual inspection. These detectors provide no image, but simply indicate how many counts were detected per certain time, such as *counts per sec*, per min, per 5 min, etc. This relative unit (e.g., count/min) is directly proportional to the radioactivity in the emitting source.

A *gamma camera* is essentially an array of probes that line a flat detector and is capable of capturing the distribution of the gamma-emitting RF within the body in a 2-dimensional (2-D) image, called a planar image (*scintigraphy*). Those images can be acquired in a *static* mode (single image, or a *spot* image, obtained for either a set time or number of counts) or *dynamic* mode (sequential frames – same as spot images, but set for a same amount of time each and acquired in uninterrupted succession), as exemplified in gastrointestinal NM chapter (Figs. 37.1, 37.2, and 37.3). The static mode can be adapted for the *whole-body imaging* obtained by slowly moving the camera head along the long axis of the body and capturing the image along its path (Fig. 8.2).

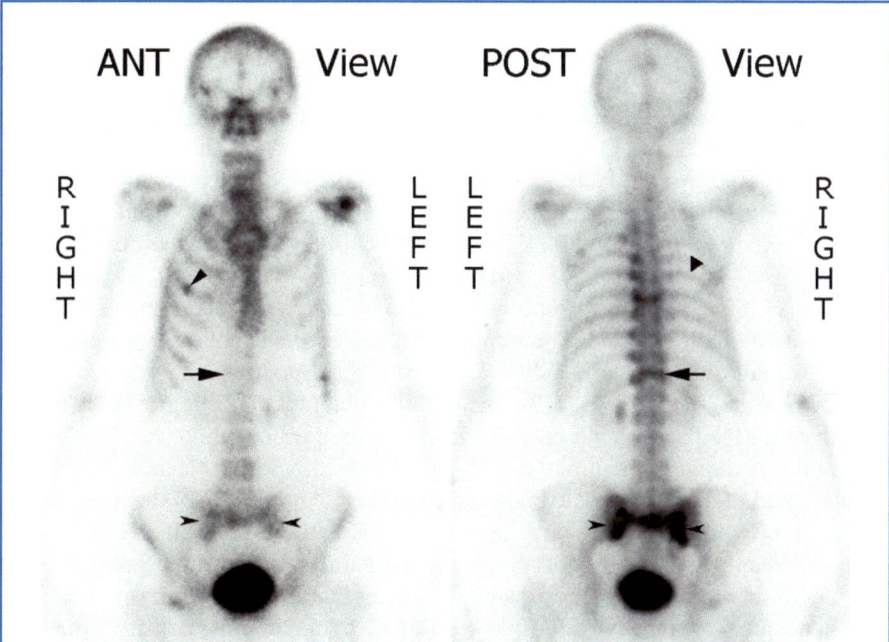

FIGURE 8.2 - BONE SCAN
Planar bone scan obtained in whole-body mode (lower extremities excluded) in anterior (*ANT*) and posterior (*POST*) views. Note the letter "H" shaped, intensely increased tracer uptake on POST view over the upper sacral bone (*concave-base arrowheads*). This is called the Honda sign and is typical for sacral insufficiency fracture. The same finding is much less intense on the ANT view due to the attenuation of a significant percent of photons. A linear, mildly increased tracer uptake seen on POST view (*arrow*) corresponds to a twelfth thoracic vertebra superior endplate compression fracture, not seen on ANT view due to attenuation. Similarly, a focal area of mildly increased uptake in the right anterior third rib (*straight-base arrowhead*) on ANT view cannot be seen on the POST view as a result of attenuation

Specific to NM is the concept of emission imaging whereby imaged gamma rays (photons originating from the nucleus) are emitted from within the body. Some of those rays will be absorbed (attenuated) in the surrounding tissues. The less tissue that stands between the organ of interest and the camera detector, the fewer photons are lost and more of them make it to the detector, creating an informative image. For example, to image the sacrum during bone scanning, the detector would be optimally positioned closest to the patient's back – called *posterior view* (Fig. 8.2). If the image of anterior ribs is desired, the front of the patient would be facing the detector – called *anterior view*. The posterior view would be less useful in depicting the anterior portion of the ribs, as most of the photons would be attenuated. In conventional radiology (refer to conventional radiology chapter in the introduction section), x-rays (photons originating from de-excitation of electrons) are emitted from the tube that is outside the patient and transmitted through the imaged part of the body. Unlike NM imaging, there is a small difference if the tube is facing the patient's front with the detector at the back or vice versa.

The same camera can obtain multiple 2-D static images from evenly spaced angles around the body. A computer algorithm can then reconstruct a 3-dimensional (3-D) depiction of the RF biodistribution. This is called *single-photon emission computed tomography* (SPECT). Newer cameras combine SPECT with CT on one gantry (called SPECT/CT), which takes both SPECT and CT images. This enables the fusion of the two modalities into one blended image called a *fusion image*. The positron-emitting isotopes are imaged using another 3-D imaging technique, called *positron emission tomography* (PET), which is routinely combined with a CT on the same gantry – called PET/CT camera and imaging. The newest advance is to combine PET with MRI, but only a few PET/MR cameras are in practice today. These 3-D modalities provide tomographic slices in the standard three planes for physiological/molecular tests (SPECT or PET), corresponding anatomical (usually CT or MRI) and fused slices. This type of molecular and physiological information displayed on the background of exquisite anatomy has been more recently termed *molecular imaging*. A simplified display of the physiological/molecular 3-D images (SPECT and PET) of the whole body can be achieved by projecting the most intense activity along parallel tracks piercing through the entire 3-D stack of slices onto a perpendicular 2-D plane. This is similar to the parallel rays of light going through the film of an old movie projector and displaying that image on a screen. Owing to this conceptual similarity, this imaging is called maximum intensity projection (MIP). This projection can be done from any angle. Creating MIP images from evenly spaced angles all around the body (360°) produces a rotating object as if one is looking at the spinning whole body. This technique was invented by a nuclear medicine physician for the display of SPECT information and now is used in most 3-D imaging techniques (MRI, CT, ultrasound), particularly PET.

Description of the imaging (scintigraphic) findings is based on relative intensity as compared to expected normal activity. It can be either increased (often called "hot spot") or decreased (termed "photopenic"). It is customary to describe the severity of the scintigraphic findings as showing intensely or severely, moderately, mildly, and slightly increased or decreased radiotracer uptake. The pattern of the finding(s), such as fusiform or linear, focal or diffuse, is important in the consideration of a likely cause. Location is described using standard anatomical terms.

The organs of interest can be evaluated for dynamic handling of the RF by drawing regions of interest and creating curves of radioactivity over time (called *time-activity curves*). Those curves can be qualitatively described or mathematically analyzed (the most common metric is halftime of exponential activity disappearance). The activity of RF deposited in the paired organs (such as kidneys or lungs) according to their functions can be quantified as the percent each side contributes to the total function, which is called differential function. Such analyses are standard in renal scanning and quantitative lung function scintigraphy (see Chap. 39, "Pulmonary Nuclear Medicine").

S: Unlike other modalities where the radiation or energy source is external, nuclear medicine imaging and therapy occur from injecting radioactive material into the patient who is therefore radioactive to themselves and potentially people they get close to. Health physicist and nuclear medicine physicians are trained to minimize the exposure to the patient and to the surrounding community, including health care providers.

A: Nuclear medicine imaging and therapy are unique modalities in which physiology is as important a component as anatomic detail.

F: Data from physiology such a wash-out data of radioactive pharmaceuticals to assess renal or thyroid function and cardiac activity and metabolic activity (positron portion) coupled to CT anatomic detail of a PET-CT are unique features of nuclear medicine imaging.

E: Nuclear medicine imaging is not commonly used in emergency situations. Rarely health physics emergencies, such as a vomiting patient who has been treated with oral radioactive iodine for thyroid cancer, may require expeditious intervention by health physicists and nuclear medicine physicians.

9 CARDIOVASCULAR AND INTERVENTIONAL RADIOLOGY

Objectives:
1. Review the types of imaging utilized in Cardiovascular and Interventional Radiology (CVIR).
2. Understand the concept behind digital subtraction angiography (DSA).
3. Be able to list the types of procedures performed in CVIR.

In Cardiovascular and Interventional Radiology (CVIR), needles, wires, catheters, balloons, and stents are used to perform a wide variety of minimally invasive procedures through small access points in the skin. Access to a vascular structure or organ is accomplished with the use of real-time x-rays (i.e., fluoroscopy), ultrasound, computed tomography, and least commonly MRI. Once access to a vessel, organ or body cavity is achieved, a contrast agent (e.g., iodinated contrast, gadolinium-based contrast, CO_2, or air) is injected for further diagnosis and to aid in the intervention.

Digital Subtraction Angiography (DSA)

Imaging for the purpose of diagnosis or intervention is often performed with digital subtraction angiography (DSA). In DSA, images are processed with the help of a computer. The initial image has no contrast and is called the "mask." The X-ray images are then obtained in rapid sequence while contrast is injected. The computer then digitally "subtracts" the mask from the subsequent images leaving only the contrast, thereby yielding finely detailed imaging of the vasculature (Fig. 9.1).

© Springer Nature Switzerland AG 2020   45
J. Kissane et al. (eds.), *Radiology Fundamentals: Introduction to Imaging & Technology*, https://doi.org/10.1007/978-3-030-22173-7_9

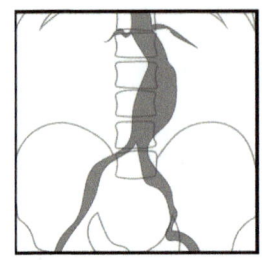 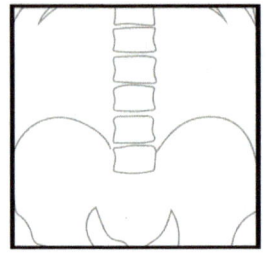 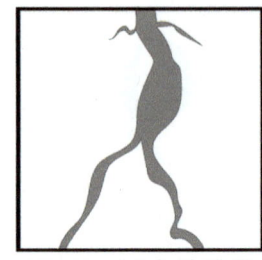

FIGURE 9.1 - DIGITAL SUBTRACTION ACQUISITION (DSA)
Contrast is injected in the patient's aorta, and images are acquired. Just before the contrast is injected, the computer acquired a mask, as seen in the *center*. As the contrast images are acquired, the computer subtracts the mask from the images, leaving the only portion which has changed between the two: the intravascular contrast

Interventional Radiology Procedures

Arteriograms are used to diagnose changes in vasculature associated with disease (most commonly atherosclerosis and vasculitis) or injury (either iatrogenic or traumatic). After primary access is obtained (most commonly via the femoral, brachial, or radial artery), a catheter is advanced into the branch arteries requiring imaging, and contrast is injected. If an area of narrowing is identified, it can be treated using percutaneous transluminal angioplasty (PTA), with or without the use of a metallic stent. If blood flow cessation is required in an area of bleeding (e.g., after trauma) or as preoperative embolization to reduce operative blood loss at subsequent surgery, various materials can be delivered into the artery to stop flow including metallic coils, Gelfoam®, polyvinyl alcohol particles (PVA, which is fixed-size particulate material), alcohol, chemotherapeutic material, autologous clot, biocompatible glue, and other agents.

Central venous access can be accomplished in many different ways. There are catheters used for short-term to intermediate-term access such as the peripherally inserted central catheter (PICC) and the nontunneled central line. Long-term access catheters include tunneled infusion catheters and subcutaneous ports. Dialysis access catheters, such as tunneled hemodialysis catheters, are also inserted in Interventional Radiology. Access is obtained with ultrasound and with the use of real-time imaging (fluoroscopy), placement of the line can be quick, accurate, and safe. Difficult access pathways can be potentially treated with angioplasty (balloon dilation) if necessary as well.

Gastroenteric access can be performed entirely percutaneously. The placement of gastrostomy tubes (G-tubes) or gastrojejunostomy tubes (G-J tubes) is accomplished with fluoroscopic guidance in a multi-planar fashion (many X-ray angles).

The use of fluoroscopy allows the quick, accurate, and safe placement of gastroenteric tubes.

Placement of inferior vena cava filters can be performed through several access points, most often via the internal jugular or common femoral veins. Careful evaluation of the inferior vena cava prior to filter placement should be performed to evaluate for variant anatomy and ensure proper filter size and positioning.

Genitourinary procedures are commonly performed in Interventional Radiology, including percutaneous nephrostomy tube placement, gonadal vein embolization, uterine fibroid embolization, and fallopian tube recanalization.

Biliary procedures are commonly performed on patients who are clinically ill as a result of biliary obstruction. Percutaneous drainage with placement of an internal/external drainage catheter can be a precursor to surgical resection of a biliary or pancreatic mass. The biliary system frequently needs to be decompressed on a long-term basis, so biliary tube maintenance is also conducted by interventional radiology. If the patient is not an operative candidate, the interventional radiologist can place metallic stents (similar to those used in the arterial system) into the biliary system. This palliates symptoms and improves quality of life without the need for external drains.

These are many types of imaging studies and additional procedures that are performed by interventional radiologists:

1. Abscess drainage (using CT, ultrasound, and/or fluoroscopy)
2. Intraoperative cases (e.g., thoracic and abdominal aortic stent grafts)
3. Noninvasive cardiac and vascular imaging (e.g., cardiac MRI, coronary CT angiography, and duplex ultrasound)
4. Percutaneous oncologic interventions (e.g., transarterial chemoembolization, transarterial ^{90}Y radioembolization, radiofrequency ablation, and cryoablation)
5. Percutaneous biopsies (using CT, ultrasound, and/or fluoroscopy)
6. Minimally invasive venous procedures (e.g., endovenous laser or radiofrequency ablation, sclerotherapy, and phlebectomy)

The scope of interventional radiology is quite extensive and diverse. The various interventional procedures expand the diagnostic and therapeutic armamentarium for the clinical care team.

S: The fundamental principle of interventional radiology is to investigate, diagnose, and treat diseases utilizing image guidance and therefore begins with a history and physical examination (including a thorough evaluation of current medication, medication allergies, and laboratory panels). This enables the interventionalist to carefully develop a periprocedural plan that ensures increased probability of successful intervention and decreased radiation exposure and complication mitigation, in essence, effecting a safe and positive clinical patient outcome.

A: Despite the expansive and diverse scope of interventional radiology and the armamentarium it offers the clinical team in addressing complex diseases, ensuring an intervention is indicated and following recommended guidelines help ensure that patients undergo procedures for appropriate reasons. Procedural contraindications vary with respect to disease entities and their comorbidities; however a procedure is absolutely contraindicated if the information sought can be obtained by a less/noninvasive method or will not change management. Relative contraindications are addressed before procedure on a case-by-case basis, for example, severe hypertension, hypotension, coagulopathy, renal insufficiency, congestive heart failure, left bundle branch block, connective tissue diseases (such as Ehlers-Danlos syndrome), etc.

F: The evolution of multi-detector CT and multiphasic MR has allowed for highly sensitive and specific detection of visceral and vascular abnormalities, predominantly serving as the primary and preferred pre-/post-interventional disease evaluative imaging modalities. However since the core of interventional radiology is image-guided procedures, other imaging modalities (mainly, fluoroscopy, ultrasound, and CT) are used intra-procedurally to evaluate anatomy and pathology as well as guide therapeutic intervention. Therefore, it is of vital importance that the images (dedicated views and orthogonal obliquities) obtained during an interventional procedure are of adequate diagnostic quality.

E: Image guidance during an interventional procedure offers the opportunity to diagnose and treat diseases (catheter-directed therapy) intra-procedurally, and as such, a positive disease finding and concomitant instituted therapy warrants that the patient and clinical team be informed of the procedure performed and advised on post-procedural management and follow-up recommendations.

PART II
THORACIC RADIOLOGY

10 HEART AND MEDIASTINUM

Objectives:
1. Identify the structures that form the left and right mediastinal borders on a PA chest radiograph.
2. Know how cardiac size is assessed on a PA chest radiograph as well as technical factors that may affect this assessment.
3. Identify the radiographic divisions of the mediastinum and the differential diagnosis of abnormalities arising from each division.

Cardiac Contours

When evaluating the cardiopericardial outline and mediastinal contours, it is easiest to follow the right and left borders that these structures make with the aerated lung. Although the mediastinum is optimally visualized by various cross-sectional imaging techniques, the initial evaluation is often made on plain chest radiographs.

Review Fig. 10.1. The first convex segment along the left mediastinal border is formed by the aortic arch. The segment inferior to the aortic arch represents the main pulmonary artery. The large convex border inferiorly is formed by the left ventricle, with a small contribution from the left atrium. On the right, the superior vena cava is visualized superiorly. The right lateral border of the right atrium forms the convexity seen inferiorly. These contours can vary with age and technique and can change dramatically in abnormal situations. A review of the cardiomediastinal silhouette should begin with an evaluation of these contours.

© Springer Nature Switzerland AG 2020
J. Kissane et al. (eds.), *Radiology Fundamentals: Introduction to Imaging & Technology*, https://doi.org/10.1007/978-3-030-22173-7_10

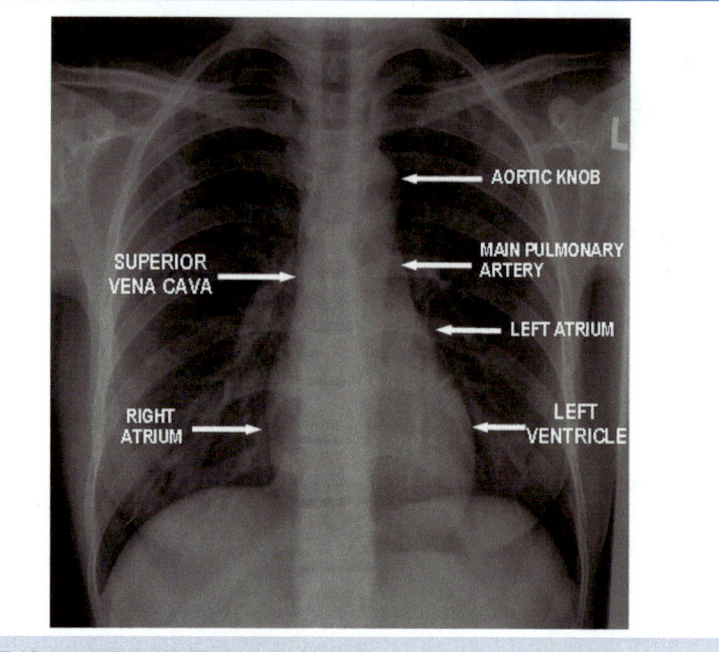

FIGURE 10.1 - MEDIASTINAL CONTOURS

Heart Size

The largest structure occupying the mediastinum is the heart. Recall from an earlier chapter that the cardiac size may vary depending on the projection of the radiograph (PA vs. AP). On an upright PA radiograph, the heart is said to be normal if its transverse diameter is no greater than 50–55% of the transverse diameter of the internal bony thorax. This will not hold true on AP radiographs, since the heart will be artificially magnified and where a diameter of 60% of thoracic diameter is considered normal. It may also not hold true in cases where the radiograph has been taken with a less than adequate inspiratory effort. Figure 10.2 demonstrates both a normal and an enlarged heart and shows examples of the points of measurement for both the heart and thoracic dimensions.

Mediastinal Structures and Compartments

In addition to the heart, great vessels, esophagus, and central airways, lymph nodes are present in the mediastinum. Lymph node enlargement can change the appearance of the mediastinum on a chest radiograph as seen in Fig. 10.3b. Figure 10.3a shows

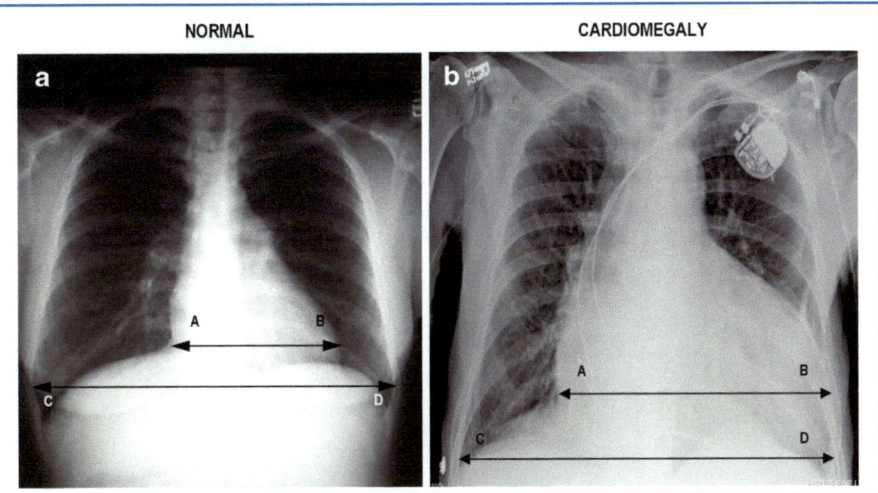

| NORMAL | CARDIOMEGALY |

FIGURE 10.2 - MEASURING THE HEART
(**a**) When evaluating the size of the heart, *AB* (maximum heart size) should be 50–55% of the measurement of *CD* (the maximum internal transverse thoracic diameter). (**b**) There is marked enlargement of the cardiac silhouette. Note how the ratio of *AB* to *CD* is greater than 50%

where mediastinal lymph nodes are located. Figure 10.3c is an axial CT image demonstrating enlarged lymph nodes around the aorta and superior vena cava.

Figure 10.4 shows a lateral view of the chest demonstrating the division of the mediastinum into three compartments: anterior, middle, and posterior. This method, recommended by the International Thymic Malignancy Interest Group (ITMIG), is one of several methods that can be used to divide the mediastinum. These are not true compartments, but are useful in locating a mediastinal abnormality on the radiograph for a differential diagnosis.

The anterior compartment of the mediastinum is bounded anteriorly by the sternum and posteriorly by a line drawn along the anterior margin of the heart, ascending aorta, and arch branches. Normally, fat, thymic tissue, and lymph nodes are present in this region. The middle compartment lies posterior to this. It is defined posteriorly by a line drawn 1 cm posterior to the anterior margin of the vertebral bodies. Middle mediastinal structures include the central airways, heart and great vessels, esophagus, and lymph nodes. The posterior mediastinum lies posterior to this and contains the thoracic spine and paravertebral soft tissues. Refer to Table 10.1 for mediastinal abnormalities by compartment.

The differential diagnosis for mediastinal masses is not as important as having a systematic method for reviewing conventional radiographs to identify normal or abnormal mediastinal contours. CT is almost universally employed as the next imaging step when a mediastinal abnormality is seen on a chest radiograph. In some cases, MRI is used for evaluation of mediastinal abnormalities.

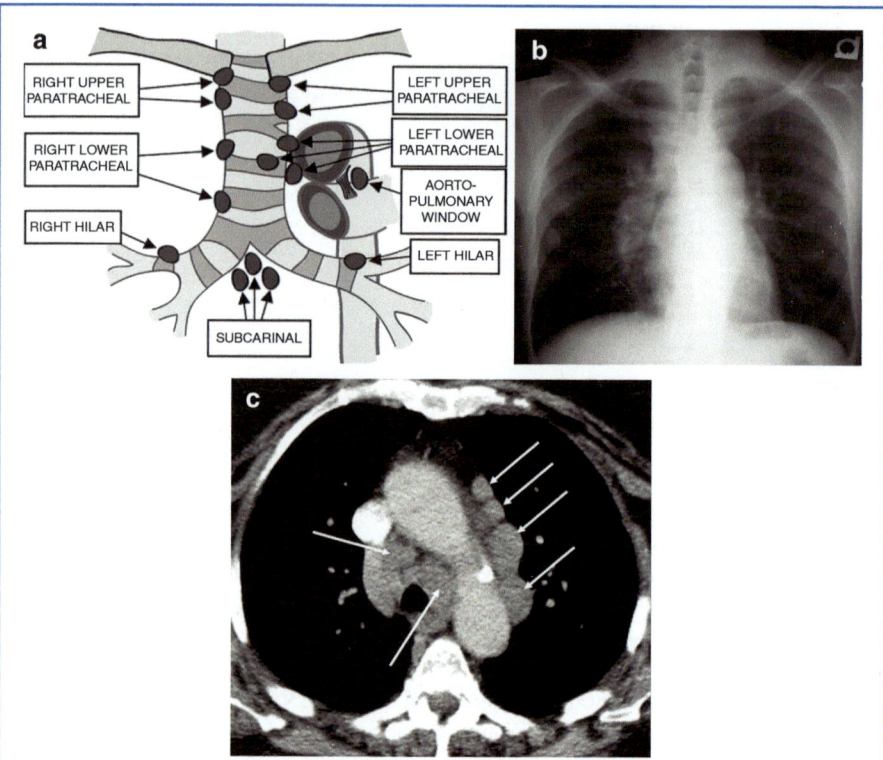

FIGURE 10.3 - LYMPH NODES OF THE MEDIASTINUM
In (**a**), the location of the lymph nodes in the chest are shown. Enlargement of these nodes can change the appearance of the mediastinum on a chest radiograph as seen in (**b**). In (**c**), mediastinal lymphadenopathy on an axial CT slice is demonstrated

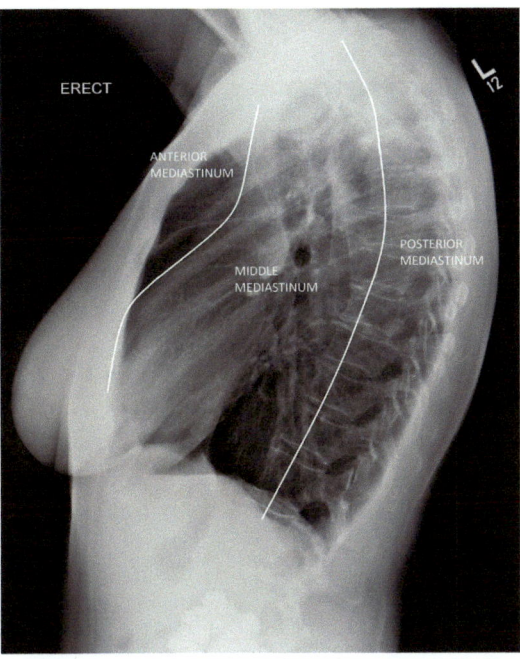

FIGURE 10.4 - MEDIASTINAL COMPARTMENTS
The subdivisions are the anterior, middle, and posterior mediastinum. These are important to the differential diagnosis of mediastinal pathology

Table 10.1 Mediastinal masses. A differential diagnosis of mediastinal masses may be made by the primary site of origin of the mass

Mediastinal division	Differential diagnosis
Anterior mediastinum (prevascular compartment)	Lymphadenopathy/lymphoma
	Retrosternal thyroid
	Thymic tumors
	Germ cell tumors
Middle mediastinum (visceral)	Lymphadenopathy
	Aortic aneurysms
	Esophageal neoplasms
	Thyroid goiter
	Bronchogenic and pericardial cysts
Posterior mediastinum (paravertebral)	Neurogenic tumors
	Soft tissue tumors
	Spinal infections and neoplasms

S: Evaluating cardiac and mediastinal contours by chest radiograph is an essential skill to help guide patient treatment and/or additional imaging. Normal and abnormal contour features are recognizable and identified on frontal and lateral chest radiograph with only more complex cases requiring the increased exposure to ionizing radiation of CT.

A: The frontal and lateral radiograph can be used to guide further imaging management by identifying the location of an abnormality and its origination. From these clues, the type and necessity for subsequent imaging can be determined.

F: Obtaining a chest x-ray requires significant attention to exposure, breath hold, rotation, etc. – all part of "technique." Uniform acquisition techniques help in rapid assessment of the radiograph and identification of pathology.

E: Urgent mediastinal findings can prompt emergent subsequent studies such as a change in the aortic contour in a patient with impending aortic rupture or a mass causing SVC syndrome. The quick identification of a contour abnormality can lead to prompt communication of the findings and action by the care team.

11   CARDIAC CTA

Objectives:
1. Understand a typical indication for coronary CTA.
2. Be able to describe the steps in a coronary CTA exam.
3. Describe other possible imaging uses in the heart for a gated CT scan.

CT scanners are now able to acquire images rapidly enough to "freeze" the heart in time and clearly delineate the coronary arteries. Their utility has been focused on the differentiation of patients with cardiac and noncardiac chest pain with an emphasis on those patients who have low to intermediate risk for coronary artery disease without EKG changes or enzyme elevation.

The patients are optimized for the coronary CT scan including the placement of a large-bore IV in the right arm (why the right arm?) and given oral or IV beta-blockers. Beta-blockers are contraindicated in patients with the following:

- Known or suspected sick sinus syndrome
- Unexplained presyncope or collapse
- Current use of other antiarrhythmics
- Depressed left or right ventricular function
- History of bronchospastic disease, severe COPD
- Allergy to β-blockers

Finally, 800 mcg of sublingual nitroglycerin (SL NTG) is given just prior to contrast injection. Contraindications to the NTG include the following:

- Pronounced hypovolemia
- Inferior wall MI with RV involvement
- Elevated intracranial pressure

© Springer Nature Switzerland AG 2020   57
J. Kissane et al. (eds.), *Radiology Fundamentals: Introduction to Imaging & Technology*, https://doi.org/10.1007/978-3-030-22173-7_11

- Cardiac tamponade
- Constrictive pericarditis
- Severe aortic stenosis
- Hypertrophic obstructive cardiomyopathy
- Severe systolic hypotension

Contrast is usually injected at 6–8 mL/sec for a total of 65–75 mL of nonionic contrast after bolus tracking technique (Fig. 11.1). Images are acquired during *diastole*, when the heart is filling passively but also has the least amount of motion (Fig. 11.2). If there is any ectopy, using certain imaging acquisition protocols, there can be significant artifact (Fig. 11.3) on the images. The images acquired are then viewed in both standard planes and on a 3D workstation (Fig. 11.4). Description of any plaque should include whether the plaque is noncalcified versus calcified versus mixed. Sensitivity and specificity for the 128 slice CT scanners are ~92% and 95%, respectively. It has a very good negative predictive value, and in that sense, it is very useful for the patient in the ED with convincing chest pain and significant risk factors and no objective evidence of cardiac ischemia.

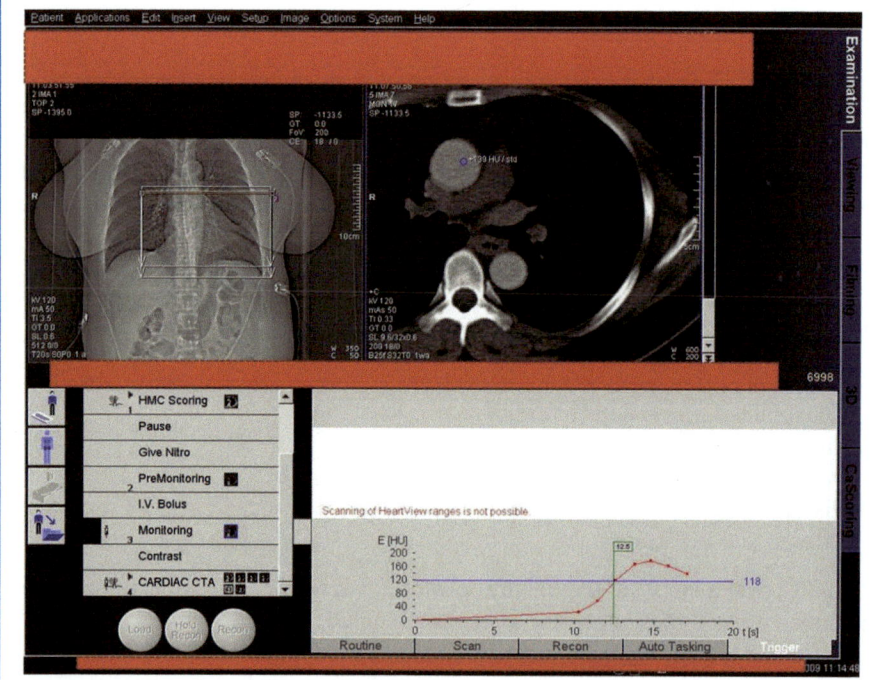

FIGURE 11.1 - CARDIAC CTA PLANNING
Image from the planning screen of a cardiac CTA demonstrating the field of view (*upper left image*), the bolus tracking area in the ascending aorta (*upper right image*), the actual steps in the protocol (*lower left*), and the contrast-density curve (*lower right image*)

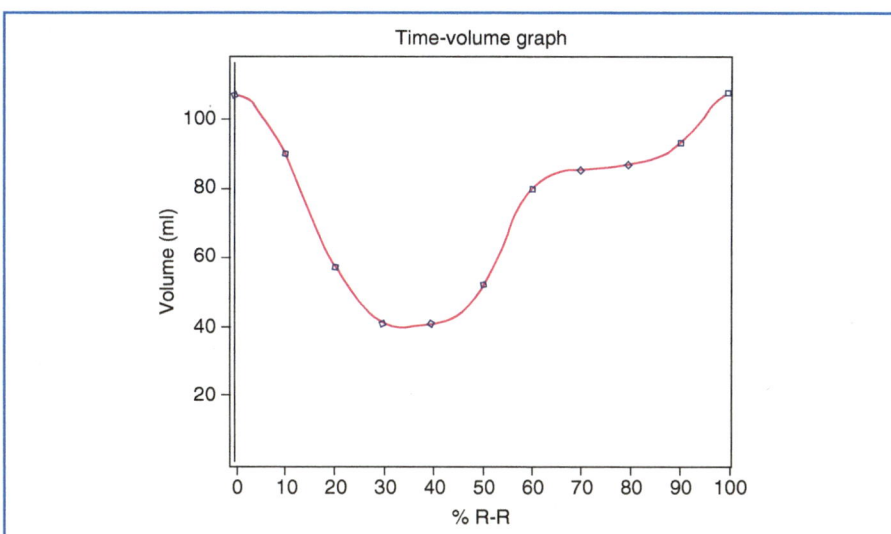

FIGURE 11.2 - R-R INTERVAL DIVISION
Time-volume graph with the R-R interval divided into 0–100% on the x-axis and the volume on the y-axis. Note that the volume does not change from ~65% to ~75%, coinciding with diastole and the optimal time in the cardiac cycle to obtain images

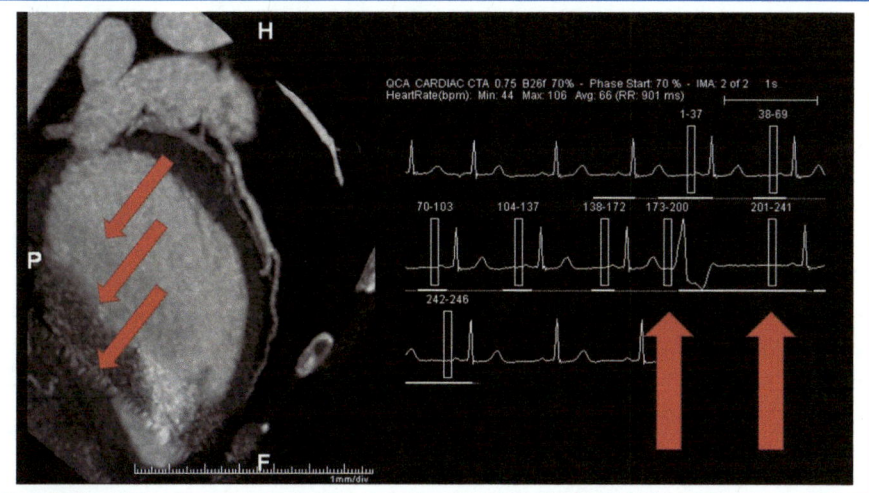

FIGURE 11.3 - PVC ARTIFACT
In this image from a cardiac CTA scan, it is noted on the image to the *right* that acquisition times (*the rectangular boxes*) are all appropriate except in the region of the PVC (*arrows*). That corresponds to the imaging artifact noted on the image to the *left* (*smaller arrows*)

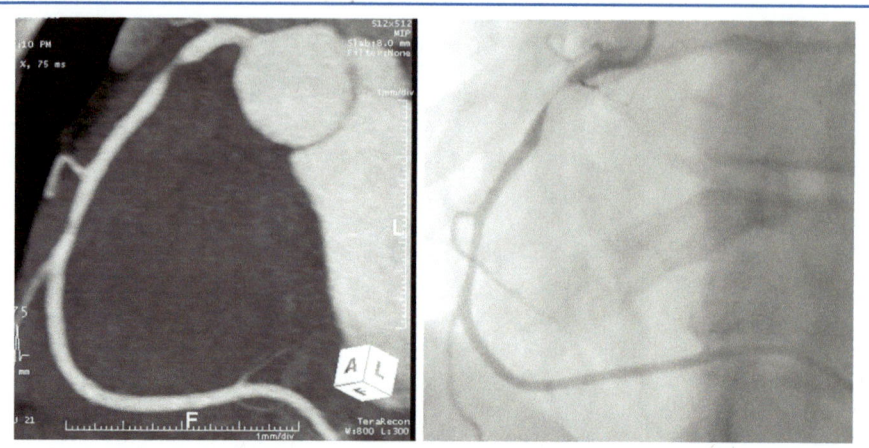

FIGURE 11.4 - CORONARY CTA VS CATHETERIZATION
Coronary CTA of the RCA (image on the *left*) and the subsequent cardiac catheterization image of the same segment (image on the *right*). There is strong correlation between the images

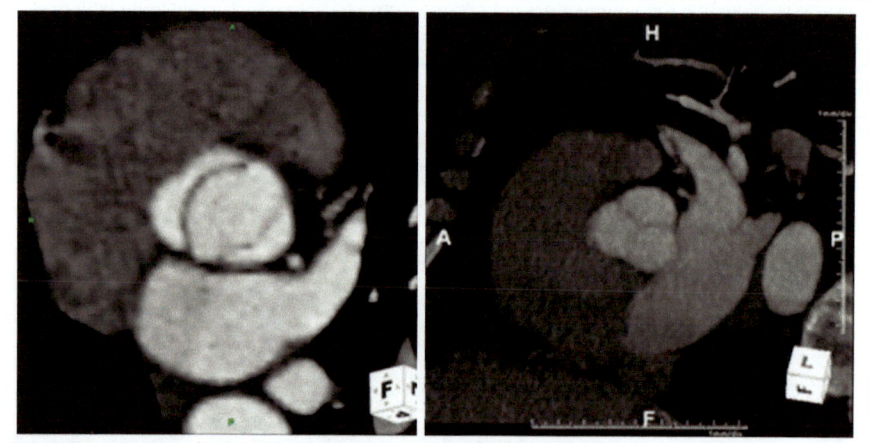

FIGURE 11.5 - BICUSPID VS TRICUSPID VALVES ON CARDIAC CTA
En face images of the aortic valve in a patient with a bicuspid aortic valve (image on the left) and a patient with a normal, tricuspid aortic valve (image on the *right*)

Although the other indications for cardiac CTA are beyond the scope of this textbook, one indication for the use of cardiac CTA is the evaluation of the cardiac structures, such as the aortic valve (Fig. 11.5).

Additionally, there is increased utilization in the pre-procedure planning for transfemoral aortic valve replacement (TAVR) as well as for mitral valve replacement (Fig. 11.6).

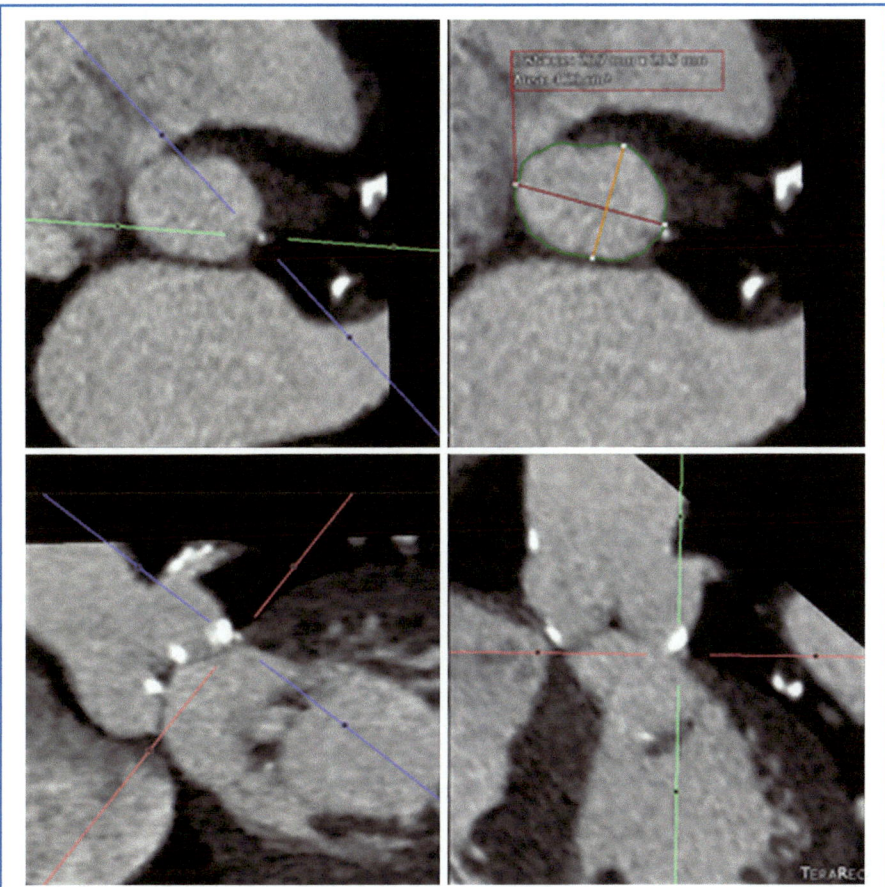

FIGURE 11.6 - TAVR PLANNING ON CARDIAC CTA
En face images of the aortic valve in a patient scheduled for TAVR (images on *top*) and a coronal plane imaging demonstrating extent and location of calcifications around the valve (images on *bottom*)

S: The use of coronary CTA in patients presenting with typical chest pain but no objective evidence of cardiac ischemia has been a useful adjunct in the diagnosis, preventing the unnecessary catheterization of patients with chest pain.

A: The acquisition of a cardiac CTA is very dependent on the patient's heart rate and rhythm. These should be optimized prior to scanning including a heart rate in the upper 50's to upper 60's. Additionally, a right arm IV should be placed so that the contrast bolus does not cause artifact across the mediastinum for imaging.

F: Viewing the images on a post-processing workstation is critical. The ability to look at the coronary arteries in a stretched vessel view as well as a cross-section view is essential to the evaluation of the artery's patent lumen and to characterize the plaque. Additionally, reconstructed views of the mitral and aortic valve plane are needed to plan implanted valve parameters.

E: For the patient in the ED with chest pain, a timely evaluation of the coronary artery patency expedites the management of these patients to discharge home or possible cardiac catheterization. Many studies have recognized the utility of the coronary CTA in the Emergency Department.

12 LATERAL CHEST RADIOGRAPH

Objectives:
1. Learn to use a systematic method for review of the left lateral chest radiograph.
2. Identify major structures (heart, aorta, central airways, pulmonary arteries, and hemidiaphragms) and recognize normal areas of lucency on the lateral view.
3. State how the silhouette sign and magnification can be used to differentiate the left and right hemidiaphragms on the lateral view.

Lateral View: Systemic Approach

The lateral chest radiograph is obtained in conjunction with a frontal (PA or AP) chest radiograph and contains valuable information. This chapter describes the systematic review of the lateral radiograph. Begin by reviewing the systematic approach to the left lateral chest radiograph in Fig. 12.1.

Start by reviewing the major structures including the heart, aorta, and pulmonary arteries at the hilum, central airways, and the right and left hemidiaphragms. Follow this with a review of the areas of lucency in the retrosternal region, retrotracheal triangle, the large rectangular area extending inferiorly from the retrotracheal triangle to the diaphragms (with a gradual gradation of density from lighter to darker as one moves inferiorly), and the costophrenic angles. Lastly, review the upper abdomen, bones, and soft tissues. If you proceed in this manner on each x-ray, you will develop a consistent method for detecting abnormalities. This takes considerable practice.

The importance of the lateral view cannot be underestimated. The lateral view helps to add information about an abnormality (or apparent abnormality) seen on the PA view, see small effusions, determine the position of an abnormality, give a

© Springer Nature Switzerland AG 2020
J. Kissane et al. (eds.), *Radiology Fundamentals: Introduction to Imaging & Technology*, https://doi.org/10.1007/978-3-030-22173-7_12

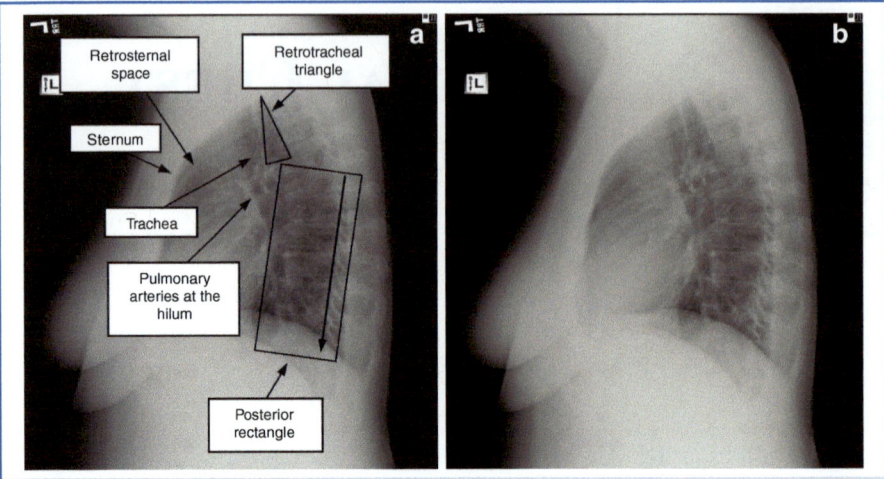

FIGURE 12.1 - THE LATERAL CHEST
(a) Normal lateral view. Use this image to identify structures and spaces on the image (b)

Labels in figure (a): Retrosternal space, Retrotracheal triangle, Sternum, Trachea, Pulmonary arteries at the hilum, Posterior rectangle

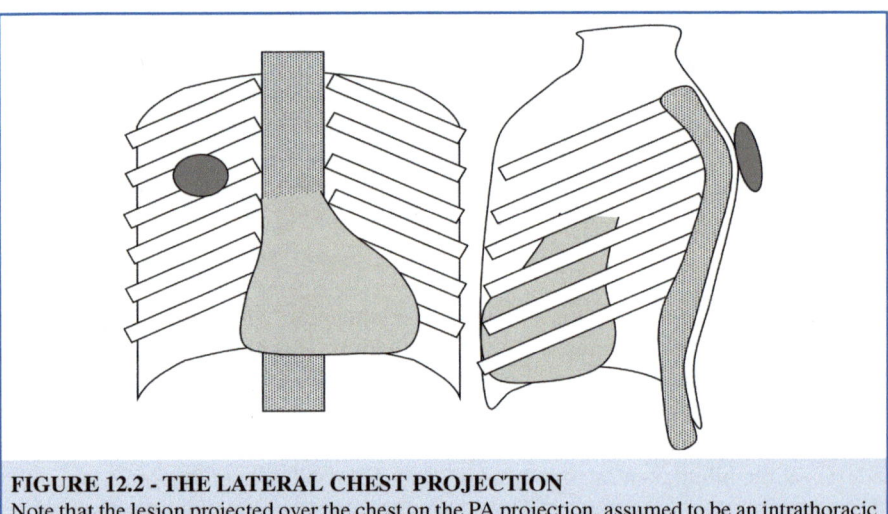

FIGURE 12.2 - THE LATERAL CHEST PROJECTION
Note that the lesion projected over the chest on the PA projection, assumed to be an intrathoracic mass, is actually in the soft tissues of the back

better estimate of lung volume, and uncover the hilum. Without a lateral view, the position of any abnormality projected over the lungs cannot be determined with certainty, in most cases.

Figure 12.2 is a schematic of a skin lesion arising from the soft tissues of the back that is projected over the right lung on the frontal view. The lateral view can be useful in ascertaining whether a structure lies within or outside the patient. Figure 12.3

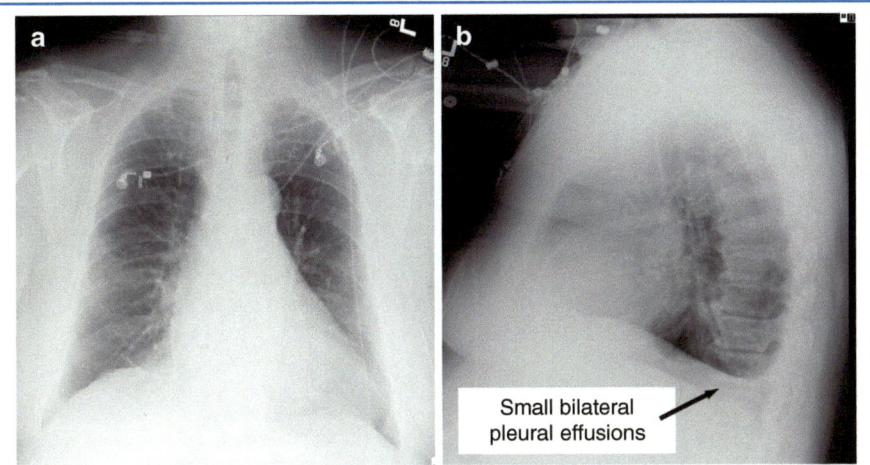

Small bilateral
pleural effusions

FIGURE 12.3 - BILATERAL PLEURAL EFFUSIONS
Frontal and lateral views of a patient with suspected bilateral pleural effusions. Note that although bilateral pleural effusions are clearly evident on the lateral projection (**b**), the costophrenic angles are clear and sharp on the frontal view (**a**)

demonstrates frontal and lateral views of a patient with suspected bilateral pleural effusions. The bilateral pleural effusions are clearly evident on the lateral projection as curved menisci. However, the costophrenic angles are clear and sharp on the frontal view. This is a good example of how small pleural fluid accumulations that may be of clinical significance can be overlooked if one relies only on the frontal (AP or PA) projections. Similarly, patients with small areas of consolidation or nodules in the lower lobes may not be correctly diagnosed if one does not carefully review the lateral projection, as a portion of the lower lobes is obscured by the hemidiaphragms on the frontal view.

Hemidiaphragms

There are several ways to determine which hemidiaphragm and which costophrenic angle is the left versus the right on the lateral view (see Fig. 12.4 for correlation).

1. Since the anterior portion of the left hemidiaphragm comes into contact with the inferior aspect of the heart, it is often obscured or silhouetted anteriorly – another example of the silhouette sign. For this reason, the left hemidiaphragm cannot usually be traced as far anteriorly as the right hemidiaphragm.
2. Lateral chest radiographs are usually performed in the left lateral position. This means the patient's left side is placed against the cassette, and the beam traverses

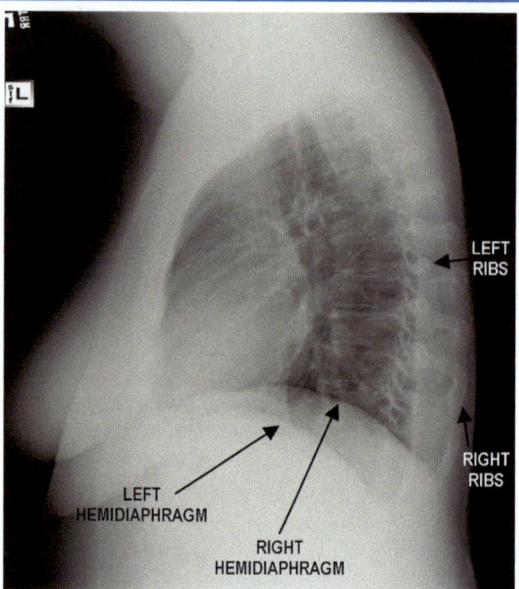

FIGURE 12.4 - HEMIDIAPHRAGMS
Lateral chest with well-visualized hemidiaphragms

the patient from right to left. This is noted by an "L" marker somewhere on the radiograph. You will recall that objects that are further from the radiograph are magnified more. If one looks at the posterior portion of the left lateral chest radiograph, two sets of ribs, a large set and a corresponding smaller set, can be seen. One can reason that the larger set of ribs must be located further from the radiograph and must represent the right ribs. The hemidiaphragm that can be traced to this set of ribs must be the right hemidiaphragm. This also allows separating the right and left costophrenic angles.

3. Since the left hemidiaphragm lies directly above the stomach, the left hemidiaphragm can be seen to have the stomach beneath it on the lateral view, if the left hemidiaphragm is slightly higher than the right in this region.

4. By correlating the height of the hemidiaphragm on the frontal projection with the highest point of the hemidiaphragm on the lateral projection, one may be able to distinguish left from right on the lateral view.

Think about these relationships, since they represent a recapitulation of two important principles presented earlier – the silhouette sign and the principle of magnification.

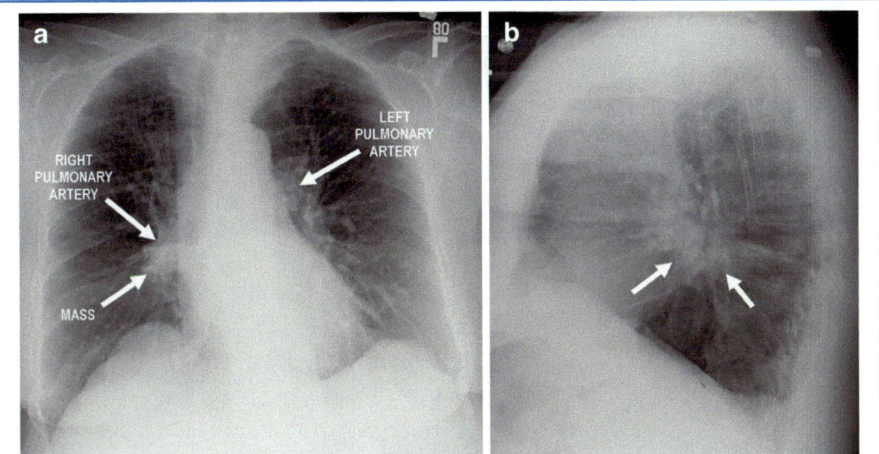

FIGURE 12.5 - HILAR MASS
AP (**a**) and lateral (**b**) chest radiographs show a patient with a right hilar mass. *Arrows* seen on the lateral (**b**) radiograph indicate the margins of the mass inferior to the pulmonary arteries

Hilar Enlargement

Review Fig. 12.5a. The arrows on this PA view indicate the right and left interlobar pulmonary arteries. On the right side, there is increased density overlying the vessel. On the lateral view (Fig. 12.5b), one can clearly separate the right and left pulmonary arteries from an irregular mass. This was a lung adenocarcinoma. The lateral view may be useful in distinguishing hilar enlargement from enlarged pulmonary arteries (due to pulmonary hypertension) from hilar adenopathy.

S: Skillful evaluation of the lateral chest radiograph can add value and prevent needless further exposure to ionizing radiation. Important lucencies such as the retrotracheal triangle, the retrosternal clear space, and the posterior rectangle should be used to find space-occupying lesions. Occasionally, a lesion presumed to be intrathoracic on frontal view can be proven to be subcutaneous with the use of a lateral view, preventing needless further workup.

A: When a lesion is located on the frontal radiograph, sometimes it is advantageous to request a lateral radiograph for localization rather than CT. Examples include extrathoracic pathology or normal structures which mimic a lesion. The lateral view is also useful to find pleural fluid which may be occult on frontal view. A CT is appropriate as further workup for suspected malignancy and in many clinical situations.

F: It is important to adopt a systematic method of viewing the lateral chest radiograph, for example, starting with the major structures including the heart, aorta, and pulmonary arteries; then ensure that the retrosternal clear space, retrotracheal triangle, and the posterior rectangle are intact. This way, subtle abnormalities can be identified and localized.

E: The lateral radiograph can be used to expedite care by preventing further evaluation of a benign finding or by finding a cause of the patient's symptoms that is impossible to view on frontal projections. It is also useful for directing the clinical team, for example, by identifying a hilar opacity which could be ill-defined on the frontal view due to overlying structures but easily discerned as a mass on the lateral view.

13 PULMONARY NODULES OR MASSES

Objectives:
1. Understand the need for pulmonary nodule characterization on a chest radiograph. Remember to assess the following characteristics of the lesion: size, location, margin characteristics, involvement of contiguous structures, calcification or cavitation, solitary versus multiple, time course of growth from old radiographs, and other chest radiograph findings.
2. List four differential diagnoses for a solitary pulmonary nodule.
3. Discuss the significance of calcification within a pulmonary nodule or mass.

A pulmonary nodule is a well-circumscribed opacity (typically spherical) measuring up to or equal to 3 cm in diameter. A mass is a lesion more than 3 cm in diameter. The principles of evaluation are the same for nodules and masses, and so for the rest of this chapter, the term nodule is used.

Nodules within the lung are commonly suspected and/or appreciated on the conventional chest radiograph. There are several criteria which must be used to arrive at a list of potential differential diagnoses for a lung nodule.

Evaluation of a Pulmonary Nodule

1. *Is it pulmonary?* Make sure the nodule is in the lung and not a superimposed structure related to the chest wall, as would be the case in a patient with a skin or breast lesion or other external density (Fig. 13.1 below, and Fig. 12.2 from Chap. 12). Healing rib fractures can also simulate lung nodules.

© Springer Nature Switzerland AG 2020
J. Kissane et al. (eds.), *Radiology Fundamentals: Introduction to Imaging & Technology*, https://doi.org/10.1007/978-3-030-22173-7_13

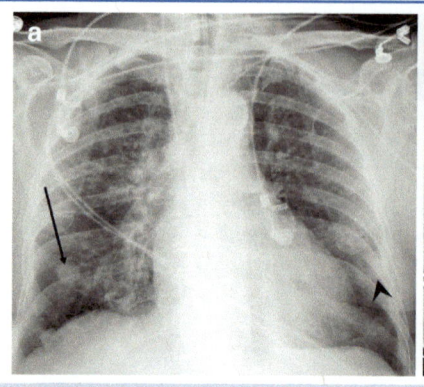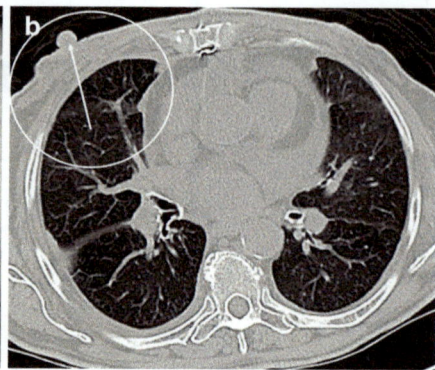

FIGURE 13.1 - NIPPLE SHADOWS

Image (**a**) depicts what appears to be a right lower lung nodule on a frontal chest x-ray (*black arrow*). The *arrowhead* shows a similar "nodule" on the right chest wall indicating these represent the nipples. Note the appearance on the corresponding CT slice, image (**b**), (*arrow* inside of *circle*)

2. *Compare with old studies*: The "cancer" you have just diagnosed may be a benign nodule which has been present for many years. If old studies are not available at your institution, you should check with the referring clinician or patient if old studies are available. A nodule that is new compared with a recent radiograph (from one to a few weeks earlier) is more likely to be infectious or inflammatory.

3. *Size*: Larger lesions are more likely to be malignant; however, bigger lesions are not always malignant, and smaller lesions are not always benign. Interval growth is also important.

4. *Location*: Assess the location of the nodule with respect to the pulmonary lobes and pulmonary segments (if possible). This requires frontal (preferably PA) and lateral views. Computerized tomography (CT) is used to more accurately characterize and localize a nodule.

5. *Margin characteristics*: Assess whether the margins of the lesion are smooth or irregular. Obviously, the more irregular the margins of the mass, the more suspicious we are that we are dealing with a malignant process. Keep in mind, though, that many infectious and inflammatory lesions have quite irregular margins. This should be correlated with the patient's symptoms. If there are clinical features of infection, a follow-up radiograph after treatment should be considered. Metastatic lesions may be very smoothly demarcated. Although the contours of a lesion should be evaluated, they are not absolute indicators of a benign versus malignant lesion.

6. *Involvement of contiguous structures*: This may be an important indicator of the etiology of the lesion. A mass that is close to the chest wall and destroys a rib is very likely to be malignant.

7. *Presence or absence of cavitation or calcification*: Cavitation may be seen both benign and malignant processes. Calcification that is diffuse or laminated is generally benign. Central, dense calcification occupying a significant portion of the nodule is also often benign. Metastatic osteosarcoma, however, may be densely ossified.
8. *Solitary or multiple lesions*: Multiple pulmonary nodules often have a different connotation and differential diagnosis than a solitary lesion. For this reason, when one pulmonary nodule is seen, a careful search for other nodules should be made. Computerized tomography, because of its sensitivity for detection of nodules, is useful in this regard.
9. *Other findings*: Once you have found a nodule, do not stop your search for other abnormalities: "satisfaction of search" is a common problem. Additional findings such as mediastinal adenopathy, hilar adenopathy, or destructive rib lesions suggest malignancy and warrant early CT evaluation.

In addition to these findings, take into account the age and clinical history to guide your recommendations. Assess the temporal evolution, if prior imaging is available. The differential diagnosis of a solitary pulmonary nodule includes granulomatous disease (such as old tuberculous and histoplasma infection), primary lung malignancy, and post-inflammatory parenchymal scarring. Other less common causes of solitary pulmonary nodules include hamartoma, solitary metastasis, carcinoid tumors, round pneumonia, arteriovenous malformations, and cysts.

Cases to Review

The following series of radiographs depict various causes of pulmonary nodules or masses. Try to describe each in terms of the criteria provided and arrive at a brief differential diagnosis.

As always, the point is not to memorize the many possible diagnoses for each abnormality. You should however be fastidious in employing these criteria and remembering the pitfalls for all cases of pulmonary nodules.

Case 1: Figure 13.1 demonstrates an approximately 1 cm, soft tissue nodule projected over the lower right chest. While this may be confused with a pulmonary nodule, its smooth margins (it is unusually well outlined because it is surrounded by air), classic position, and the presence of a corresponding similar density on the left side indicate that this represents the nipple. When a questionable nodule is suspected to be a nipple shadow, a repeat study with small metallic markers taped to the nipples may be performed for confirmation.

Case 2: Figure 13.2 demonstrates a solitary pulmonary nodule in the left lower lung behind the heart. This is the so-called coin lesion, even though it is a three-dimensional sphere. This lesion turned out to be a granuloma, but there are no distinguishing characteristics on the radiograph that would allow you to make this diagnosis. A biopsy was necessary to make this diagnosis.

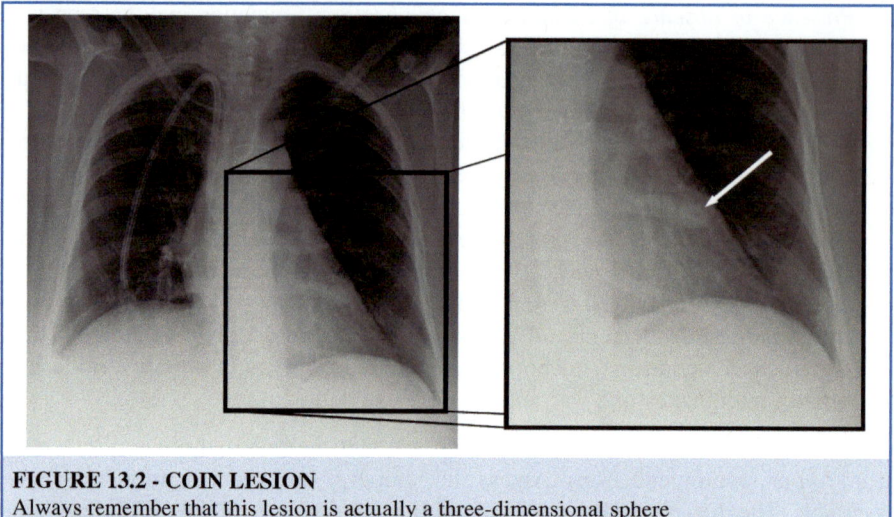

FIGURE 13.2 - COIN LESION
Always remember that this lesion is actually a three-dimensional sphere

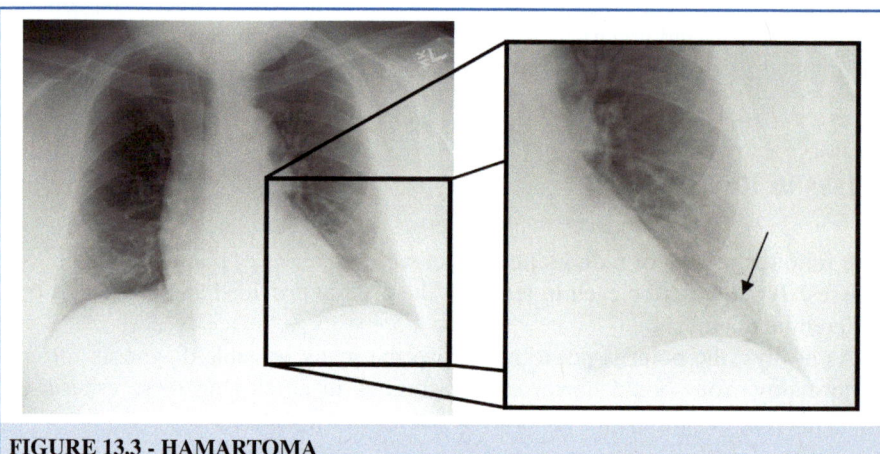

FIGURE 13.3 - HAMARTOMA
Hamartoma in the left lower lobe. Note the typical "popcorn" calcification within the lesion

Case 3: Figure 13.3 demonstrates a large smoothly marginated solitary lesion without evidence of cavitation in the left paracardiac region. Mottled densities may be seen within the mass representing "popcorn"-like calcifications. Although calcification within a lesion does not guarantee that it is of benign etiology, this pattern of calcification is often associated with a particular benign neoplasm of the lung, a hamartoma. Comparison with old studies also showed the mass to be unchanged in size. In this case, detection of this pattern of calcification and stability compared with prior imaging made surgical removal or tissue sampling for diagnosis unnecessary.

Case 4: Figure 13.4 was obtained from a 60-year-old man with a history of heavy smoking who now presents with weight loss and hemoptysis. The left mid-lung mass demonstrates obvious cavitation. It is also contiguous to the left lateral chest wall, but it does not erode or destroy the ribs and does not produce a pleural effusion on this view. The hilum on the left side has a relatively normal appearance without definite evidence of lymphadenopathy. Again, as in so many disease processes of the chest, CT scans would better evaluate lymphadenopathy. The differential diagnosis of this cavitary lesion includes a primary lung neoplasm. Cavitation is most common in the squamous cell type of primary lung carcinoma. A lung abscess could give a similar appearance if the patient's symptoms related more to an inflammatory process than this patient's obviously malignant symptomatology. Cavitation may be artifactually simulated by a number of conditions, and before cavitation is accepted as a finding, it must be clearly present. Often, debris or soft tissue density will be seen within a cavity. This can represent clotted blood, inflammatory exudate, a "fungus ball" (due to an aspergilloma), or necrotic debris from the inner wall of the neoplasm. This lesion was a squamous cell carcinoma on biopsy.

Case 5: Figure 13.5 demonstrates multiple pulmonary nodules in both lungs that are highly suspicious for metastases. It is their size and multiplicity, which strongly suggests their etiology. Any time one nodule is found, carefully search for others. Because metastases to the lungs are essentially an embolic process, metastases are more common in the lower lobes, because of the normally increased blood

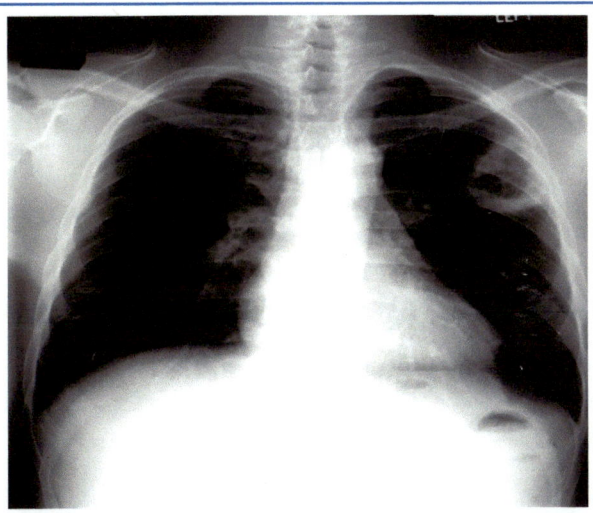

FIGURE 13.4 - CAVITARY LESION
Note the area of decreased density within the well-defined left upper lung mass

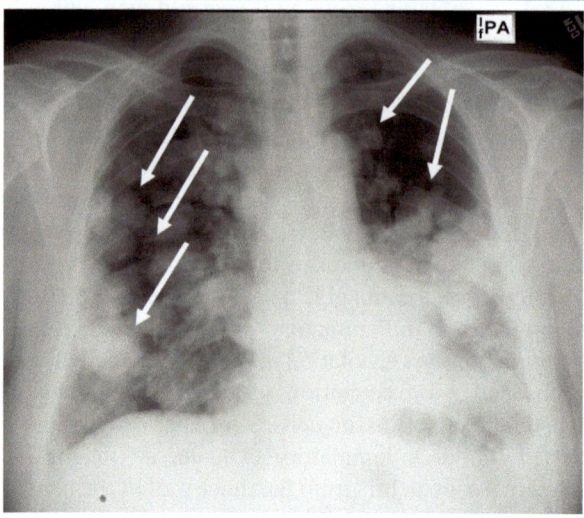

FIGURE 13.5 - PULMONARY NODULES
A chest radiograph demonstrating numerous pulmonary nodules throughout both lungs

flow to this region. Computerized tomography (CT) is the most sensitive test for detecting early metastatic disease. Other processes such as granulomatous disease can also demonstrate multiple nodules.

Case 6: Figure 13.6 is a frontal chest radiograph of a young adult patient with a small amount of blood-tinged sputum and a fever of 101°. Obviously, the presence of the fairly well-marginated mass lesion in the right mid-lung is of concern for possible malignancy. However, because this patient's age and symptoms favor pneumonia, a trial of antibiotics for 2 weeks was performed. There was no cavitation to indicate a lung abscess. A follow-up radiograph at that time showed significant resolution of the opacity. This is an example of "round pneumonia." Although more commonly seen in children, round pneumonia can also occur in adults, as in this case. Inflammatory exudate spreads from alveolar unit to alveolar unit through the pores of Kohn, opacifying the lung in an expanding manner from a central focus. In certain cases, the pattern of expansion and flow of exudate can be very well defined and simulate a mass lesion. It is important to pay attention to the clinical presentation of the patient, in addition to the radiographic findings, when evaluating a pulmonary nodule or mass.

Case 7: Figure 13.7a demonstrates a well-defined density projected over the right mid-lung. The lateral view (Fig. 13.7b) demonstrates that this density has a lentiform (or lens-like) configuration and lies within the right major fissure. This density represents the so-called pseudotumor, caused by fluid loculated within a

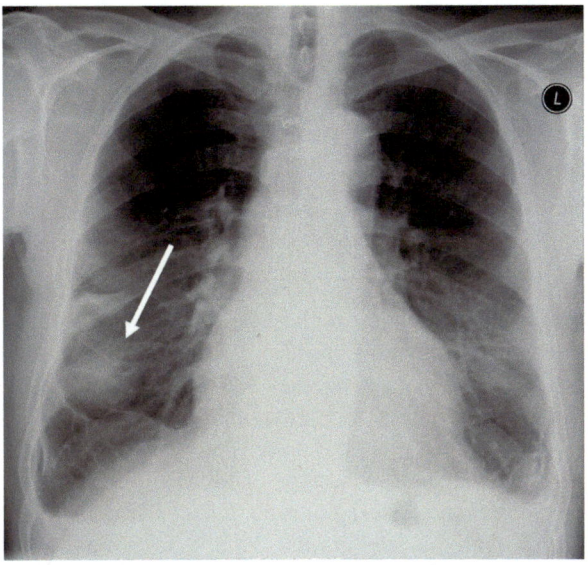

FIGURE 13.6 - ROUND PNEUMONIA
Round pneumonia in the right lower lung (*arrow*)

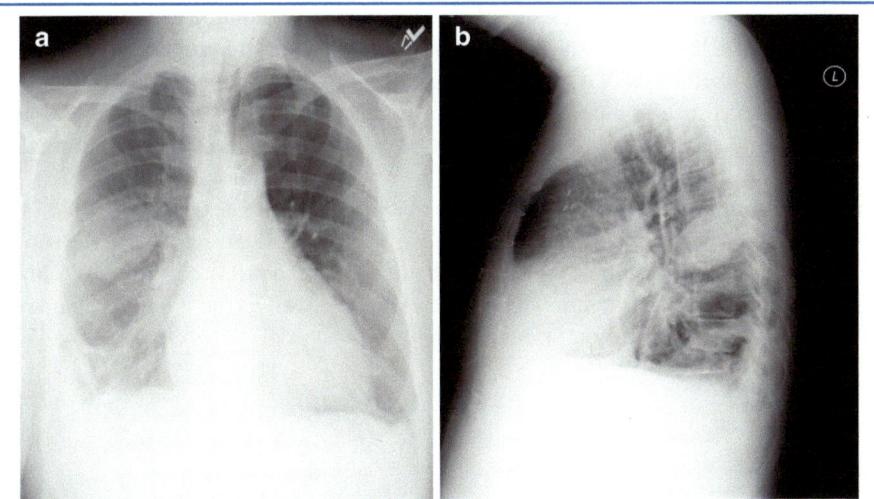

FIGURE 13.7 - PSEUDOTUMOR
Frontal (**a**) and lateral (**b**) chest radiographs demonstrating a pseudotumor in the right mid-lung along the right major fissure

fissure. Clues to the diagnosis include location in the area of the fissure, ovoid shape with long axis in the plane of the fissure, and association with a pleural effusion either on the same radiograph or on prior studies.

In summary, the differential diagnosis of solitary and multiple pulmonary nodules is long. There is considerable overlap between the appearance of benign and malignant conditions. Time and expense may be saved through careful observation and analysis of the plain radiographs, comparisons with old radiographs, as well as correlation with the patient's clinical presentation. If the abnormality is not clearly benign or acute on chest radiographs, chest CT is often the next step in evaluation.

S: Detecting a pulmonary nodule on chest radiograph can lead to a multitude of downstream examinations and exposure to ionizing radiation. Therefore, it is important to realize that many processes do not require CT evaluation such as a benign hamartoma seen on prior imaging, nipple shadow, or even round pneumonias.

A: It is imperative to understand what type of follow-up imaging is appropriate for lesions that are noted on chest radiograph. Clearly, it is important not to miss a finding, but it is equally as important to be able to explain whether a nodule is malignant or benign. Using clues such as lesion location and time course are important factors in determining the appropriate further use of ionizing radiation.

F: A systematic search pattern can identify small or subtle nodules by radiograph. Often, CT is an appropriate exam when no priors are available to demonstrate the stability of a lesion or if the extent is unclear. An important tool to keep in mind is also the usefulness of a follow-up examination, for example, round pneumonia that presents as a nodule. If the patient presents with symptoms of infection, a follow-up radiograph after treatment is all that is necessary if the lesion disappears.

E: Clear communication with referring providers about the next course of action is necessary when evaluating nodules since such a wide array of disease can be represented. The fact that a nodule has been present on priors can be an extremely helpful tool in evaluation and recommendation as well as the nodule's characteristics such as calcification or cavitation.

14 AIRSPACE DISEASE

Objectives:
1. Describe the radiographic finding characteristic of airspace disease.
2. List the major differential diagnostic categories for acute airspace disease.
3. List two causes of chronic airspace disease.

The purpose of this chapter is to discuss the appearance of airspace disease in the lungs. The pulmonary acinus is the basic structural unit of the lung involved in gas exchange (Fig. 14.1). It is the structural unit of lung distal to the terminal bronchiole, is supplied by respiratory bronchioles, and is 6–10 mm in diameter. It contains alveolar ducts and alveoli. The terminal bronchiole is the most peripheral airway that is purely conductive in function with no gas exchange capability. A pulmonary lobule (or secondary pulmonary lobule) is the smallest unit of lung surrounded by connective tissue septa. One lobule contains between 3 and 25 acini. Recall the four densities seen on a radiograph – air, soft tissue, fat, and bone. Disease within the airspace is manifest on the radiograph as soft tissue density. Disease may involve numerous acini or spread from one acinar unit to another. The opacified acini become confluent, producing a fluffy, homogeneous radiographic pattern characteristic of airspace disease as seen in Fig. 14.2.

Since disease, which primarily affects the airspace, often spares the larger conductive airways, these airways become visible as tubular, branching, air-filled structures surrounded by the fluid-filled acini. These air-filled structures are normally surrounded by air-filled lung and are not normally distinguished on the chest radiograph. These air-filled bronchi surrounded by opacified airspace are called air bronchograms. Air bronchograms are the radiographic hallmark of airspace disease. Figure 14.3 is an excellent example of air bronchograms in a patient

© Springer Nature Switzerland AG 2020
J. Kissane et al. (eds.), *Radiology Fundamentals: Introduction to Imaging & Technology*, https://doi.org/10.1007/978-3-030-22173-7_14

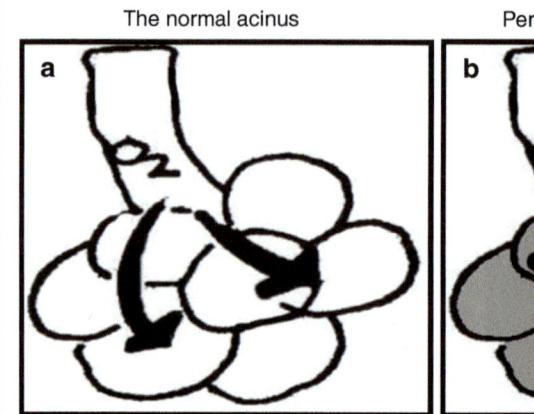
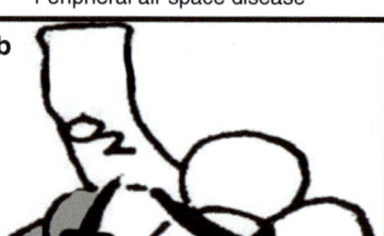

FIGURE 14.1 - LUNG ACINUS
(**a**) The normal acinus is 6–10 mm in diameter. (**b**) In the picture on the *right*, volume is unaffected and the airways remain patent

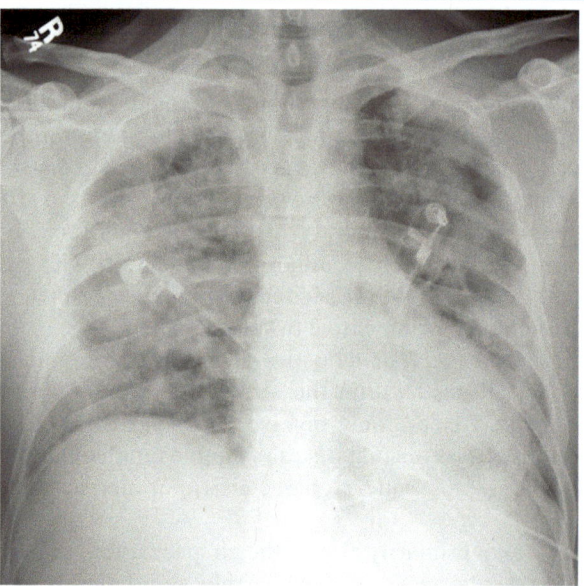

FIGURE 14.2 - AIRSPACE DISEASE
Frontal chest radiograph demonstrating perihilar predominant airspace disease, due to pulmonary edema. The radiograph 24 h after diuresis was significantly improved

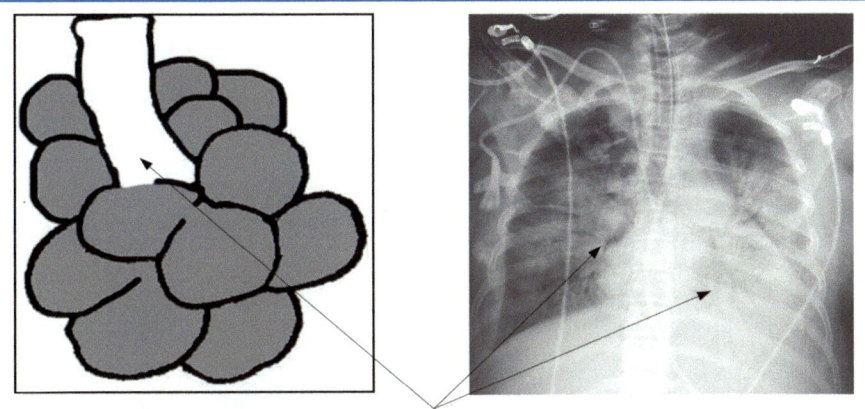

FLUID FILLED ACINI DEMONSTRATING AIR BRONCHOGRAMS

FIGURE 14.3 - AIR BRONCHOGRAMS
Schematic and radiograph of an air bronchogram. Note that the bronchi are usually not seen peripherally on a normal chest radiograph. With the acini surrounding the bronchus filled with fluid, the bronchus is outlined

with pneumonia and acute respiratory distress syndrome (ARDS). The distribution of airspace disease and time course of development may be useful in determining its etiology.

Figure 14.4 demonstrates airspace disease in the right lower lung. In a patient with cough and fever, this would be consistent with pneumonia. The right dome of the diaphragm and right heart border are preserved. A lateral view is necessary to localize this to the right middle or lower lobes.

Consider the common differentials for acute airspace disease:

1. Pulmonary edema: transudate fills the alveoli.
2. Infection: pneumonic exudate fills the alveoli.
3. Hemorrhage: blood fills the alveoli.

Within each of these major categories, however, multiple pathologies may be included:

1. Pulmonary edema – cardiogenic (CHF) or noncardiogenic (ARDS).
2. Infection – numerous organisms may cause pneumonia.
3. Hemorrhage – etiology includes pulmonary contusion, pulmonary infarctions, vasculitis, coagulopathy, and drug-induced hemorrhage.

This list does not include all possibilities. Clinical information and comparison with old studies must be utilized to narrow the diagnostic possibilities. Fever would suggest pneumonia, while hemoptysis would suggest pulmonary hemorrhage. The

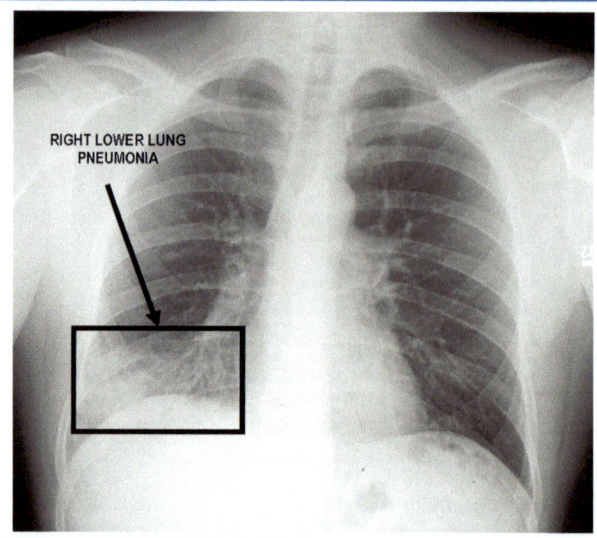

FIGURE 14.4 - PNEUMONIA
Patchy airspace disease in the right lower lung consistent with pneumonia

distribution and pattern of evolution of the abnormality may also help. Cardiogenic edema tends to be bilateral and associated with other findings (enlarged heart, pleural effusions). Pneumonia is classically more focal.

Pathologic processes involving the airspaces (alveoli) can be further subdivided into acute and chronic etiologies. The time course of appearance and regression of airspace disease is useful. Edema can come and go quickly (regression can occur within hours). Pneumonia regresses more slowly. Non-resolving airspace opacity may require evaluation for other processes such as neoplasms (including some types of adenocarcinoma and pulmonary lymphoma), hypersensitivity pneumonitis, alveolar sarcoidosis, and alveolar proteinosis.

S: Airspace disease identified on radiographs is not specific and can have many etiologies. In order to provide for the safety of the patient, an ordered differential diagnosis should be assigned based on the clinical history and relevant prior imaging.

A: To assess the appropriate study, airspace disease should be evaluated over time and re-evaluated on repeat imaging if it is obtained. Sometimes, time course or pattern can distinguish etiology between infection, edema, and hemorrhage without the need for excessive ionizing radiation. Other clinical situations require further assessment with CT, for example, to evaluate for an abscess when pneumonia does not improve.

F: Differentiating airspace disease from interstitial disease or atelectasis is at times difficult, but clues such as preservation of volume and air bronchograms can allow radiologists to be more confident with the diagnosis of airspace disease. The almost universal use of digital radiography and the ability to window and level a radiograph, like CT scans, has improved the ability to evaluate areas of pathology.

E: An appropriately interpreted radiograph with the patient's history and presenting symptoms in mind can make the difference between attempting to treat numerous etiologies and treating the appropriate etiology on the first attempt which can expedite care and save resources.

15 INTERSTITIAL DISEASE

Objectives:
1. Know the radiologic appearance and anatomic location of interstitial disease associated with Kerley lines, peribronchial cuffing, subpleural thickening, a reticular or reticulonodular pattern.
2. List three common causes of interstitial lung disease.
3. Understand the significance of the broad classification of chest radiographic abnormalities into interstitial and airspace disease.

Introduction

The pulmonary interstitium surrounds the pulmonary alveoli (which make up acini), conductive airways, and blood vessels. Figure 15.1 shows the anatomy of several secondary pulmonary lobules each containing between 3 and 25 acini. Notice that the interlobular septum defines the secondary pulmonary lobule. The peribronchovascular interstitium surrounds the pulmonary artery and accompanying bronchiole. The subpleural interstitium lines the inner aspect of the pleura. The interstitium is a continuum of dense elastic tissue and collagen throughout the lung that merges into the elastic component of the alveolar walls. It is not normally separately defined on the plain radiograph and becomes visible when disease increases its volume and/or radiographic density.

The anatomic subdivisions of the interstitial space are useful since the involvement of various subdivisions give rise to the specific radiographic findings associated with interstitial disease. These radiographic findings are Kerley lines, peribronchial thickening or cuffing, reticular or reticulonodular opacities, and subpleural thickening. Most disease processes involve the airspaces and the interstitium. Even diseases that are called "interstitial diseases" often have some airspace involvement.

© Springer Nature Switzerland AG 2020
J. Kissane et al. (eds.), *Radiology Fundamentals: Introduction to Imaging & Technology*, https://doi.org/10.1007/978-3-030-22173-7_15

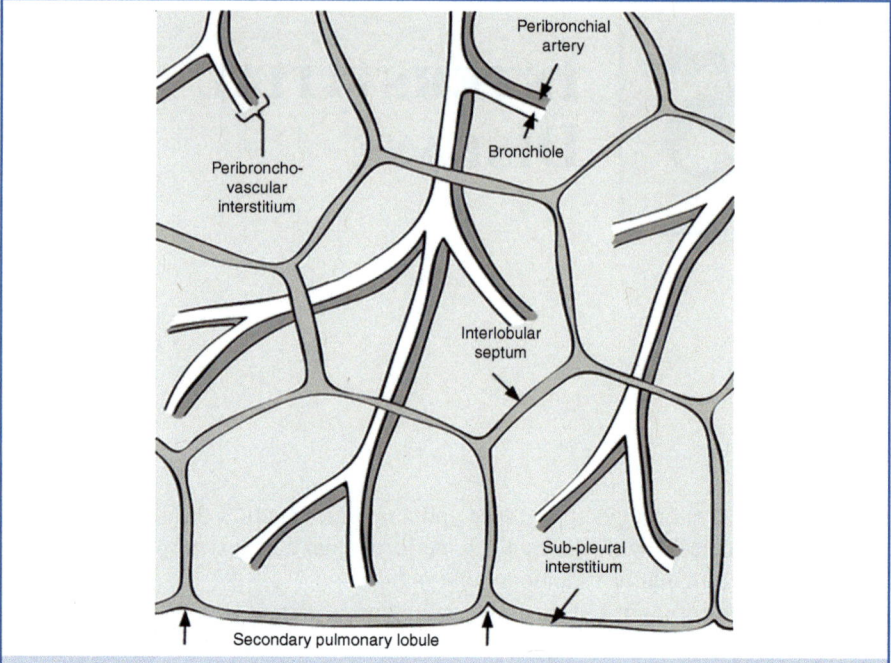

FIGURE 15.1 - SECONDARY PULMONARY LOBULES
Note the components of the interstitium and their relationship to the secondary pulmonary lobule

However, the broad categorization into airspace or interstitial disease (based on the predominant pattern of involvement), in combination with the clinical presentation, allows a more accurate differential diagnosis.

Kerley Lines

The lung is subdivided into numerous secondary pulmonary lobules by connective tissue septa. It is the thickening of these septa that produces Kerley lines, identified by and named for Dr. Peter Kerley, an Irish radiologist. The septa contain lymphatics and pulmonary venules. The short, 1–2 cm horizontal lines in the inferolateral aspect of the lungs are called Kerley B lines (Fig. 15.2). These are typically described in congestive heart failure but can be seen in a number of other conditions. The less commonly seen 2–6 cm septa visualized radiating from the hila to the upper lobes cast shadows known as Kerley A lines when thickened. Kerley also described C lines that have no distinct anatomic correlate and are due to superimposition of A and B lines into a weblike pattern.

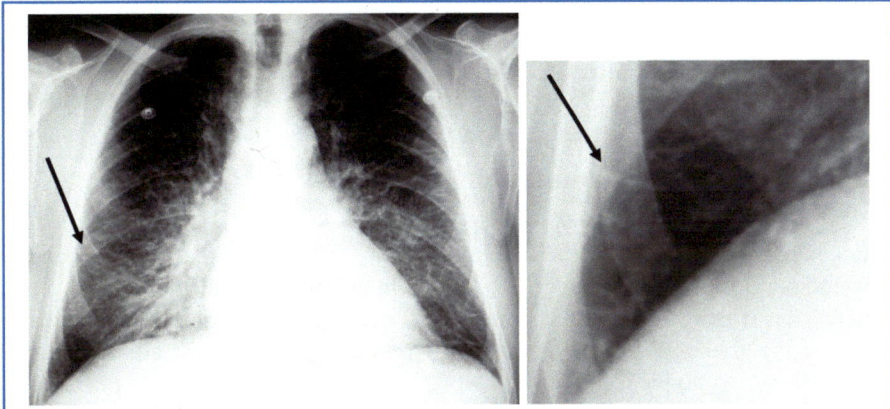

FIGURE 15.2 - KERLEY B LINES
Kerley B lines in a patient with congestive heart failure. Image on the right is a magnified view at the right CP angle

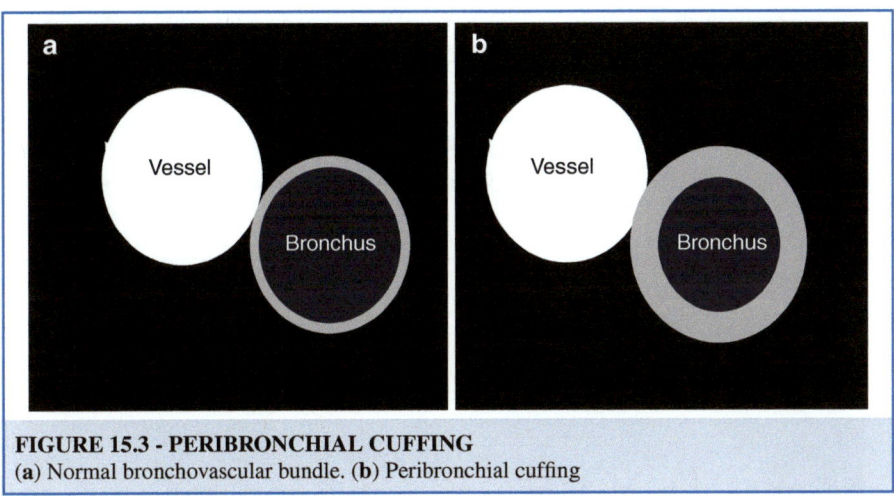

FIGURE 15.3 - PERIBRONCHIAL CUFFING
(**a**) Normal bronchovascular bundle. (**b**) Peribronchial cuffing

Peribronchial Cuffing

Bronchi, when seen on end, cast thin-walled ring shadows on the normal chest radiograph. These are usually seen in the perihilar region. Remember that the bronchus and pulmonary artery travel together and bifurcate to the terminal bronchial-pulmonary arterial level. When the peribronchovascular component of the interstitial space becomes thickened, the normally "paper thin" bronchial wall becomes more visible (Fig. 15.3 and 56.3). Causes of peribronchial thickening are varied and include CHF and infection. Diseases that thicken the bronchial wall on an inflammatory basis chronically, such as chronic bronchitis or cystic fibrosis, may also lead to thickened bronchial walls.

Reticular and Reticulonodular Patterns

Thickening or nodularity of the interstitium may result in increased linear and/or fine nodular opacities in the lungs (Fig. 15.4). In this situation, the descriptive terms reticular or, if there is a nodular component, reticulonodular may be employed to describe the findings. Common causes of reticular opacities include congestive heart failure and atypical infections. More chronic causes of reticular or reticulonodular opacities include sarcoidosis and interstitial fibrosis.

Subpleural Thickening

When the accumulation of fluid or thickening of the subpleural interstitial space occurs, increased radiographic density that outlines the fissures is produced. This occurs frequently in early pulmonary edema and is commonly attributed to "fluid within the fissure." Any process affecting the subpleural interstitial space will give this appearance of thickened fissures. Hence, thickening of the visceral pleural line can be seen in patients with early interstitial pneumonia or evolving interstitial disease from any cause.

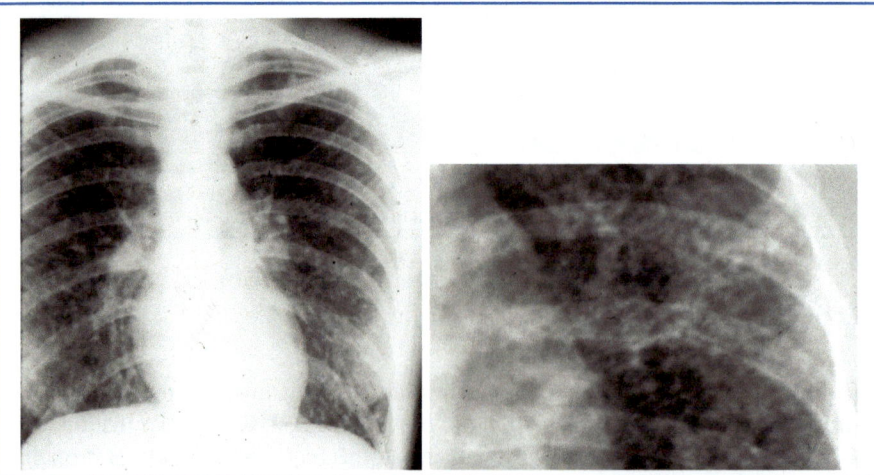

FIGURE 15.4 - RETICULONODULAR DISEASE
A radiograph and close-up of the same patient showing the "lines and dots" of reticulonodular lung disease

Summary

There are many causes of interstitial disease. Common acute causes include pulmonary interstitial edema and atypical infections. Chronic causes include sarcoidosis, fibrotic lung disease, occupational lung disease, and the distinctly interstitial form of metastatic disease (as seen in carcinoma of the lung, breast, and stomach) called lymphangitic carcinomatosis. It is important to be able to recognize the radiographic findings of interstitial disease and correlate it with the clinical information for the best differential diagnosis.

S: Interstitial lung disease can have a number of appearances and etiologies, so it is important to keep an open differential diagnosis unless specific signs or history can aid in diagnosis. This will help the radiologist to prevent errors in diagnosis which could happen if an incorrect assumption is made.

A: Simple interstitial patterns are easily identified on radiograph such as bronchial wall thickening, Kerley B lines, and reticular patterns, but it's best to keep in mind that these processes can be combined and often are better illustrated by CT which should be reserved to evaluate the more complex interstitial lung cases. As noted in a previous chapter, digital radiography has helped in evaluating more subtle changes on a radiograph such as interstitial lung disease.

F: Imaging of interstitial lung disease is commonly performed with radiographs and can be identified commonly as Kerley B lines, peribronchial thickening, or a reticular pattern which can help to determine etiology. While nonspecific, certain patterns can point to a diagnosis of etiology such as cystic fibrosis, congestive heart failure, atypical infection, or sarcoidosis.

E: Radiologists can expedite the diagnosis and treatment for causes of interstitial lung patterns of disease by identifying secondary signs that can narrow the differential diagnosis such as an enlarged heart with interstitial disease which can often be seen with congestive heart failure.

16 ATELECTASIS

Objectives:
1. Define "atelectasis."
2. Define and give examples of postobstructive atelectasis, cicatrization atelectasis, adhesive atelectasis, and passive atelectasis.
3. Explain why the loss of lung volume does not always lead to increased radiographic density.
4. Learn the characteristic patterns of lobar atelectasis.

Introduction

Many chest radiographic reports include the term atelectasis. Atelectasis means incomplete lung expansion. It is important to think about the underlying pathophysiology any time the term atelectasis is employed in describing a chest radiograph finding. Pneumonia and atelectasis are often considered in the differential diagnosis of airspace opacities. It can be difficult to differentiate between the two processes without examining the patient for signs of pneumonia (fever, elevated WBC, lung auscultation findings, etc.).

Atelectasis is defined as diminished volume affecting all or part of a lung. Loss of volume does not imply increase radiographic opacity. The normal lung is so transparent to X-rays that it does not increase in opacity until it has lost *90–95% of its volume*. Hence, the small areas of atelectasis seen on chest radiographs represent small foci of lung parenchyma, which have lost nearly all of their air.

There are four basic mechanisms that lead to atelectasis or loss of lung volume. These can occur individually or in combination and are listed below:

1. Postobstructive atelectasis
2. Passive (compressive) atelectasis
3. Adhesive atelectasis
4. Cicatrization (scarring) atelectasis

Postobstructive Atelectasis

When a bronchus is obstructed, due to external or internal causes, the air within the alveoli and the bronchi distal to the obstruction is reabsorbed. This leads to volume loss, as depicted in Fig. 16.1. Extrinsic compression of a bronchus by a mass, or internal causes such as mucus plugging, endobronchial tumor or a foreign body, can lead to postobstructive atelectasis.

In situations in which the inspired gas contains an elevated proportion of oxygen in comparison to room air, postobstructive atelectasis is more likely to occur. This is because alveoli will rapidly absorb gas that is rich in oxygen. Hence, postobstructive atelectasis, especially on the basis of mucous plugging, is a commonly observed phenomenon on portable radiographs obtained in the operating room or in the intensive care units where patients often breathe gas mixtures with a greater percentage of oxygen than found in room air.

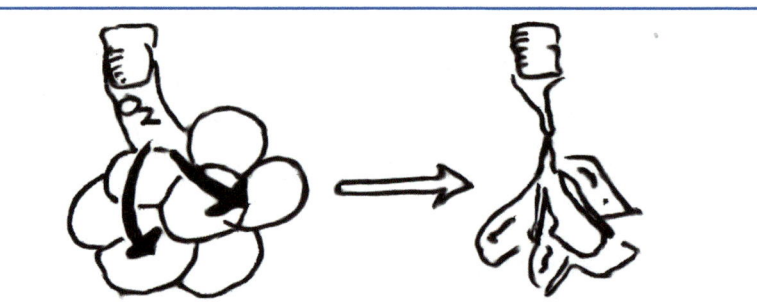

FIGURE 16.1 - POSTOBSTRUCTIVE ATELECTASIS
An airway obstruction results in collapse (incomplete expansion) of the airway and air spaces distal to the obstruction

Adhesive Atelectasis

When type II pneumocytes lining the alveolus decrease their surfactant production, the alveolus can no longer remain inflated, and adhesive atelectasis occurs. Collapse results, according to the law of Laplace. Laplace's law states that the pressure (P) required to keep an alveolus open is directly proportional to the wall tension (T) and inversely proportional to its radius (r). Hence, for any given tension, the smaller the radius, the larger the pressure required to keep that alveolus open. Surfactant decreases the surface tension, helping reduce the pressure required to keep small alveoli open (and maintain smaller alveoli open at a lower pressure) (Fig. 16.2).

The prototype of adhesive atelectasis is the respiratory distress syndrome of prematurity, which occurs in infants whose type II pneumocytes have not matured enough to produce surfactant. Atelectasis is commonly seen following surgery, especially thoracic chest and abdominal procedures. The cooling of the heart performed to decrease the heart's metabolic requirements while on bypass also decreases the metabolic rate of type II pneumocytes in the adjacent lung. The most common location for this is in the left lower lobe.

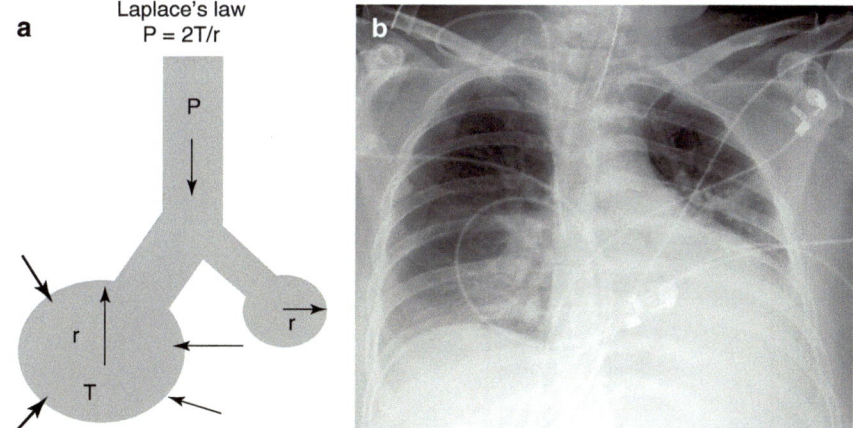

FIGURE 16.2 - ADHESIVE ATELECTASIS
(a) Figure illustrating Laplace's law. (b) AP post-operative chest x-ray showing left lower lobe atelectasis

Passive Atelectasis

The lung is highly elastic and normally exists at a volume "greater than it desires to be." The chest wall is also elastic and exists at a volume slightly "less than it desires to be." The equilibrium between the lung and chest wall establishes these relative volumes as you may recall from physiology. When something is introduced to change the equilibrium, the lung and chest wall also change volume in a predictable manner.

Anytime the lung loses volume due to a manifestation of its propensity for elastic recoil, this is termed passive atelectasis. The most obvious example of this is a pneumothorax, but similar changes occur when fluid is introduced into the pleural space as in a pleural effusion (Fig. 16.3).

Cicatrization Atelectasis

Cicatrix is a medical word for scar or replacement of normal tissue by fibrous tissue. This form of atelectasis occurs secondary to healing of inflammation from infection, radiation therapy, etc. It is characterized by marked perialveolar fibrosis with resultant loss of volume as noted in Fig. 16.4.

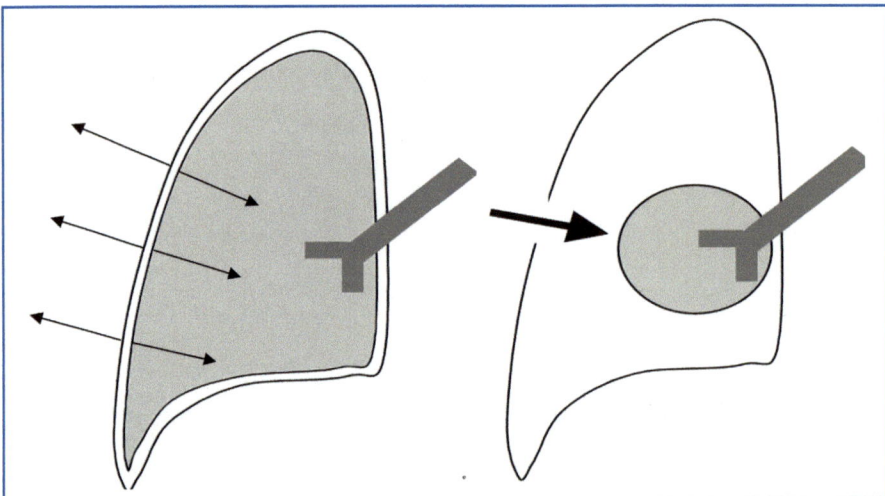

FIGURE 16.3 - NORMAL AND ABNORMAL FORCES ON THE LUNG
The normal elastic forces between the chest wall and the lung oppose each other, resulting in equilibrium as noted in the picture on the *left*. With a pneumothorax, as seen on the *right*, when the chest wall is compromised, air enters the thorax, allowing the lung to collapse

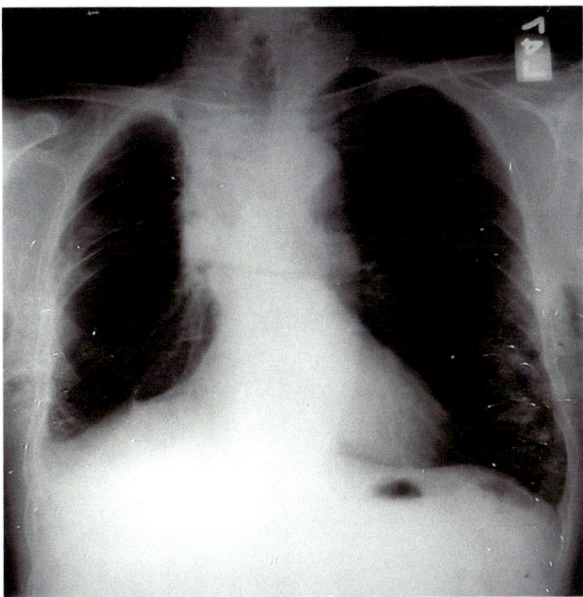

FIGURE 16.4 - RIGHT PARAMEDIASTINAL FIBROSIS (CICATRIZATION)
Replacement of normal tissue by fibrous tissue in the right middle and upper lobes, post radiation

Lobar Atelectasis

Atelectasis may involve an entire lung. It can also be lobar, segmental, or subsegmental. Lobar atelectasis (or lobar collapse) causes specific appearances. *Lobar collapse may be due to bronchial obstruction.* Common etiologies would include an endobronchial mass and significant mucus plugging of a large airway. The atelectatic lobe usually appears as a white dense triangle or pyramid with its apex pointing to the hilum.

With right upper lobe atelectasis (Fig. 16.5), the frontal view shows an opacity in the right upper hemithorax, merging with the right superior mediastinal border. Elevation of the right hilum and the minor fissure indicate volume loss. The lateral view showed superior displacement of the minor fissure as well as anterior displacement of the right major fissure (not included).

With left upper lobe atelectasis (Fig. 16.6a, b), the frontal view shows an ill-defined opacity in the left hemithorax and a crescent of air between the aortic arch and the ill-defined opacity. The lateral view shows increased opacity adjacent to and

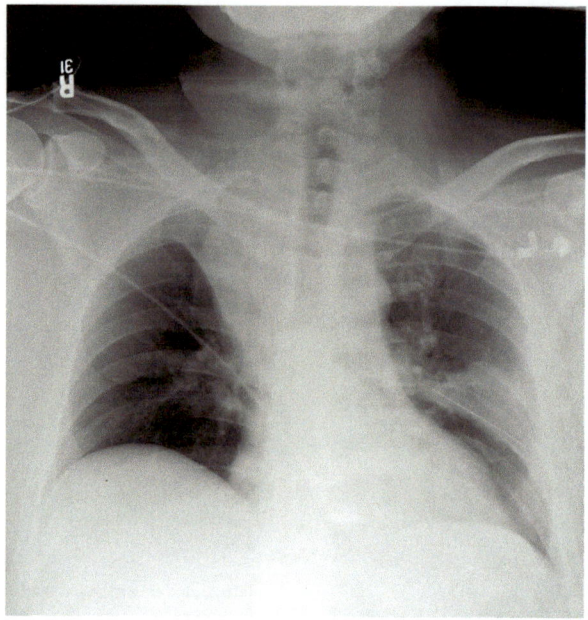

FIGURE 16.5 - RIGHT UPPER LOBE COLLAPSE
AP radiograph. Note the opacity in the right upper hemithorax, merging with the superior mediastinum. There is elevation of the right hilum, and superior displacement of the minor fissure

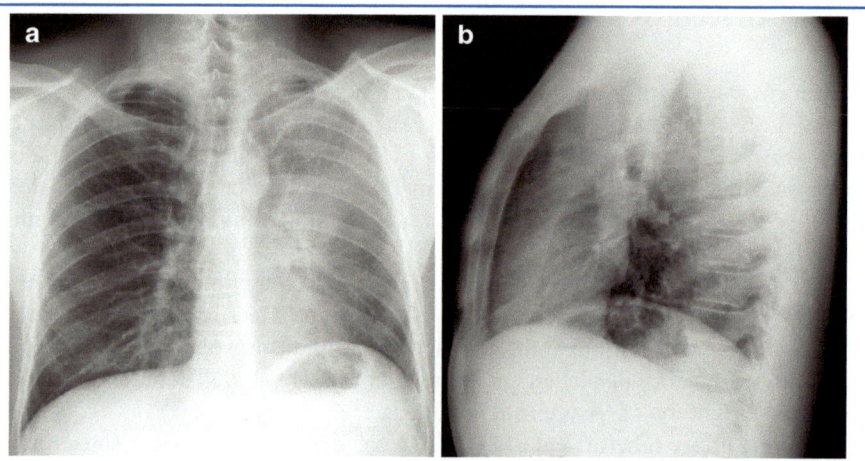

FIGURE 16.6 - LEFT UPPER LOBE COLLAPSE
(**a**) PA radiograph. Note the ill-defined opacity in the left hemithorax and a crescent of air between the aortic arch and the ill-defined opacity. (**b**) Lateral radiograph. Note the increased opacity adjacent to and parallel to the anterior chest wall

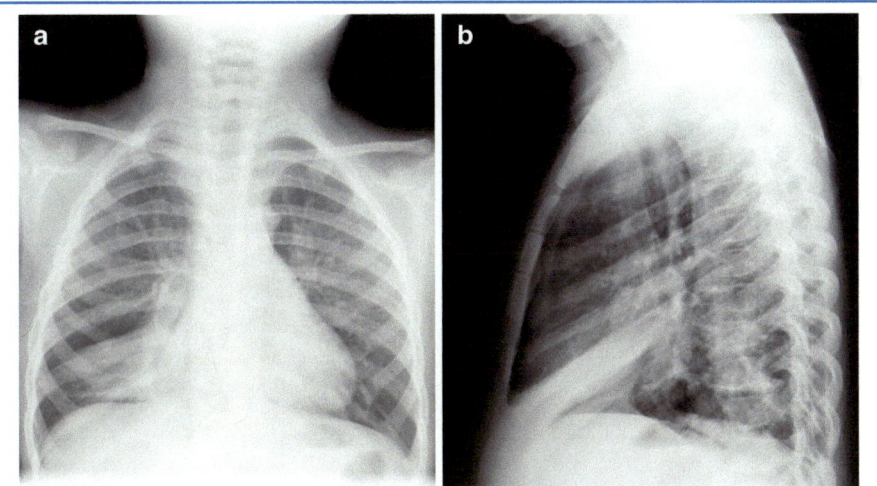

FIGURE 16.7 - RIGHT MIDDLE LOBE COLLAPSE
(**a**) PA radiograph. Note the right lower lung opacity causing silhouetting of the right heart border. (**b**) Lateral radiograph. Note the wedge of increased opacity between the inferiorly displaced minor fissure and the anteriorly displaced right major fissure

parallel to the anterior chest wall, as well as anterior displacement of the left major fissure.

Right middle lobe atelectasis (Fig. 16.7a, b) may cause silhouetting of the right heart border, disappearance of the minor fissure, and increased right lower lung opacity on the frontal view. The lateral view will show a wedge of increased opacity between the inferiorly displaced minor fissure and the anteriorly displaced right major fissure.

Lower lobe atelectasis (Fig. 16.8a–c) shows in the frontal view as an inferomedial triangular opacity silhouetting the diaphragm of the affected side. The lateral view will show increased opacity overlying the inferior spine and posterior bowing of the corresponding major fissure.

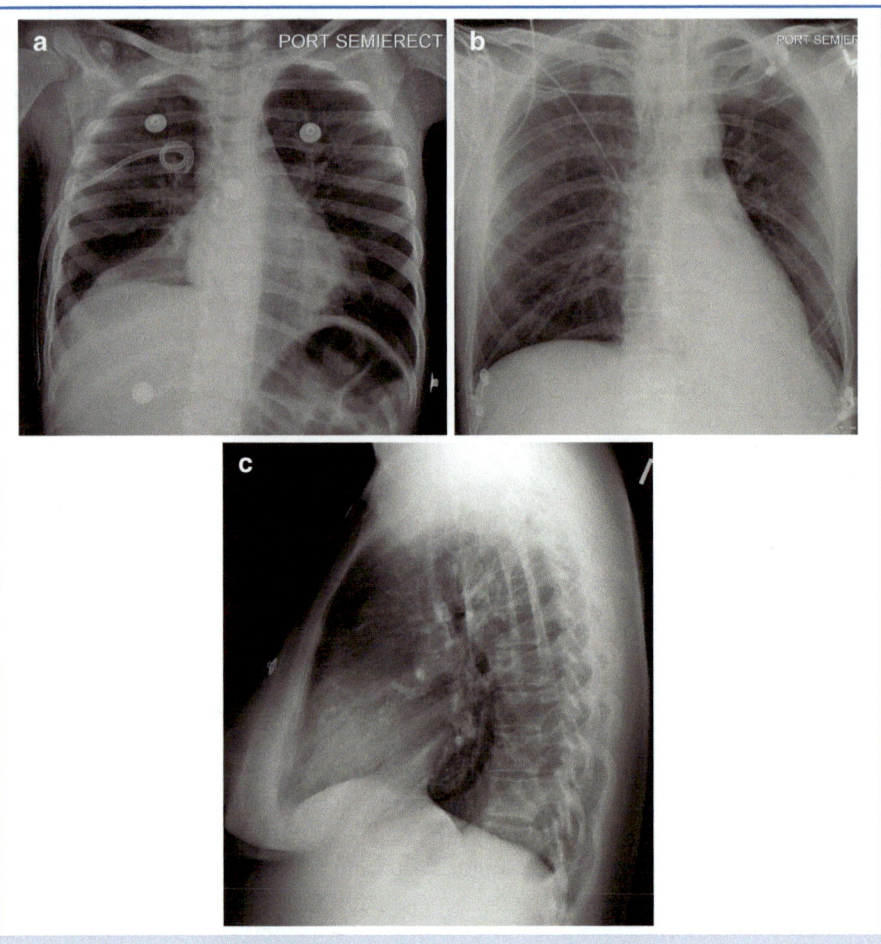

FIGURE 16.8 - LOWER LOBE COLLAPSE
(**a**) AP radiograph of right lower lobe collapse. Note the right lower lung triangular opacity silhouetting the right hemidiaphragm. (**b**) AP radiograph of left lower lobe collapse. Note the subtle triangular opacity overlying the heart, with silhouetting the left hemidiaphragm. (**c**) Lateral radiograph of left lower lobe collapse (different patient). Note the increased opacity overlying the inferior spine and posterior bowing of the left major fissure

S: Evaluation of atelectasis is often carried out by chest radiograph and analysis of the pattern of atelectasis can determine the location. While etiology may not be as easily determined, knowing the patterns of atelectasis can reduce the use of CT in patients with various forms of atelectasis.

A: The radiologist's role in evaluating atelectasis is not necessarily to determine the exact etiology since atelectasis can be due to mucus plugging, bronchial compression, lack of surfactant, or other causes. Appropriate use of resources includes evaluating by chest radiograph and follow-up exams with a keen knowledge of the patient's presentation. If an etiology is unclear and treatments are not progressing as planned, CT can be utilized to search for alternative diagnosis.

F: PA or AP and lateral radiographs are very important to properly localize the pathology, in this case, increased density from atelectasis.

E: Atelectasis due to a pleural effusion, a compressing mass, or lack of full inspiration due to pain will appear peripherally and does not usually affect an entire lobe, whereas mucous plugging will often collapse an entire lobe. This concept is important when it comes to recommending the course of treatment. Incentive spirometry may be used to help with the former while bronchoscopy will be more effective for the latter. Communicating these highly disparate findings is critical to expediting the appropriate care. It is also important to remember that, depending on the confirmation of the suspected atelectasis, there is a differential to the finding including pneumonia, so correlation with clinical information such as elevated white blood cell count and fever is key.

17 PULMONARY VASCULATURE

Objectives:
1. Give three examples of technical factors that may make pulmonary vessels look more prominent.
2. Describe the physiology in pulmonary perfusion between the cephalad and more caudal portions of the lung in an upright patient.
3. List the components of the hilar shadow on a conventional chest radiograph.
4. State which hilum is usually higher on the upright chest radiograph.

Pulmonary Vessel Distribution in the Lung

Several factors can affect the appearance of the pulmonary vessels. Imaging in expiration, under penetration and supine positioning, can make the vessels look artifactually prominent.

In Fig. 17.1, note the difference in the number and size of blood vessels within the lung as one moves from the lung apex to the lung base. The vessels are larger and more numerous in the lung base because the force of gravity augments the hydrostatic force generated by the right ventricle. In the apices, the hydrostatic force generated by the right ventricle is diminished by gravity. In effect, the right ventricle is pumping "uphill" to the apices of the lung. Of course, when the patient changes position, this relationship is also changed.

In general, the greatest perfusion will be to the portion of the lung that is most dependent. Certain pathologic situations can change this normal perfusion gradient, as we will see later in this section.

© Springer Nature Switzerland AG 2020
J. Kissane et al. (eds.), *Radiology Fundamentals: Introduction to Imaging & Technology*, https://doi.org/10.1007/978-3-030-22173-7_17

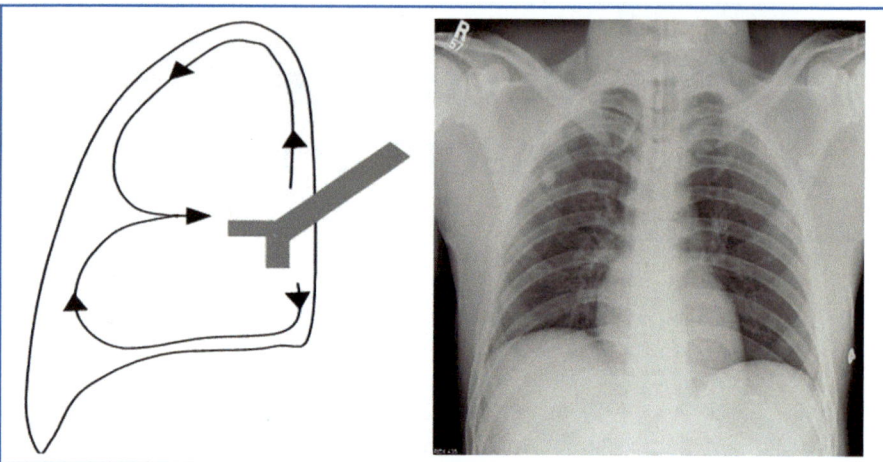

FIGURE 17.1 - PULMONARY VASCULAR FLOW
Pulmonary arteries tend to run in a vertical fashion, while pulmonary veins are more horizontal. Note the difference in number and size of blood vessel within the lung from apex to base

Identifying Pulmonary Vessels

Pulmonary vasculature may appear tubular (when seen along the length of a vessel) or nodular (when seen end-on). Vessels are larger close to the hilum and get smaller in size toward the periphery of the lungs. There is paucity of markings in the peripheral lungs, due to small vessel size.

Since bronchi and pulmonary arteries travel together, look for a bronchus that is on end adjacent to the suspected vessel on end. A bronchus is air filled and thus will have a black center, while the vessel will be uniform in opacity (Fig. 17.2).

A true nodule is spherical and should appear round on both PA and lateral views. A vessel on end will only have a round ("on end") appearance on one view, having the tubular appearance of a vessel on the other projection.

Another way to identify vessels is by noting the hila. The hila as seen on a chest radiograph are composed primarily of the pulmonary arteries and superior pulmonary veins, although there is a slight contribution from the bronchial structures. The left hilum is normally higher than the right in approximately 97% of patients. This is because the left pulmonary artery must pass over the left main bronchus in its proximal course, while the right pulmonary artery travels adjacent but not over the right main bronchus. The right hilum is never higher than the left in a normal patient.

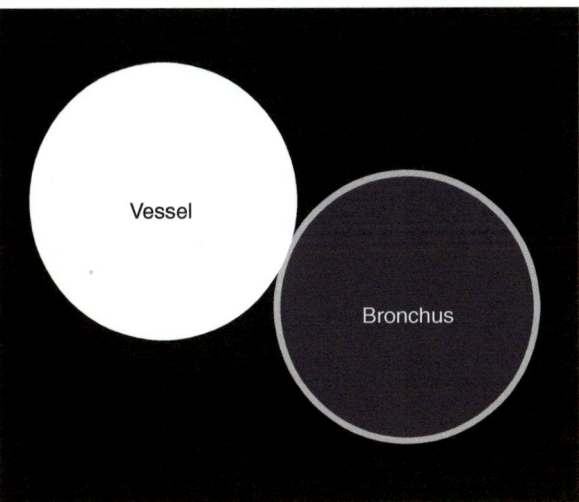

FIGURE 17.2 - VESSEL AND BRONCHUS
Note that the pulmonary artery and accompanying bronchus should be of relatively equal size and that the bronchial wall should be thin and sharp

Pulmonary Arterial Hypertension

Pulmonary hypertension is defined as pulmonary artery pressures above the mean value of 25 mmHg at rest or 30 mmHg on exercise. Figure 17.3 shows the radiographic appearance of pulmonary arterial hypertension. In this condition, pulmonary artery pressure in the lungs is elevated. Note the enlargement of the main and central pulmonary arteries. In this case, note also the rapid tapering of the pulmonary arteries peripherally causing the lungs to have a relatively oligemic (hypovascular) appearance. This was due to an atrial septal defect with Eisenmenger syndrome (reversal of shunt due to chronic elevation of pulmonary vascular resistance).

Pulmonary arterial hypertension has many causes. The World Health Organization has classified these into five groups. The most common etiologies of pulmonary hypertension are most often secondary to left heart disease, lung disease, and chronic hypoxia. Pulmonary diseases causing pulmonary hypertension could be due to lung involvement (such as interstitial fibrosis and COPD) or on the basis of restriction related to the chest wall (including severe kyphoscoliosis, morbid obesity, chronic fibrothorax, and neurologic disorders that impair the

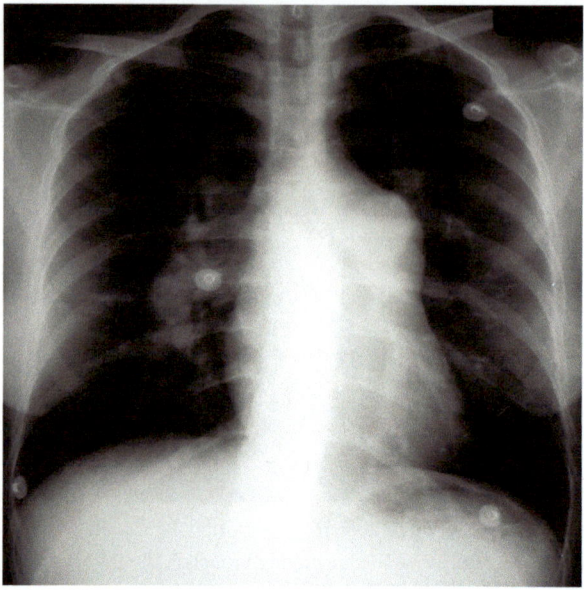

FIGURE 17.3 - PULMONARY HYPERTENSION
Note the enlarged central pulmonary arteries with "pruning" of the vessels more peripherally. This appearance was due to an atrial septal defect with Eisenmenger syndrome

respiratory muscles). Less common causes are thromboembolic disease, connective tissue disorders, and left to right intracardiac shunts (such as atrial septal defects or ventricular septal defects).

Shunt Vascularity

Figure 17.4 may at first appear identical to the radiograph on the previous patient. The enlargement of the hilar and main pulmonary artery segments is similar. However, note that the pulmonary vasculature is much more prominent in the periphery of the lung than on the previous study.

This patient has a large atrial septal defect producing a left to right intracardiac shunt, thereby increasing pulmonary blood flow. The other left to right shunts (ventricular septal defect, patent ductus arteriosus) could give a similar appearance although both would be considerably less likely in an adult.

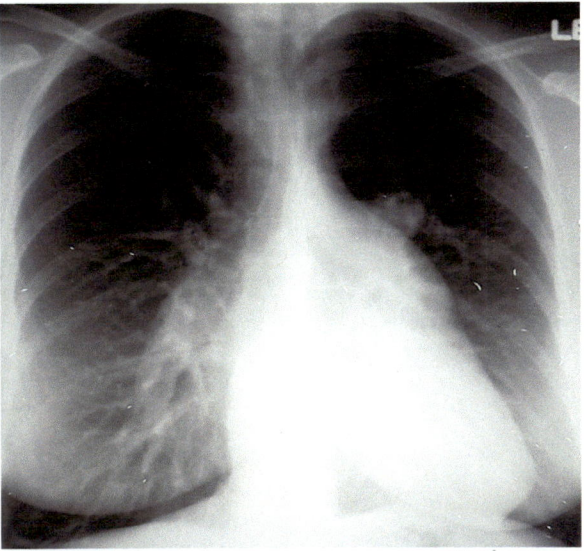

FIGURE 17.4 - SHUNT VASCULARITY
Note the enlargement of the central pulmonary arteries and the more peripheral vessels, a pattern consistent with shunt vascularity

Pulmonary Venous Hypertension

Figure 17.5 is from a patient with pulmonary venous hypertension. Although the central pulmonary vasculature is prominent, it is not nearly as prominent as in pulmonary arterial hypertension or as in patients with left to right shunts. This patient had mitral stenosis. There is a convexity along the left cardiac border, which is similar to that seen in the previous two examples; however, it is located slightly more inferior with respect to the aortic arch. This represents a dilated left atrial appendage. The left atrium is not normally a border forming structure on the frontal radiograph; however, with dilation due to increased left atrial pressure, it may become visible. There is prominence of the upper lobe vasculature relative to the lower lobes (cephalization) representing redistribution of blood flow to the upper lobes. There may also be Kerley B lines and peribronchial cuffing, as well as thickening of the fissures on the lateral view. All of the latter findings should sound familiar to you as radiographic components of interstitial disease. The interstitial findings relate to the increased pulmonary venous pressure that leads to transudation of fluid into the interstitium.

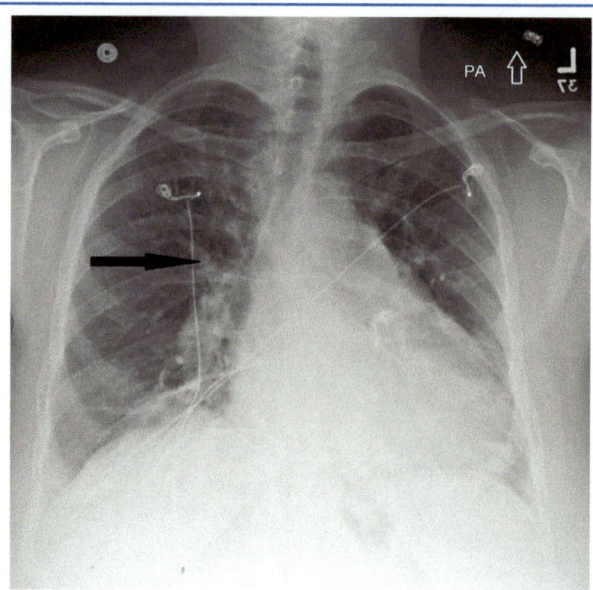

FIGURE 17.5 - PULMONARY VENOUS HYPERTENSION
The chest radiograph shows cardiomegaly. Note the enlarged right superior pulmonary vein

		Pulmonary vessels	
		Central	Peripheral
Vascular Pattern	Shunt vascularity (overcirculation)	Increased (caliber)	Increased
	Pulmonary arterial hypertension	Large	Small, decreased
	Pulmonary venous hypertension	Increased	Increased

FIGURE 17.6 - RADIOGRAPHIC DIFFERENCES BETWEEN SHUNT VASCULAR-ITY, PULMONARY ARTERIAL HYPERTENSION, AND PULMONARY VENOUS HYPERTENSION
By examining the caliber of the central and peripheral pulmonary vessels, one can determine the vascular pattern

Any obstructive lesion on the left side of the heart (where blood coming from the lungs is headed) can produce this appearance. Hence, processes that cause left ventricular failure, mitral stenosis, or obstruction to flow of blood into or out of the left atrium such as left atrial myxoma could produce the findings of pulmonary venous hypertension.

Findings of pulmonary venous hypertension are much more common than the other two categories described since left ventricular failure is such a common clinical problem. The chest radiograph is useful in distinguishing the less common, but by no means rare, causes of increased pulmonary vascularity (Fig. 17.6).

S: Appropriate technique and patient positioning to ensure adequate evaluation of pulmonary vasculature on radiography can reduce unnecessary ionizing radiation and other risks to the patient from repeat imaging, use of other advanced imaging, or more invasive evaluation, especially in pediatric patients.

A: In patients with risk factors for or suspected pulmonary arterial hypertension or cardiac shunt, radiography is recommended for initial evaluation.

F: Differentiation of shunt vascularity versus pulmonary arterial hypertension can be made by the vascularity in the periphery. In shunt vascularity, the pulmonary vasculature is more prominent in the periphery versus pulmonary arterial hypertension which has relatively decreased peripheral vascularity or "pruning." Digital radiography's ability to window/level the image can help in the evaluation of the peripheral lung.

E: Differentiating patterns of vascularity on radiography can help direct the patient care team to appropriate evaluation and management of many cardiopulmonary pathologies.

18 PULMONARY EDEMA

Objectives:
1. State the chest radiograph findings of left ventricular failure.
2. Name conditions that may mimic cardiogenic pulmonary edema.

Pulmonary edema secondary to left ventricular failure is one of the more common problems encountered in clinical medicine. The term congestive heart failure (CHF) is often applied both clinically and radiographically. Technically, CHF is a clinical diagnosis with a constellation of findings, some of which are radiographic. Nevertheless, the terms cardiogenic pulmonary edema, left ventricular failure, and CHF are often used synonymously in informal discussion.

The chest radiograph is an excellent tool for the early diagnosis of pulmonary edema and for assessing the effectiveness of treatment. This is because the chest radiograph may be reflective of minute-to-minute changes in cardiopulmonary function and circulating blood volume. A detailed description of the physiologic aspects of chest radiographic interpretation is beyond the scope of this discussion. We will emphasize the changes in radiographic appearance on the chest x-ray only (Fig. 18.1).

Blood Flow Redistribution (Cephalization)

Figure 18.2 shows a normal and abnormal appearance of the pulmonary vasculature. As discussed in Chap. 17, the upper lobe vessels are normally smaller than those in the lower lobes due to the effect of gravity on the pulmonary

© Springer Nature Switzerland AG 2020   107
J. Kissane et al. (eds.), *Radiology Fundamentals: Introduction to Imaging
& Technology*, https://doi.org/10.1007/978-3-030-22173-7_18

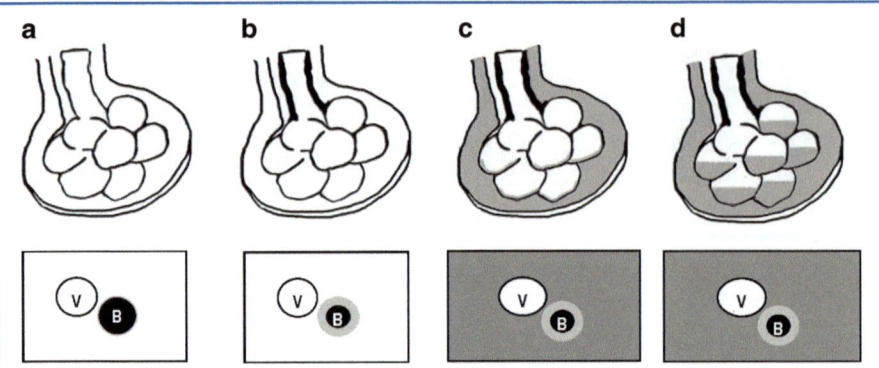

FIGURE 18.1 - PULMONARY EDEMA

In (**a**), the normal alveolus and vessel/bronchus relationship is noted. (**b**) Shows peribronchial cuffing. In (**c**), as the edema worsens, fluid starts to spill into the alveoli. (**d**) Shows the alveoli filled with fluid, markedly interfering with gas exchange

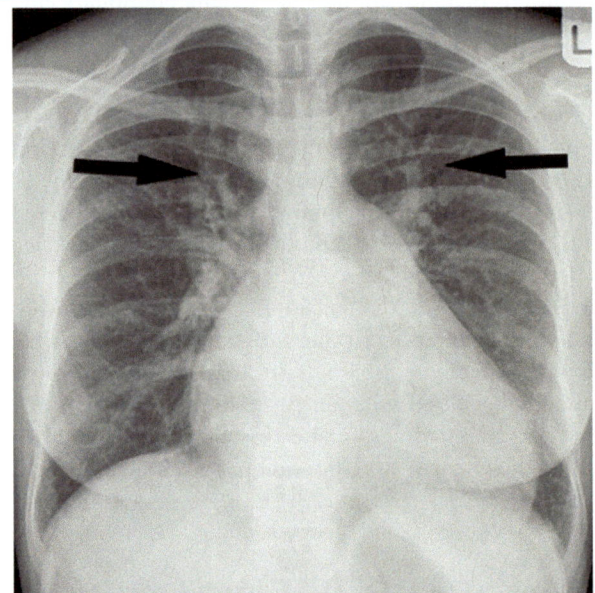

FIGURE 18.2 - REDISTRIBUTION OF VASCULAR FLOW (CEPHALIZATION)

The heart is enlarged. The double density seen in the right retrocardiac region is due to an enlarged left atrium, in this patient with mitral stenosis and mitral regurgitation. Note the enlarged vessels at the hilum, including the significantly enlarged upper lobe veins (*arrows*)

circulation. The first abnormality detected in patients with early stages of left ventricular failure may be the redistribution of pulmonary blood flow to the upper lung zones, so-called cephalization. With cephalization, the upper lobe vessels become engorged and larger than the lower lobe vessels. Cephalization may be a subtle finding for those not used to scrutinizing the pulmonary vasculature closely. Remember that in the supine patient, the normal craniocaudal gradation of perfusion due to gravity will no longer be present. Hence, cephalization may not be present on supine radiographs and therefore is lost as a useful diagnostic sign. Crowding of vessels on supine radiographs limit assessment of vessel caliber. This is another reason for obtaining an upright radiograph of the chest whenever possible.

Interstitial Edema

The next observable abnormality is the accumulation of fluid within the lung interstitium. This is the earliest stage at which there is radiographically detectable "extravascular lung water." Because this fluid is confined to the interstitium, it may not seriously compromise gas exchange. The findings (peribronchial cuffing, Kerley A and B lines, and subpleural interstitial thickening) are also seen in other forms of interstitial disease.

The transition from cephalization to interstitial edema to airspace edema may be quite rapid in many circumstances, and all the described phases may not be discreetly observed. These changes correlate with pulmonary capillary wedge pressures measured with a pulmonary artery (Swan-Ganz) catheter (Fig. 18.3).

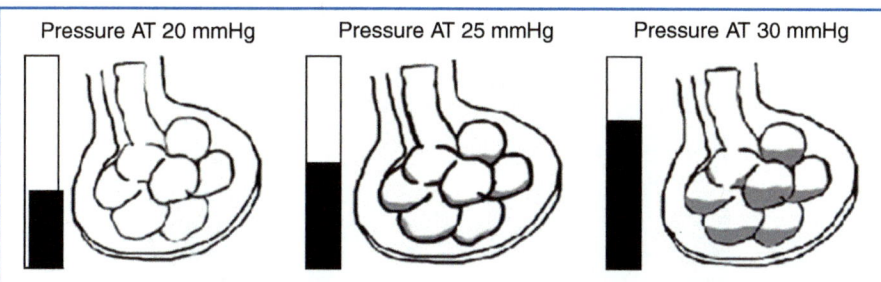

FIGURE 18.3 - PULMONARY EDEMA AND CAPILLARY WEDGE PRESSURE
Cephalization occurs when the pulmonary capillary wedge pressure is about 15–20 mm of mercury (mmHg). Between 20 and 25 mmHg, one will observe predominantly interstitial edema. Alveolar edema occurs at capillary wedge pressures greater than 25 mmHg

Alveolar Edema

Figure 18.4 shows the most severe form of pulmonary edema. This is airspace or alveolar edema. Fluid spills into the alveoli, forming a barrier to gas exchange causing clinically evident respiratory impairment. The radiographic findings will be those of airspace disease with air bronchogram and confluent acinar shadows producing a fluffy white appearance.

While pulmonary edema may be distinguishable from other forms of airspace disease radiographically by temporal evolution and the typical bilateral and fairly symmetric distribution, there is often an overlap with other causes of airspace opacification including pneumonia, noncardiogenic pulmonary edema, and pulmonary hemorrhage. Pulmonary edema may have a fairly rapid onset and resolution (in comparison to pneumonia, which usually develops and resolves more slowly). Of course, the diagnosis is best made by correlating the radiograph with an accurate medical history, physical examination, and appropriate laboratory data.

Finally, noncardiogenic pulmonary edema, seen as a part of the adult respiratory distress syndrome (ARDS), is commonly seen in intensive care unit patients as the result of various etiologies such as sepsis and head trauma. Although the radiographic

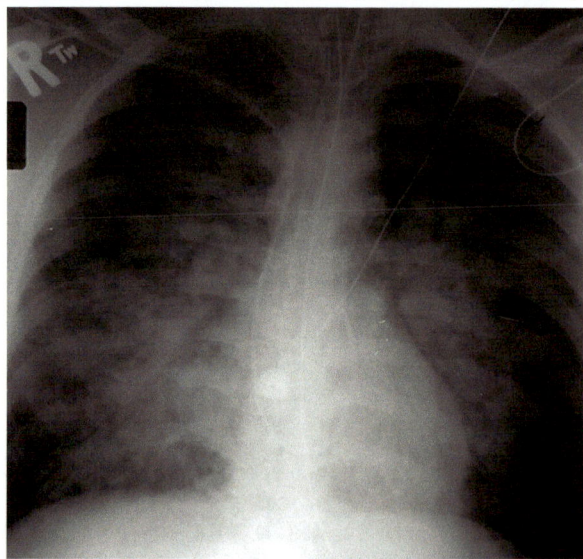

FIGURE 18.4 - AIRSPACE/ALVEOLAR EDEMA
Airspace with air bronchogram and confluent acinar opacities producing a fluffy white appearance

appearance of ARDS is similar to that of cardiogenic edema, the two are not totally identical, reflecting their very different physiological derangements. ARDS does not have the cardiomegaly or pleural effusions usually seen in CHF.

S: If CT is necessary for a patient with pulmonary edema for further evaluation of other chest pathology, non-contrast CT should be used when possible, especially in patients with renal failure who present with fluid overload.

A: The use of follow-up radiographs for patients with known pulmonary edema is not necessarily required on a routine basis but should be guided by the patient's clinical status, specifically a worsening of clinical signs or symptoms.

F: When evaluating for cardiomegaly in the setting of edema on radiographs, it is important to remember that on an AP view a normal cardiothoracic ratio can be up to 0.6 versus 0.5 on a PA view.

E: While imaging findings can be helpful in distinguishing pulmonary edema on radiographs, there may still be an overlap of findings with other disease processes. Communication with the patient care team can be helpful in correlating with primary clinical concerns and suggesting possible further evaluation when appropriate.

19 PULMONARY EMBOLISM

Pulmonary Embolism

The etiology of pulmonary embolism is often multifactorial. Risk factors include surgical procedures, cancer, immobilization, pregnancy, oral contraceptive pills, and some coagulation disorders. Pulmonary embolism has an increased incidence in hospitalized patients in general, in part due to immobilization. The chest radiograph is usually normal or shows nonspecific findings (such as atelectasis and small pleural effusion) in most patients with pulmonary embolism. The primary purpose of a chest radiograph in suspected pulmonary embolism is to rule out other causes of chest symptoms. Rarely, patients with large or extensive pulmonary emboli will have decreased perfusion of the affected lung (relative oligemia) or an enlarged pulmonary artery evident on chest x-ray. Figure 19.1 shows peripheral wedge-shaped opacity due to an infarct. This sign is known as Hampton's hump and is infrequently seen.

Catheter pulmonary arteriography, performed in the Interventional Radiology Department, was the gold standard for diagnosing pulmonary emboli but is now rarely used. For further information regarding pulmonary arteriography and IVC filter placement, refer to the CVIR section of this book.

Computed tomographic (CT) pulmonary angiography has become the standard of care in the evaluation for pulmonary emboli, due to the less invasive nature of the test and the wide availability of multidetector CT scanners. To make the diagnosis

© Springer Nature Switzerland AG 2020
J. Kissane et al. (eds.), *Radiology Fundamentals: Introduction to Imaging & Technology*, https://doi.org/10.1007/978-3-030-22173-7_19

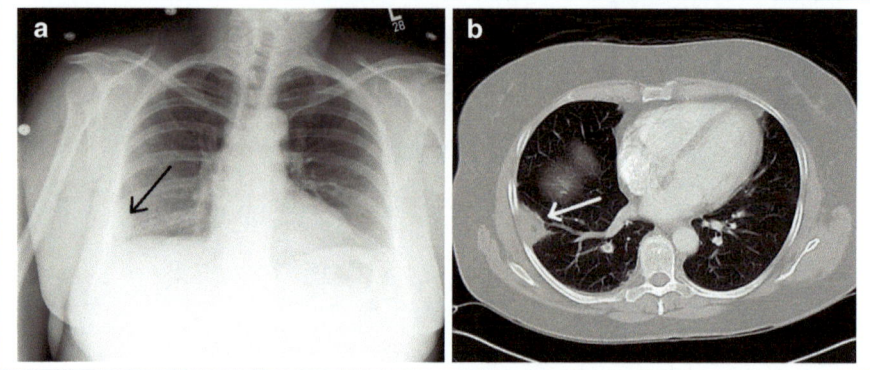

FIGURE 19.1 - HAMPTON'S HUMP
The chest radiograph (**a**) demonstrates Hampton's hump (a peripheral wedge-shaped opacity) in the right lung base (*black arrow*) just above the costophrenic angle. CT (**b**) confirms the presence of a pulmonary infarct (*white arrow*)

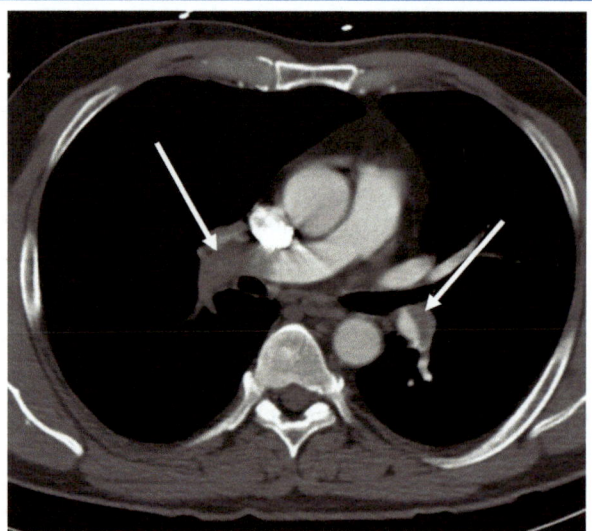

FIGURE 19.2 - PULMONARY EMBOLISM
Axial CT image showing large filling defects (*white arrows*) in both the distal right pulmonary arteries and left interlobar pulmonary arteries representing bilateral pulmonary emboli

of pulmonary embolism on a CT scan, IV contrast is administered, and the examination is timed in a way that maximizes the opacification of the pulmonary arteries. The CT scan is then reviewed for filling defects (gray) within the opacified (white) pulmonary arteries (Fig. 19.2).

If a patient cannot receive IV contrast (most commonly due to renal insufficiency or moderate to severe allergy), a lung ventilation/perfusion (V/Q) scan can be performed by the Nuclear Medicine Department. Refer to the pulmonary chapter in the Nuclear Medicine section of this book for a discussion on lung VQ scan.

S: In patients with suspected pulmonary embolism, evaluation should start with a chest radiograph. Radiographs can accurately diagnose many conditions that may have overlapping symptoms and may decrease unnecessary radiation dose from CT or V/Q scan, especially in pregnant women.

A: Use of clinical tools such as the Wells' Criteria for Pulmonary Embolism should be encouraged as a guide for clinicians in deciding the necessity of advanced imaging for the diagnosis of pulmonary embolism.

F: Acute versus chronic pulmonary embolism can be distinguished on CT pulmonary angiography by the presence of a central (acute) vs peripheral (chronic) filling defect within the pulmonary artery.

E: It is important to identify not only the distribution and extent of pulmonary embolism on CT pulmonary angiography but also any evidence of right heart strain, which should be promptly communicated to the patient care team.

20 PNEUMOTHORAX

Objectives:
1. Define "pneumothorax."
2. Learn to distinguish a pneumothorax from a skinfold overlying the chest.
3. Discuss the findings you would expect to see in a tension pneumothorax.
4. Discuss the most common location for pneumothorax in an upright patient, supine patient, and patient in the decubitus position.

Pneumothorax is the presence of air in the pleural space. Normally, the visceral and parietal pleura are in contact with each other except for a very thin layer of intervening fluid, which is not visible radiographically. Air is not normally present in this space. Clinical presentation of pneumothorax can vary from asymptomatic to life-threatening respiratory distress. The expected appearance of a pneumothorax can be anticipated by using the basic principles that have already been introduced (Fig. 20.1).

Radiographic Appearance of a Pneumothorax

As pneumothorax is composed of air, it is less dense (darker) radiographically than the lung which has a small soft tissue component in addition to its airspace component. Since air rises, the pneumothorax will occupy the least dependent (highest) position anatomically possible within the chest. This, of course, will vary depending on the patient's position. For example, in the upright patient, the highest point will be in the apex of the thorax (Fig. 20.2). In a lateral decubitus position, the lateral aspect of the higher hemithorax will be least dependent. However, if the pleural space is not normal (e.g., if the visceral and parietal pleura are fused due to an old infection or trauma), then air may not be able to flow freely to the highest point in

© Springer Nature Switzerland AG 2020
J. Kissane et al. (eds.), *Radiology Fundamentals: Introduction to Imaging & Technology*, https://doi.org/10.1007/978-3-030-22173-7_20

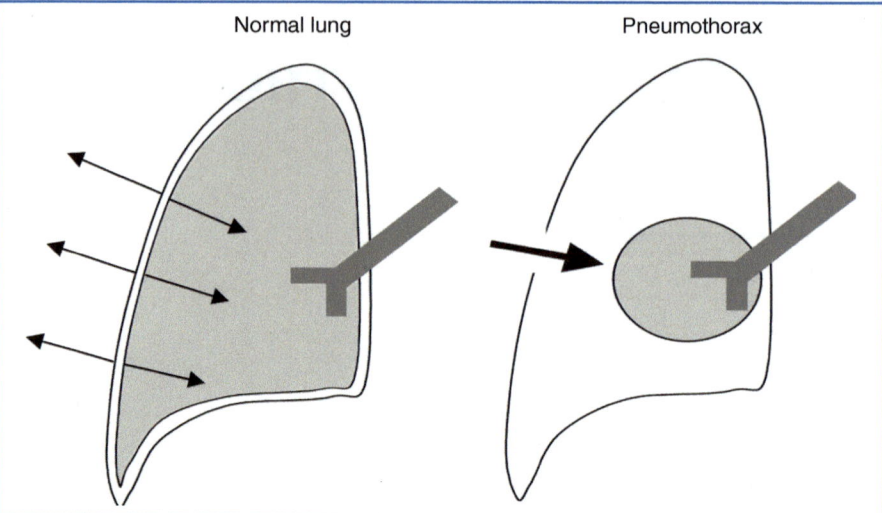

FIGURE 20.1 - NORMAL AND ABNORMAL FORCES ON THE LUNG
The normal elastic forces between the chest wall and the lung oppose each other, resulting in complete equilibrium as noted in the picture on the *left*. With pneumothorax (as depicted on the *right*), air enters the pleural space and causes the lung to collapse

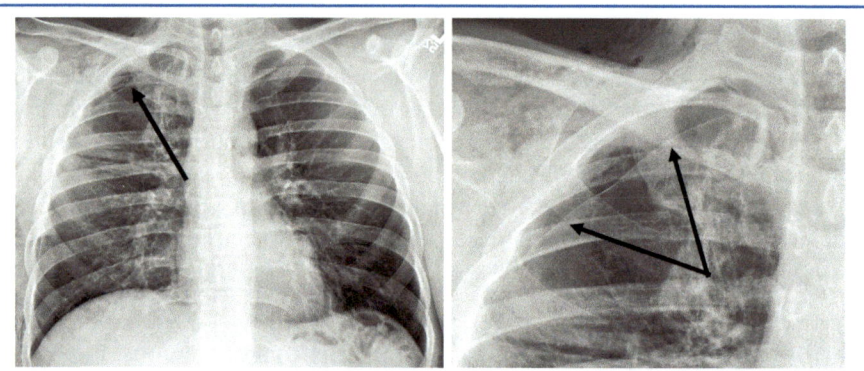

FIGURE 20.2 - PNEUMOTHORAX IN AN UPRIGHT PATIENT
Note how the edge of the right lung is delineated by a sharply demarcated thin white line (*arrows*), the visceral pleura, beyond which no pulmonary markings are identified (best seen on closeup image on *right*)

the chest. The term "loculated" is often applied to pleural air (or pleural fluid) that is constrained in such a manner. The compliance of the underlying lung may also affect the distribution of pleural air. In patients with rigid lungs (due to fibrosis, ARDS, pulmonary edema, etc.), the distribution of air in the surrounding pleural space may be altered.

Since the pleura have a small but detectable radiographic opacity, it will have the appearance of a thin white line at the edge of a pneumothorax in most cases. The pleura may become more easily visualized if it becomes thickened, in which case the white line will be more visible. The pleura will only be visualized in tangent as its density en face (head on) will not be great enough to produce a detectable shadow on the radiograph.

Indirect signs of a pneumothorax include sharp mediastinal or diaphragmatic borders and increased lucency, reflecting the location of the pneumothorax. Current digital radiographic technology allows for image manipulation that aids in the detection of pneumothorax.

Tension Pneumothorax

In certain cases, air may be trapped in the pleural space on inspiration but not released on expiration, producing a collection of air capable of exerting positive pressure on surrounding structures.

Figure 20.3 shows such a collection, termed a "tension pneumothorax." This clinical situation is potentially life-threatening since the increased intrathoracic pressure may shift the mediastinum enough to impair the function of the contralateral lung as

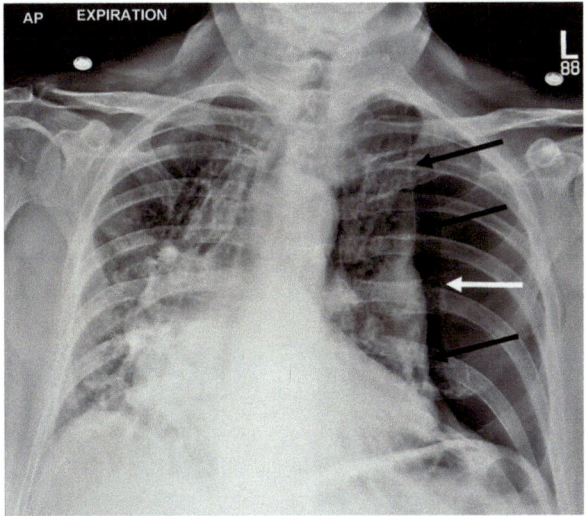

FIGURE 20.3 - TENSION PNEUMOTHORAX
Increased lucency of the left hemithorax with rightward mediastinal shift, widening of the left intercostal spaces (*white arrow*), and inferior displacement of the left hemidiaphragm, consistent with a left tension pneumothorax

well as to impair venous return to the heart. Signs indicating a tension pneumothorax include a mediastinal shift away from the side with the pneumothorax and depression of the ipsilateral hemidiaphragm. Chest tubes (thoracostomy tubes and pleural tubes) are inserted to evacuate some pneumothoraces.

Deep Sulcus Sign

Figure 20.4 shows a radiograph obtained portably in a supine patient. Notice a collection of air in the right costophrenic sulcus. When the patient is supine, this may be the least dependent position of the chest.

This finding constitutes what is called a "deep costophrenic sulcus sign." The deep costophrenic sulcus sign may be seen in supine patients who have a pneumothorax. The "deep sulcus sign" reflects the pneumothorax that is anterior and lateral. In this case, if one looks closely, the pleural line can be observed.

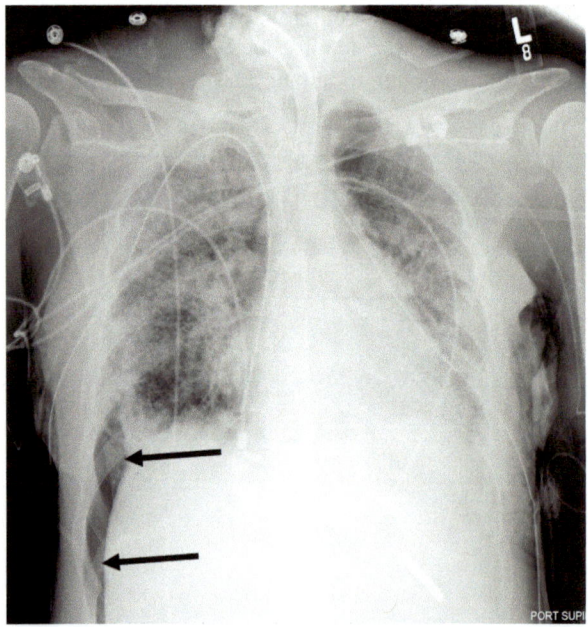

FIGURE 20.4 - DEEP SULCUS SIGN
Note the collection of air (*arrows*) in the right costophrenic sulcus in this supine patient

S: In an evaluation of suspected pneumothorax or follow-up of known pneumothorax that is not well seen on a supine radiograph, an upright radiograph should be obtained before CT as it is more cost-effective and results in lower patient radiation dose.

A: Chest radiograph should be the primary evaluation for suspected pneumothorax or in the setting of trauma for early diagnosis and intervention, if required.

F: A skinfold, which can mimic a pneumothorax on supine chest radiograph, can be distinguished from a true pleural border by the presence of vascular markings on either side of the line as well as discontinuity of the line or extension beyond normal pleural anatomic borders.

E: It is important to recognize other findings that can be associated with a pneumothorax, including evidence of tension pneumothorax (mediastinal shift), flail chest deformity (multiple contiguous segmental rib fractures), and/or pleural effusion/hemothorax.

MISCELLANEOUS CHEST CONDITIONS

Objectives:
1. Describe the radiologic appearance and etiology of calcific pericarditis.
2. Describe three distinct radiological appearances of intrathoracic tuberculosis.
3. State the relationship between asbestos exposure and bronchogenic carcinoma of the lung.
4. List the differential diagnosis of an opacified hemithorax.

The following radiographs show examples of entities with diagnostic radiographic presentations. By seeing the "classic" examples of these entities, you will hopefully gain enough familiarity to make the diagnosis should you encounter them clinically.

Calcific Pericarditis

Figure 21.1 shows a frontal radiograph and axial CT image of the chest in a patient with the diagnosis of calcific pericarditis. Note the rim of calcium surrounding the cardiac-pericardial silhouette. In severe cases, this may cause decreased diastolic filling of the cardiac chambers and require surgical removal of the pericardium.

Currently, the most common etiology for calcific pericarditis is a viral infection, often Coxsackie B virus. In the older population, granulomatous pericarditis secondary to tuberculosis is the most common cause of calcific pericarditis. Any

© Springer Nature Switzerland AG 2020
J. Kissane et al. (eds.), *Radiology Fundamentals: Introduction to Imaging & Technology*, https://doi.org/10.1007/978-3-030-22173-7_21

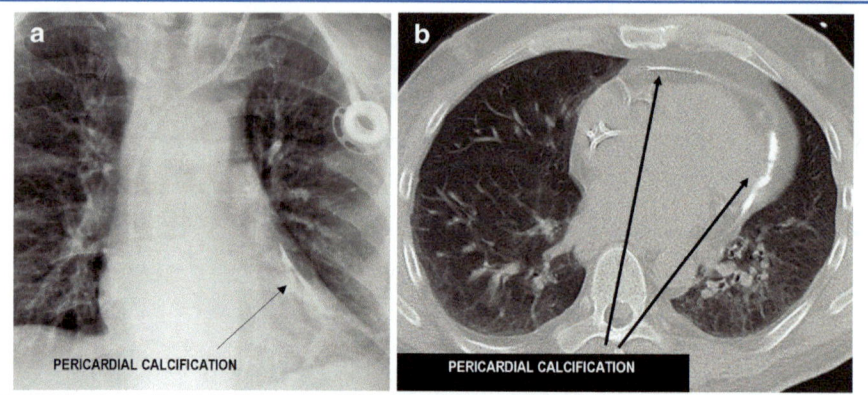

PERICARDIAL CALCIFICATION

PERICARDIAL CALCIFICATION

FIGURE 21.1 - CALCIFIC PERICARDITIS
Figure (**a**) is a cropped chest radiograph that shows a rim of calcium along the left heart border (*arrows*). Figure (**b**) is an axial CT slice from the same patient showing the rim of calcium along the left heart border. Also seen is a rim of calcium along the anterior heart border that was not seen on plain radiograph. In severe cases, this may cause decreased diastolic filling of the cardiac chambers and require surgical removal of the pericardium

cause of pericardial irritation (uremia, radiation) can eventually lead to calcific pericarditis. Approximately 50% of these cases of calcific pericarditis will have radiographically visible calcification.

Tuberculosis

Figure 21.2a shows a thick-walled cavitary lesion in the right upper lobe with surrounding areas of inhomogeneous parenchymal consolidation. In addition, there is airspace disease in the left mid lung. This is the appearance of cavitary tuberculosis with the endobronchial spread. The air within the cavitary lesion comes from erosion of the initial focus of disease into the tracheal-bronchial tree of the right upper lobe. The necrotic caseous material within the consolidation is aspirated into the more dependent lingula, in this case, causing the spread of disease. The differential diagnosis for a cavitary upper lobe lesion should always include tuberculosis, especially if the lesion involves primarily the apical or posterior segments.

Figure 21.2b, c shows innumerable punctate nodular opacities distributed throughout both lungs on a chest radiograph and CT axial image, respectively. This is the appearance of a hematogenously disseminated infection to the lungs, in this case, miliary tuberculosis. This is an advanced case of this disease, and cavitation does not occur in this process. Healing, with proper therapy, will be completed with no radiographically visible residual abnormality within the lung.

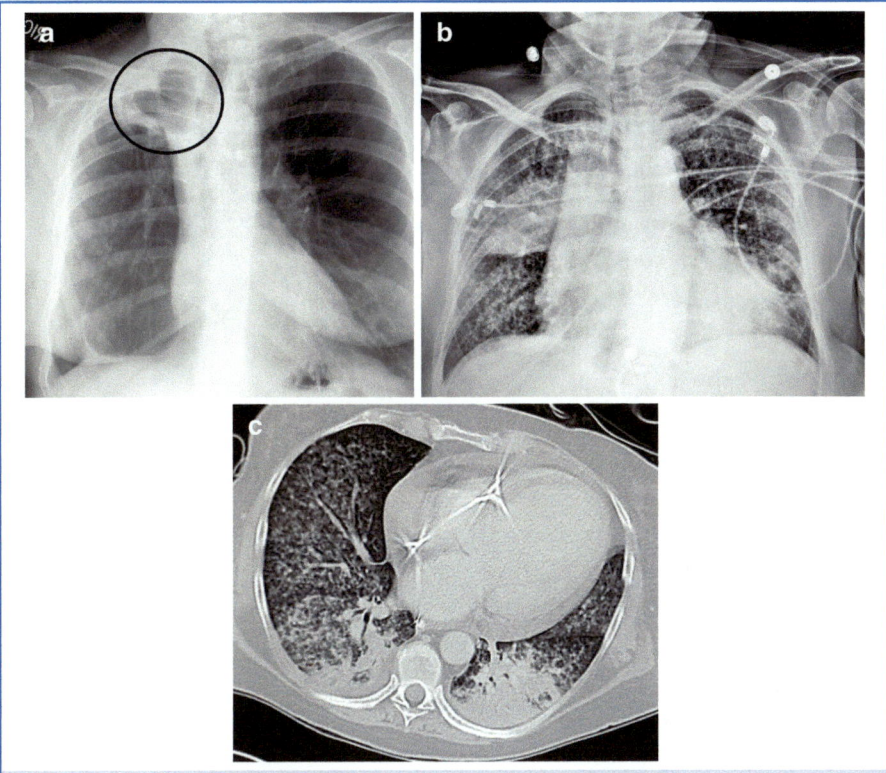

FIGURE 21.2 - TUBERCULOSIS
Figure (**a**) shows a cavitary lesion in the right upper lobe with surrounding areas of heterogeneous parenchymal consolidation from a patient with known tuberculosis. Miliary tuberculosis: Both figures (**b, c**) are from the same patient with known miliary TB. The chest radiograph shows innumerable punctate nodular opacities distributed throughout both lungs and a focal area of consolidation in the right mid lung. The axial CT image also shows innumerable punctate nodular opacities in both lungs and areas of consolidation. Though this appearance is nonspecific as it can be seen with miliary tumor metastasis, it is characteristic of hematogenously disseminated miliary tuberculosis

Mediastinal Lymphadenopathy

Figure 21.3 shows widening of the superior mediastinum in both the right and left paratracheal regions extending down to the superior aspect of both hilar and subcarinal regions. This is the appearance of mediastinal lymphadenopathy. One cause of mediastinal lymphadenopathy is the infection with *Mycobacterium avium-intracellulare* (MAI).

MAI infections may present with minimal pulmonary findings and only mediastinal and hilar lymphadenopathy, as noted in this case. Fungal disease such

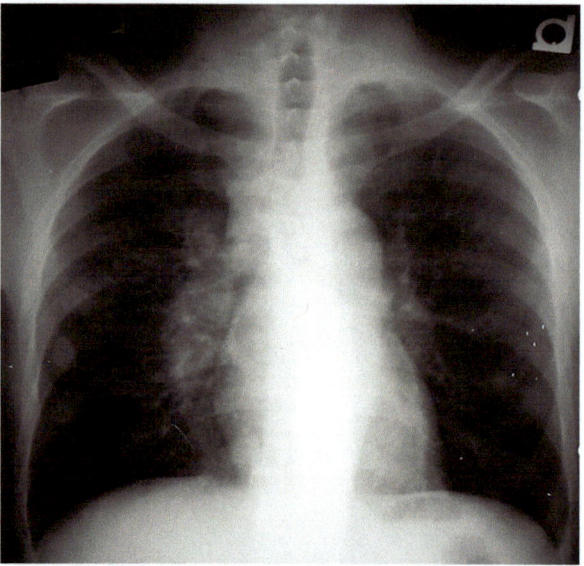

FIGURE 21.3 - LYMPHADENOPATHY
Widening of the superior mediastinum in both the right and left paratracheal regions extending down to both hilar and subcarinal regions, in a case of *Mycobacterium avium-intracellulare* (*MAI*) infection

as histoplasmosis may give a similar presentation. Of course, lymphoma and other malignant causes of lymphadenopathy and other non-malignant causes, such as sarcoidosis, would be in the differential diagnosis. Patients who are HIV positive have a considerably elevated risk for the development of all forms of *Mycobacterium* infections.

Asbestos

Figure 21.4 shows PA (a) and lateral (b) radiographs from a patient with numerous calcified and noncalcified bilateral pleural plaques. These are secondary to asbestos exposure. There is a long latent period between the time of asbestos exposure and the development of the plaques, on the order of 10–15 years in most cases. The plaques are associated with the parietal pleura, unique to asbestos plaques. Calcified pleural thickening may also be seen in patients with an old empyema or an old hemothorax. However, these characteristically primarily involve the visceral pleura and are often unilateral. Radiographically, you cannot tell between visceral and parietal pleural calcification, so clinical history is important (see Fig. 21.5).

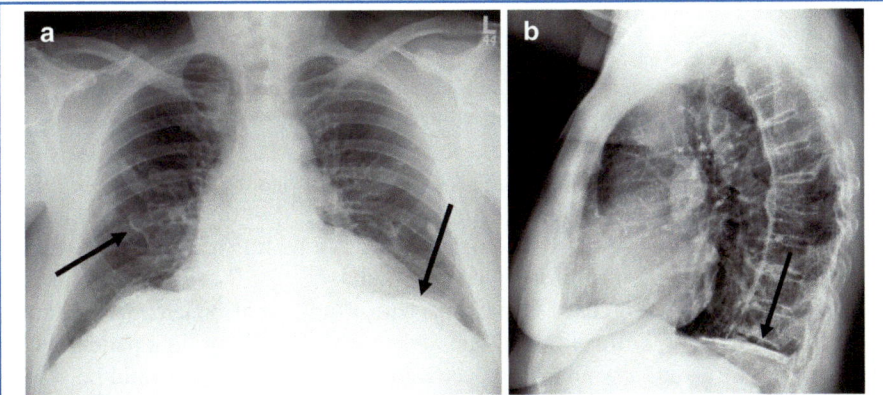

FIGURE 21.4 - PLEURAL PLAQUES

PA (**a**) and lateral (**b**) radiographs of two different patients showing calcified pleural plaques (*arrows*) secondary to asbestos exposure

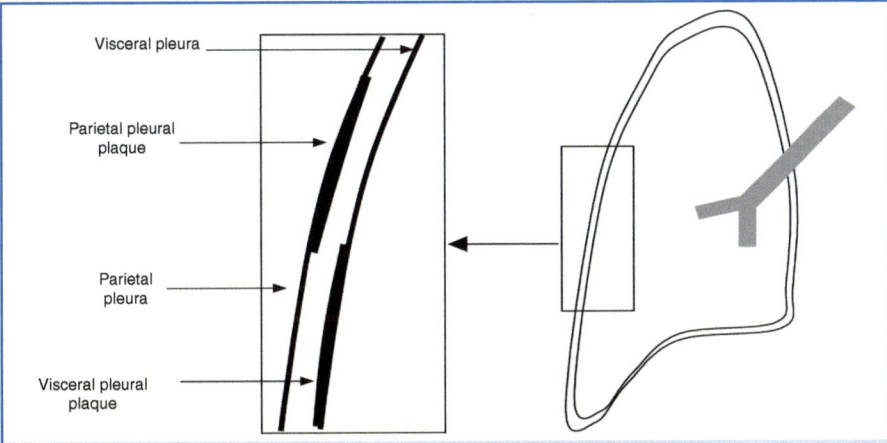

FIGURE 21.5 - PLEURAL PLAQUES

After a latent period of 10–15 years, asbestos exposure can result in parietal pleural plaques, a unique location related to asbestos exposure. Patients with a history of empyema or hemothorax will have visceral pleural plaques

Bronchogenic carcinoma is the most commonly associated malignancy in patients with a history of asbestos exposure. Mesothelioma, although more uniquely associated with asbestos exposure, is much less common. Patients with a history of asbestos exposure also have increased incidence of esophageal, gastric, and other gastrointestinal carcinomas because asbestos fibers are swallowed as well as inhaled. A patient with a history of asbestos exposure as well as significant smoking history has a very substantially increased risk of developing bronchogenic carcinoma.

Opacified Hemithorax

Figure 21.6 shows a case of homogeneously increased opacity in the left hemithorax. Note that the mediastinum is shifted toward the left side so that the heart is not clearly distinguished, obscured by the surrounding increased opacity. This patient has undergone a left pneumonectomy, the post-pneumonectomy space being filled with fluid. Note that there is still a small apical collection of air and therefore an air-fluid level. Eventually, the whole hemithorax will be filled with fluid. The right lung has undergone compensatory hyperinflation.

Other differential diagnoses in patients with a unilateral opacified hemithorax include a large pleural effusion and total atelectasis of the lung. In a patient with a large pleural effusion, it would be expected that the mediastinum would be at least in the midline or, most likely, shifted to the opposite side of the opacified hemithorax due to the mass effect of fluid in the chest. Patients with complete atelectasis of the lung or pneumonectomy will have mediastinal shift to the same side as the opacified hemithorax. A quick history and physical examination should allow one to distinguish between atelectasis and pneumonectomy. Surgical scars on the chest wall will be present with the latter.

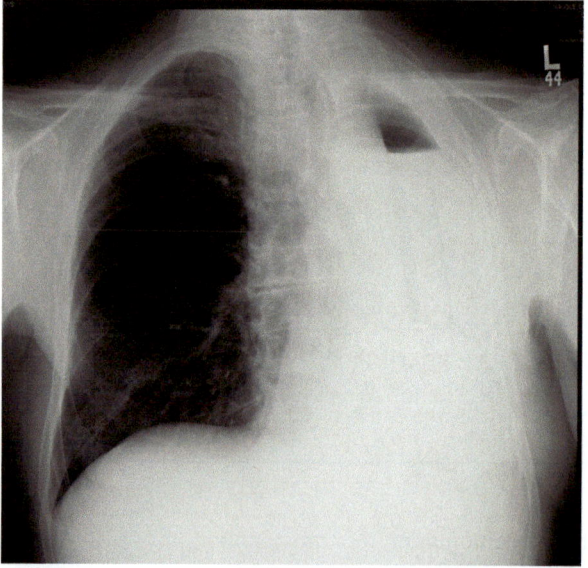

FIGURE 21.6 - OPACIFIED HEMITHORAX
Homogeneously increased opacity in the left hemithorax. Note that the mediastinum is shifted toward the left and the heart is not clearly distinguished from the surrounding increased density consistent with left hemithorax volume loss

S: Appropriate precautions should be taken if there is a strong clinical concern for active infection such as tuberculosis.

A: Opacified hemithorax can be the result of many conditions. History is key and chest CT may be necessary to help determine the cause, if the finding is new.

F: Once an etiology is determined, radiographic abnormalities can often be followed by chest x-ray, minimizing radiation exposure. However, CT may be necessary if a patient's clinical condition deteriorates.

E: Evidence of active infection or opacified hemithorax such as a large pleural effusion causing volume loss and mass effect on the contralateral lung should be communicated expeditiously with the referring clinician.

22 TUBES AND LINES

Objective:
1. State the ideal positions for the endotracheal tube, central venous catheter, and nasogastric tube.

The main point of the following radiographs is to show normal and abnormal positions of various commonly seen tubes and catheters.

The Endotracheal (ET) Tube

Figure 22.1 shows an endotracheal tube. The ideal position for an endotracheal tube is 3–5 cm above the carina. Portable radiographs, like this one, are commonly obtained to check endotracheal tube position.

The reason for positioning the ET tube 3–5 cm above the carina is that the tube moves within the trachea with changes in head position because the tube is fixed at its insertion point in the nose or the mouth. With flexion of the neck, the position of the tube moves inferiorly about 2 cm. With the extension, the tube moves superiorly approximately 2 cm. Ideal positioning assures that the endotracheal tube tip or balloon cuff will not enter one of the main bronchi inferiorly or the larynx superiorly with changes in the patient's head position. The ET tube tip should be no higher than 7–8 cm above the carina and no lower than 2–3 cm above the carina. The balloon cuff should not dilate the trachea. Its diameter should be less than 3 cm in most patients.

Figure 22.2 shows an endotracheal tube with its tip positioned in the proximal right main bronchus. Partial atelectasis (collapse) of the left lung is seen. Atelectasis

© Springer Nature Switzerland AG 2020   131
J. Kissane et al. (eds.), *Radiology Fundamentals: Introduction to Imaging & Technology*, https://doi.org/10.1007/978-3-030-22173-7_22

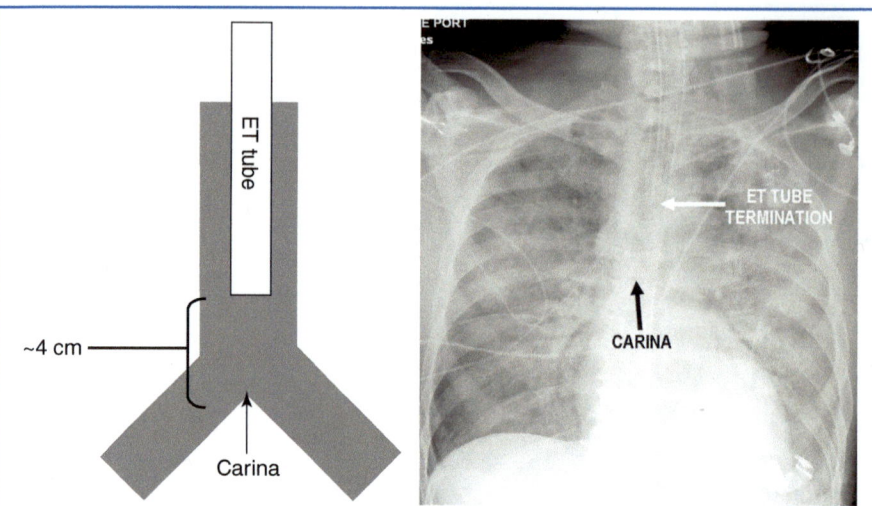

FIGURE 22.1 - PROPER ENDOTRACHEAL TUBE POSITIONING
The endotracheal tube tip should ideally be placed roughly 4 cm above the carina. The vertical radiopaque line represents a marker placed within the wall of the tube to make it visible on radiographs

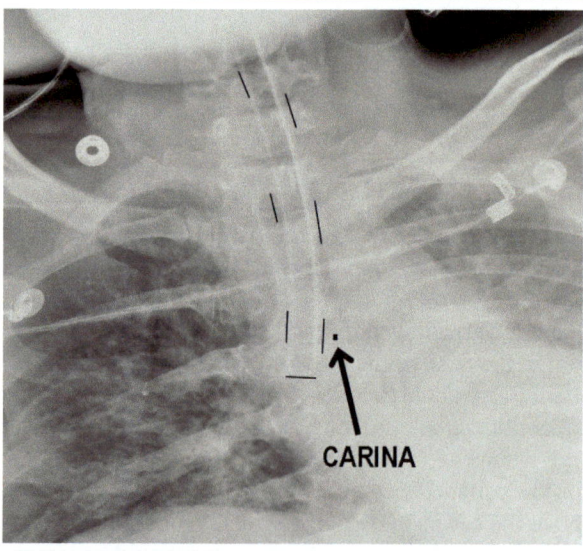

FIGURE 22.2 - RIGHT MAIN BRONCHUS INTUBATION
Endotracheal tube tip is in the right main bronchus. Diffusely increased opacity throughout the left lung is likely secondary to obstructive atelectasis, a complication of improper endotracheal tube placement

occurs because the left lung is not ventilated. This is a complication related to misplacement of the ET tube, but it readily resolves when the ET tube is appropriately repositioned.

Central Venous Catheters

Figure 22.3 shows the pathways of central venous catheters. Catheters can be inserted via the subclavian vein or the internal jugular vein. They then traverse the brachiocephalic vein to get to the superior vena cava. Ideal positioning of lines is shown. If the line is a temporary venous access such as a peripherally introduced central catheter (PICC) or a central venous access line such as an infusion catheter, the catheter tip will be in the lower superior vena cava or at the superior cavoatrial junction (#1). If the line is an exchange or dialysis catheter, either temporary or permanent, the tip will be at the mid-right atrium (#2). If the line is a pulmonary artery catheter (aka Swan-Ganz catheter) the tip will be in either the main pulmonary artery or a central pulmonary artery branch (#3).

An uncommon complication of insertion of subclavian central venous catheters is pneumothorax, since these vessels lie close to the apex of the lung. When venous access is attempted, the pleural space may be entered. For this reason, an upright radiograph should be obtained after line placement in these patients, as pneumothoraces will be more visible on an upright study. Another uncommon complication of attempted central venous placement is arterial placement or perforation.

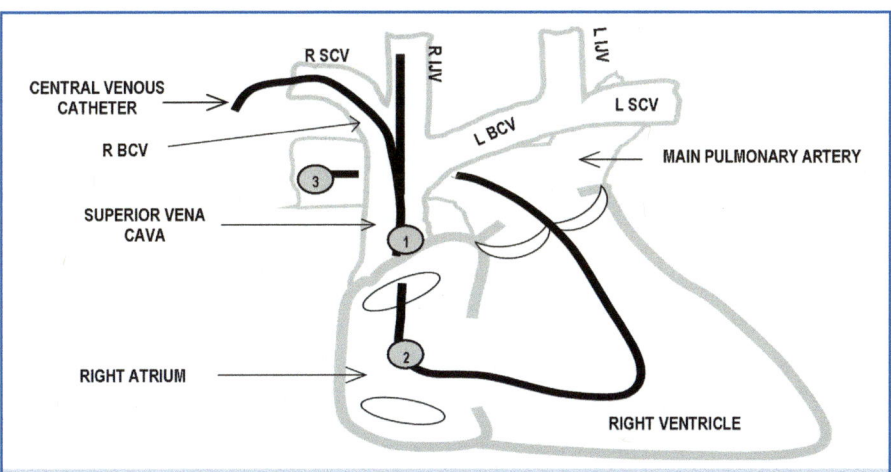

FIGURE 22.3 - COMMON PATHWAYS OF CENTRAL VENOUS CATHETERS
Nomenclature: SCV subclavian vein, IJV internal jugular vein, BCV brachiocephalic vein. The numbers denote the ideal tip placement for the following catheter types: 1. PICC or infusion catheter, 2. Dialysis catheter, 3. Swan-Ganz catheter

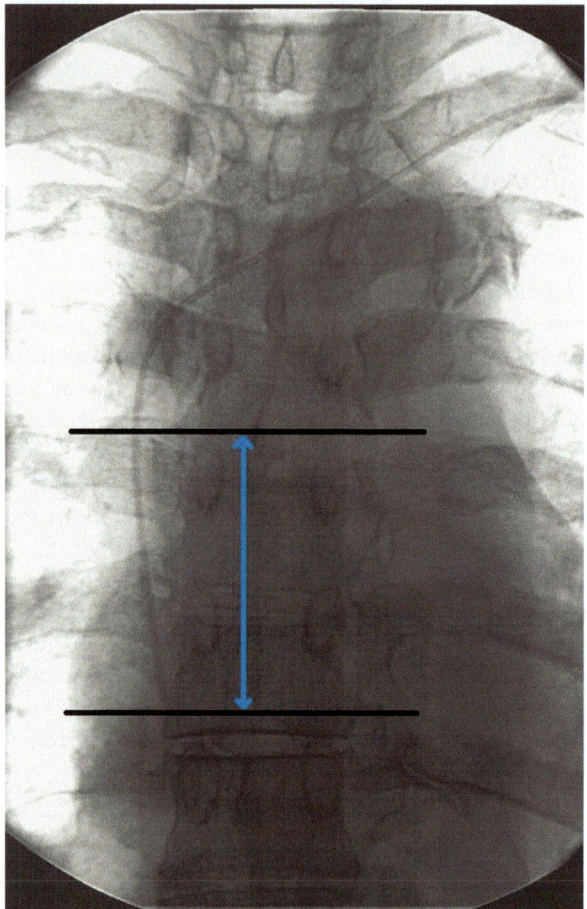

FIGURE 22.4 - PICC
A left basilic PICC line terminates at the superior cavoatrial junction, ~2 vertebral bodies below the carina; an appropriate position for the catheter tip

Figure 22.4 shows an appropriately positioned left PICC, with the tip at the superior cavoatrial junction, located two vertebral bodies below the carina. These catheters are of weak radiopacity so that proper radiographic technique must be employed to visualize them. It is routine to obtain post line placement radiographs so that problems can be detected early.

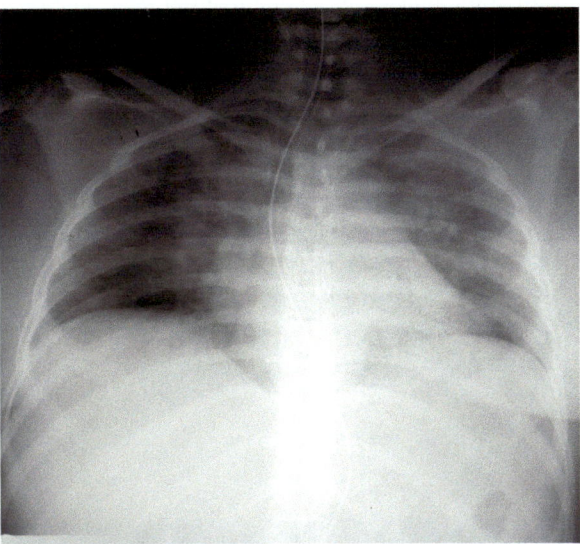

FIGURE 22.5 - NASOGASTRIC TUBE
Nasogastric tube tip is below the diaphragm, excluded from the field of view. The side port is also in the stomach, just below the GE junction

The Nasogastric Tube

Figure 22.5 shows a nasogastric tube. The tube tip should terminate in the stomach. The radiopaque marker on the tube shows a single gap in the distal portion, approximately 8 cm from the tip, denoting the location of the side hole. The side hole should also be within the stomach.

Remember: You must always ensure that a line or tube is correctly placed before using it!

S: Ultrasound guidance can greatly improve the safety and accuracy of vascular line placement and is usually readily available. Understanding the radiographic appearance of a properly positioned catheter or tube is critical to the safety of the patient.

A: A radiograph is indicated post placement of any new central venous catheter or enteric tube or repositioning of an existing line or tube to ensure appropriate placement before use.

F: Anatomic knowledge and radiographic correlates and/or relevant landmarks are crucial to the identification of line and tube positioning. For example, a central venous catheter should course through the SVC along the right side of the mediastinal silhouette and end around the level of the cavoatrial junction which is roughly at a level two vertebral bodies below the carina.

E: It is important to communicate any complication post tube or line placement. These can include pneumothorax or clinically relevant line or tube malposition such as an arterial course of a central venous line.

PART III
MAMMOGRAPHY

23 BREAST IMAGING

Objectives:
1. Understand the differences between a screening and diagnostic mammogram including the recommendations for screening mammography.
2. Describe additional imaging modalities used for evaluating the breast and the indications for each modality.
3. Understand the radiation dose of mammography in relation to other common imaging exams.
4. State the main radiographic criteria for the detection of breast carcinoma.
5. Understand the BI-RADS classification system for communication of breast imaging results to clinicians.

Breast carcinoma is the most common non-skin cancer in women, with approximately 200,000 new cases each year with the incidence of breast cancer increasing with age. Risk factors are those primarily related to hormonal history and parity. Multiple randomized controlled trials have demonstrated a reduction in mortality in women who are routinely screened with mammography compared to women who are not screened. Although there has been some controversy regarding the benefits of screening women aged 40–49, currently the American Medical Association and the American College of Radiology recommend routine screening of average-risk women beginning at age 40. The early detection of breast cancer through screening mammography has contributed to a decrease in mortality of over 40% [1]. Increased survival rates are likely due to both early detection of disease through mammography as well as improvements in the therapy for breast cancer with agents that target cancers based on their individual biology.

The sensitivity of mammographic screening is in part based on breast density, with sensitivity increasing as breast density decreases (see section "Dense Fibroglandular Breast Tissue"). However, early detection is also dependent on compliance with the recommendations for annual examinations. Annual screening increases the likelihood

© Springer Nature Switzerland AG 2020
J. Kissane et al. (eds.), *Radiology Fundamentals: Introduction to Imaging & Technology*, https://doi.org/10.1007/978-3-030-22173-7_23

Table 23.1 The ACR guidelines for screening mammography

Risk	Qualifier	Age	Modality (annual)
Average	Screening to begin at age 40 and to continue until life expectancy is 5–7 years	40	Mammogram
High	BRCA I or II mutation	30, not before 25	Mammogram and MRI
	>20% lifetime risk	30, not before 25	Mammogram and MRI
	Chest irradiation between 10 and 30 years	8 years following therapy, not before 25	Mammogram and MRI
Moderately high	Personal history of breast cancer	Annually from diagnosis; 6–12 months postradiation if breast conserved	Mammogram; consider supplemental MRI or US
Moderately high	High-risk histology: ADH, lobular neoplasia	From the age of diagnosis, not before 30	Mammogram; consider MRI
Moderately high	Increased breast density	40, unless other risks present	Mammogram; consider US

of detecting subtle changes on the mammogram. This is particularly important in women with increased parenchymal breast tissue density. The American College of Radiology guidelines for screening mammography can be found in Table 23.1 [2]. It is important to note the difference between screening and diagnostic mammography. Screening mammography is the annual routine examination performed in women who have no signs or symptoms of breast disease. Two views of each breast are obtained in the CC (craniocaudal) and MLO (mediolateral oblique) projections, described below. Diagnostic mammography is utilized to better characterize an abnormality that has been identified on a screening mammogram and is the appropriate first test for a patient over the age of 30 presenting with a breast symptom, such as a palpable lump. Diagnostic mammograms involve extra views in varied projections including specialized spot compression views of any symptomatic area and/or magnification views for better characterization of calcifications. Mammography is also the initial modality of choice in the evaluation of suspected male breast disease in patients over the age of 25.

The introduction of digital mammography has proven to be beneficial in women with dense breast tissue, premenopausal and younger women, and those at high risk for breast cancer [3]. Full-field digital mammography (FFDM) is a mammography system in which the x-ray film is replaced by solid-state detectors that convert x-rays into electrical signals. The electrical signals and unique breast-specific algorithms are used to produce images of the breast that can be viewed and manipulated on a computer workstation. This ability to manipulate the image by changing the contrast, combined with the use of specialized algorithms for displaying the mammographic images, results in a higher degree of sensitivity for digital mammography compared to analog or screen-film mammography. Results of the Digital Mammography Imaging Screening Trial (DMIST) suggest up to 30% increase in sensitivity in the detection of occult malignancies [3].

Digital breast tomosynthesis (DBT) has been introduced as a means to create and view thin reconstructed mammographic images from a finite number of two-dimensional projections at different tube angles. The STORM study (among many others) has successfully shown that the cancer detection rate is increased with the use of DBT compared with 2D mammography alone [4]. While dose is increased when DBT is used as an adjunct to 2D mammography, synthesized reconstructed planar images have come into favor to combat this dose dilemma by eliminating the need to acquire separate DBT and 2D mammograms [5].

The purpose of the following section is to acquaint you with some basic aspects of breast imaging and the early detection of breast cancer.

Standard Mammography Views: CC and MLO

Figure 23.1 demonstrates the two standard views obtained during a routine mammogram.

The craniocaudal (CC) view is obtained by placing the x-ray tube overhead and the film cassette or digital detector beneath the breast so that the beam traverses the breast from a cranial to caudal direction.

A mediolateral oblique (MLO) view is obtained by placing the film cassette or digital detector in the axilla and allowing the x-ray beam to traverse the breast from the medial upper breast to the lateral lower breast and axilla.

The breast is compressed during mammography for the purpose of decreasing the amount of tissue the x-ray beam must traverse. The act of compression functions to

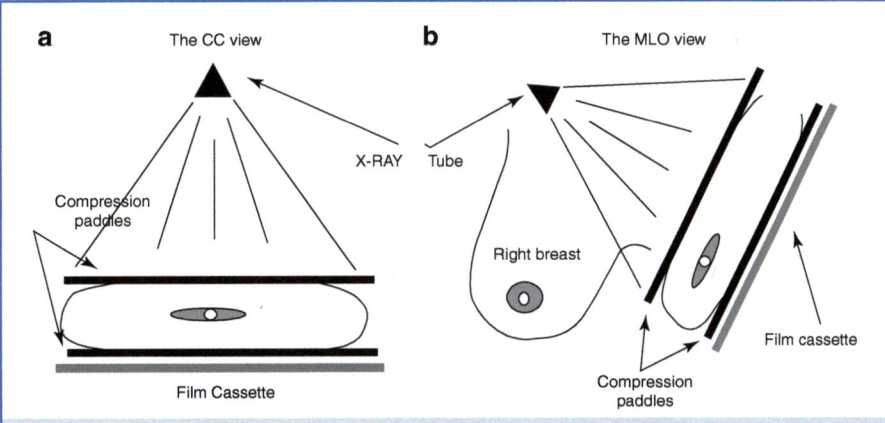

FIGURE 23.1 - THE CC AND MLO BREAST VIEWS
In the CC view (**a**), the breast is compressed between two radiolucent paddles to spread the tissue out, reducing tissue overlap and decreasing dose. In the MLO view (**b**), the breast is compressed in an oblique fashion, with the tail of breast tissue that extends toward the axilla, included on the film

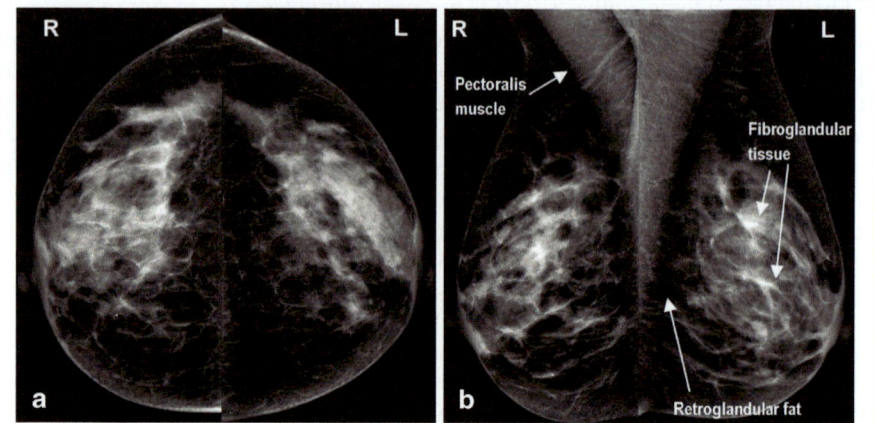

FIGURE 23.2 - THE CC AND MLO BREAST VIEWS
In the CC view (**a**), the breast is compressed between two radiolucent paddles to spread the tissue out, reducing tissue overlap and decreasing dose. In the MLO view (**b**), the breast is compressed in an oblique fashion, with the tail of breast tissue that extends toward the axilla, included on the film

stabilize the breast and reduce motion artifact as well as to spread out superimposed structures. Compression of the breast maximizes the mammogram image quality and decreases the radiation dose to the breast. This compression may be uncomfortable for some patients, but it is brief in duration and results in a mammogram with higher diagnostic quality.

Figure 23.2 shows an example of a typical mammogram consisting of CC and MLO views. The darker, more lucent areas represent fat, while the whiter, less transparent areas are composed of fibroglandular tissue. Fibroglandular tissue is comprised of the glandular tissue of the breast as well as the underlying fibrous stromal elements that add support to the overall structure of the breast.

The fibroglandular tissue is generally distributed in a "cone" with the nipple at the apex and the base closer to the chest wall. Between the posterior aspect of the cone of fibroglandular tissue and the underlying pectoral muscle is the retroglandular fat. A well-positioned MLO view should contain the fibroglandular tissue in its entirety, the retroglandular fat and a portion of the pectoralis muscle.

Dense Fibroglandular Breast Tissue

Figure 23.3 demonstrates a breast with a predominance of dense fibroglandular tissue. For comparison, Fig. 23.4 demonstrates breasts that are predominantly fatty tissue. Mammographic patterns showing mainly fatty breast tissue are typically found in older women, whereas younger, premenopausal women tend to have a greater percentage of dense fibroglandular tissue.

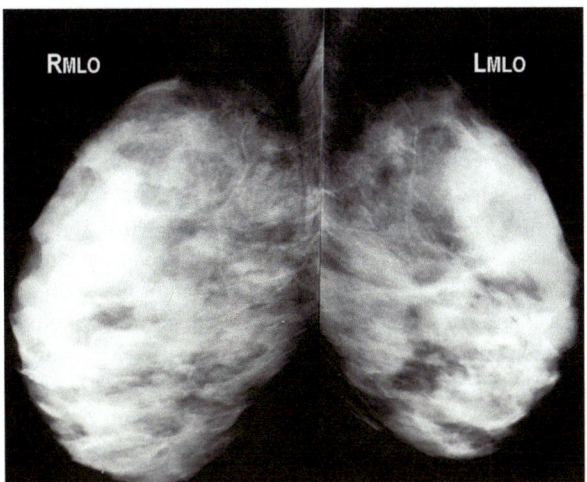
FIGURE 23.3 - DENSE BREAST TISSUE

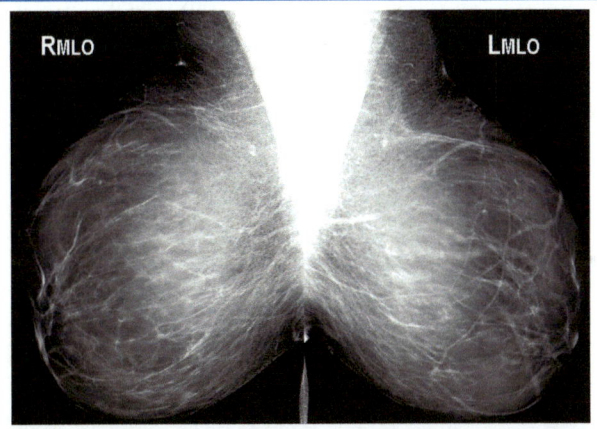
FIGURE 23.4 - FATTY BREAST TISSUE
An example of fatty breast tissue for comparison to the dense breast tissue in Fig. 23.3

Detection of a small mass is more difficult when the background mammographic density is high. This must be kept in mind when reading a mammographic report. The current BI-RADS lexicon includes the statement "increased mammographic density can lower the sensitivity of mammography" in the report to the woman's physician. Increased breast density is also associated with an increased risk of developing breast cancer, independent of the masking of small tumors. Published estimates suggest five times the risk of cancer in women with the highest breast density compared to those with the lowest breast density [6].

The young breast not only tends to be denser but also more sensitive to the potential carcinogenic effects of radiation. Therefore, unless the patient's personal risk factors indicate a higher than average risk of developing premenopausal breast cancer, screening for breast cancer should begin at age 40 [7]. It is important, however, that high-risk patients under the age of 40 also be appropriately screened. Women with first-degree relatives with premenopausal breast cancer or with known genetic mutations should be screened annually, at age 10 years younger than the age of the first-degree relative's cancer. Women who have had chest radiation for Hodgkin lymphoma are also considered high risk and should begin screening 8 years following the therapy, but not before age 25. Women under 40 years who have had biopsies showing certain pathologic findings (ductal or lobular atypia, etc.) are considered at increased risk and are advised to begin annual screening at the time of the diagnosis of high-risk histology [7].

Breast Implants

Figure 23.5 demonstrates a very dense homogeneous opacity close to the chest wall. This is the appearance of a breast implant.

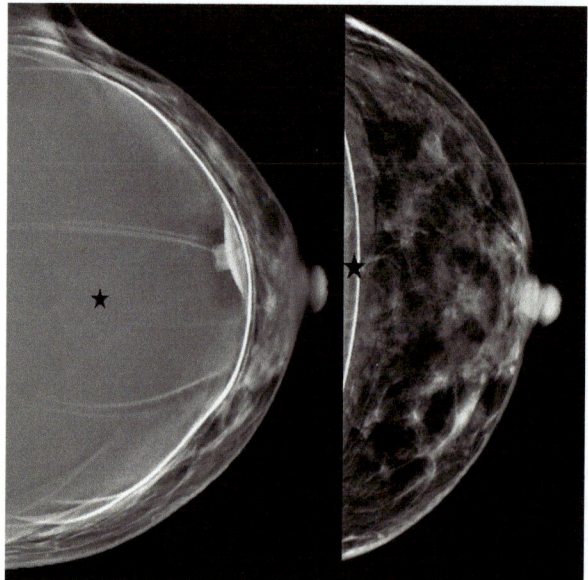

FIGURE 23.5 - BREAST IMPLANTS
The image on the *left* is a conventional CC view, while the one on the *right* is an implant displaced CC view

Implants may be surgically located either anterior or posterior to the pectoralis major muscle (described as prepectoral and retropectoral, respectively). When retropectoral, the muscle can be seen curving around the anterior surface of the implant. On standard views, implants may obscure a considerable amount of breast parenchyma and can make detection of early carcinomas more difficult. For this reason, patients with breast implants undergoing mammography get four views of each breast, rather than two views. One set is the conventional type (MLO and CC), while the other set is taken with the implant displaced against the chest wall.

Mammographic Findings

To detect breast cancer at its earliest stage, radiologists evaluate the images for subtle changes in the density and architecture of the breast tissue, new asymmetries or masses, and new or suspicious microcalcifications. If an abnormality is detected on a standard screening exam, the more specialized diagnostic exam is ordered. The margins of the masses are better characterized by spot compression views. Margins that are irregular or spiculated are suspicious for malignancy, while circumscribed margins favor the benign disease. Calcifications must be evaluated with magnification technology before a final assessment is rendered.

Calcifications occur frequently in the breast, and when the calcifications are large and coarse, they can be confidently reported as benign. However, smaller calcifications (referred to as "microcalcifications") may require biopsy for definitive diagnosis. The following four figures provide examples of both benign and malignant calcifications (Figs. 23.6, 23.7, 23.8, and 23.9).

Figure 23.10 demonstrates two examples of a well-circumscribed mass called fibroadenoma. In Fig. 23.10b, the mass contains coarse "popcorn" calcification characteristic of a degenerating fibroadenoma. Fibroadenomas are one of the most common benign tumors of the breast that may manifest as a mass on mammogram or breast ultrasound.

In contrast to the benign fibroadenomas above, Fig. 23.11a, b demonstrate a mass characteristic of carcinoma as seen on the standard two-view mammogram.

Radiation Dosage

The effective dose is the measurement of radiation that allows for the variable radiosensitivity of different tissues and for the quantification of the risk for future adverse outcomes related to the exposure. The effective radiation dose to the breast for a two-view examination (four total exposures) is approximately 0.2–0.3 mSv (200–300 millirads). The exposure is less for some digital imaging, measuring approximately 0.08–1.5 mSv (85–150 millirads). The federal limit for exposure during a mammogram is up to 0.3 mSv or 300 millirads per exposure.

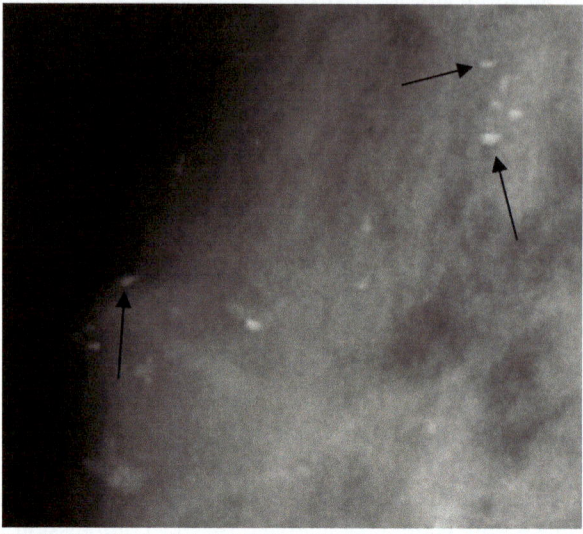

FIGURE 23.6 - BENIGN CALCIFICATIONS
Milk of calcium layering out in a gravity-dependent fashion, demonstrated with 90° positioning of the breast (*arrows*)

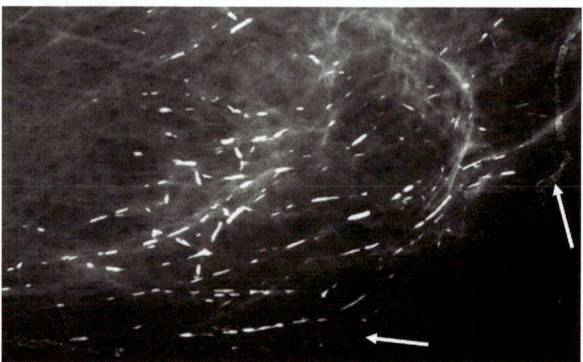

FIGURE 23.7 - BENIGN CALCIFICATIONS
Two examples of benign calcifications. First, the numerous large, *rod*-shaped calcifications scattered throughout the breast are benign calcifications within ectatic ducts. Second, vascular calcifications are common with age (*arrows*)

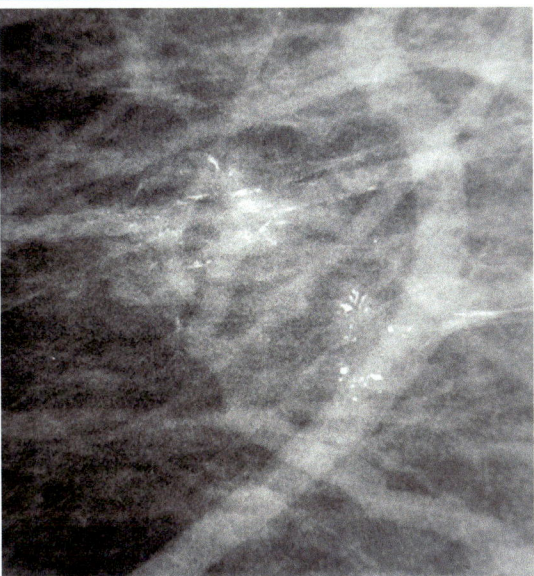

FIGURE 23.8 - MICROCALCIFICATIONS
Spot magnification compression views showing pleomorphic, fine branching microcalcifications related to DCIS

The normal background radiation is comprised predominantly of cosmic radiation and naturally occurring radiation in the ground such as Radon. For a person living at sea level, the average background radiation is approximately 3 mSv per year. Therefore, a standard mammogram is equivalent to approximately 7 weeks of normal background radiation.

At the stated dose level, mammography carries the hypothetical risk for approximately one excess cancer case per year per million women examined. If one assumes 50% breast cancer mortality, the hypothetical risk would be one excess death per two million women examined. The term hypothetical is used because, at such low increased risk, a large number of patients followed for a long period of time would be required to statistically demonstrate an effect. Because of the large population size needed for valid research, the actual research study has never been performed, and the statistics are extrapolations of patients exposed to higher dosage levels from other sources. Background radiation contributes more exposure to each of us each year, particularly those who fly frequently, due to the exposure to cosmic radiation. The airport scanners

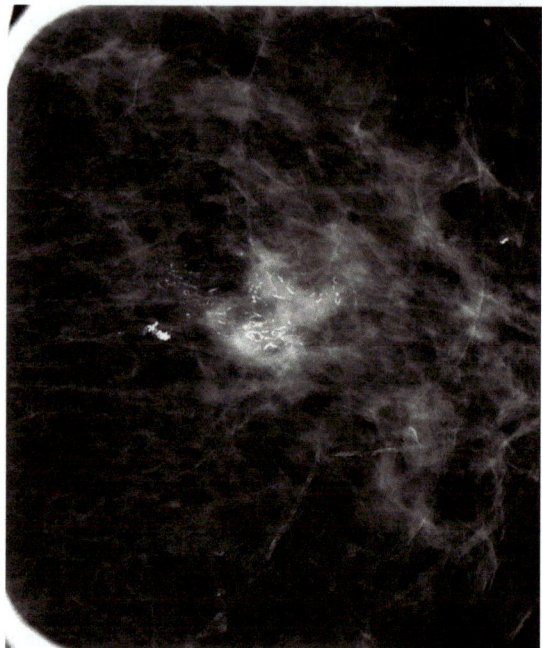

FIGURE 23.9 - MICROCALCIFICATIONS
Spot magnification compression views showing classic pleomorphic, linear branching calcifications associated with a spiculated mass in coexisting invasive ductal carcinoma and DCIS

contribute little, with 100–200 backscatter scans equal to 1 day of natural background radiation exposure. It is important to keep these relationships in mind, since you will be asked frequently by patients about the safety of mammography [8].

Ultrasound Utilization in Breast Imaging

Breast ultrasound is advocated for focused evaluations of abnormalities on physical examination, focused evaluation of abnormal mammographic findings and occasionally as a "second look" tool after an abnormal breast MRI. Ultrasound is also the modality of choice in the evaluation of masses in children and anyone (male or female) under the age of 30.

When a circumscribed (smoothly marginated) breast mass is discovered on mammography, the differential diagnosis includes breast carcinoma, benign tumor of the breast such as fibroadenoma, and simple breast cyst. To avoid performing biopsies

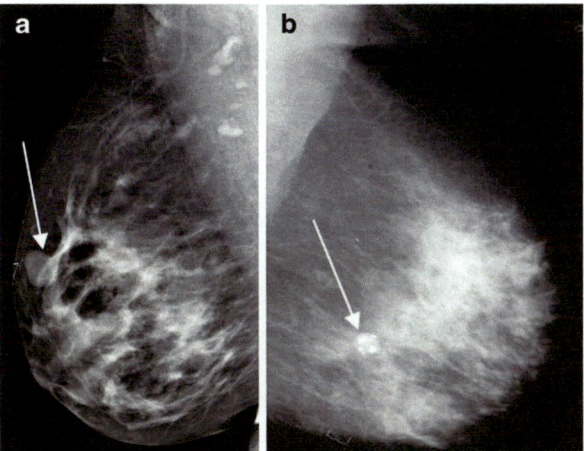

FIGURE 23.10 - FIBROADENOMA
Two different examples (**a**, **b**) of fibroadenomas. Both are smoothly marginated. Note how the one on the *right* (**b**) contains coarse calcifications, which is characteristic of a degenerating fibroadenoma

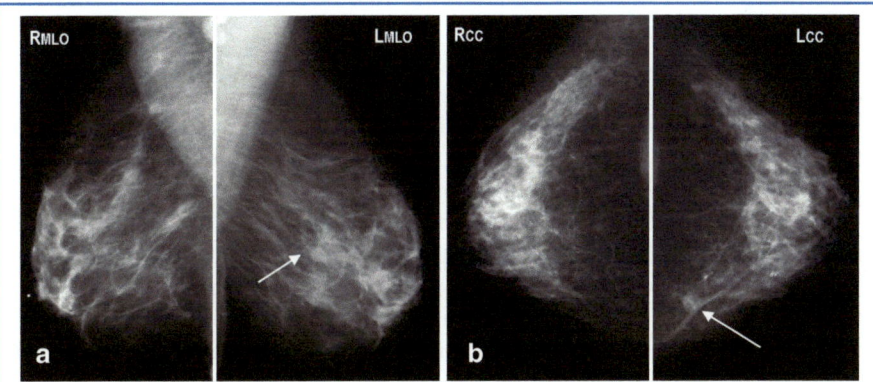

FIGURE 23.11 - (A) BREAST MASS MLO VIEWS. (B) BREAST MASS CC VIEWS
Mass in the left breast suspicious for carcinoma

on women with breast cysts and other clearly benign lesions, ultrasound is employed to discriminate cystic from solid lesions and to characterize solid masses to determine the need for biopsy.

Figure 23.12 demonstrates a mammogram of a palpable mass highlighted by a triangular marker placed on the skin over the area of concern. This lesion was subsequently imaged by ultrasound and is depicted in Fig. 23.13. The ultrasound

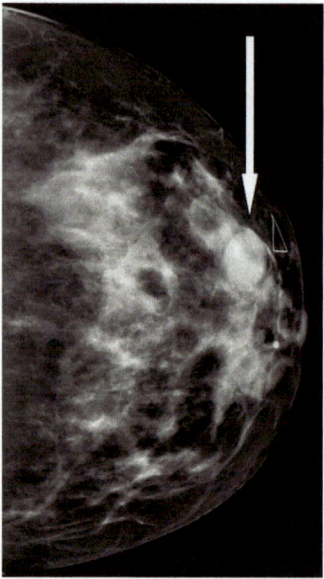

FIGURE 23.12 - PALPABLE MASS
Skin marker (the metallic triangle) used to indicate a palpable mass

shows an oval lesion that is free of echoes (anechoic) with circumscribed margins. This corresponds in location to the opacity seen on the conventional mammogram depicted in Fig. 23.12. The sonographic characteristics are definitive for a simple fluid-filled cyst, and no further evaluation is required.

Whole breast ultrasound alone has not been proven to be sensitive or efficient enough to use as a screening test for breast cancer in lieu of mammography. However, screening breast ultrasound has been shown to increase the cancer detection rate in patients at elevated risk or in patients with dense breasts [9]. Therefore, supplemental screening with US should be considered in high-risk women who are not eligible for MRI and in the intermediate-risk patient, particularly in the setting of dense breasts (https://www.acr.org/-/media/ACR/Files/Practice-Parameters/US-Breast.pdf).

Breast MRI

Breast MRI utilizes gadolinium contrast to highlight areas of increased vascularity in the breast. Therefore, MRI provides not only an anatomic evaluation of the breast but also a physiologic assessment of the vascularity of breast tissue. Because breast cancers are often associated with tumoral vascularity ("neovascularity"), and because differentiation of soft tissues is 10–100 times greater on MRI images than

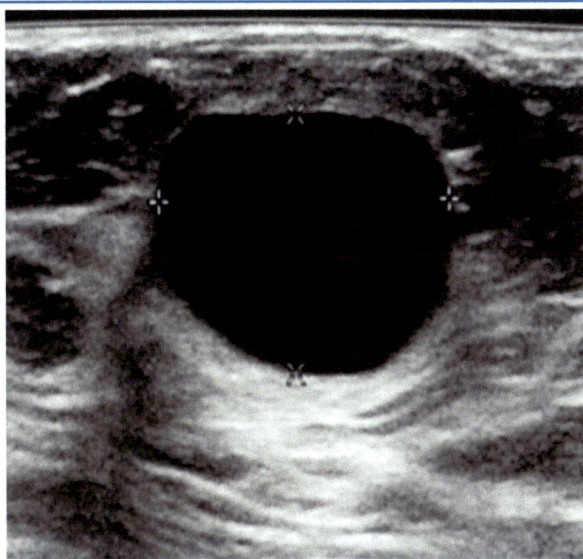

FIGURE 23.13 - SIMPLE BREAST CYST
A simple cyst is defined as anechoic, well-circumscribed, with well-defined borders, and posterior acoustic enhancement

on conventional x-ray, MRI is a highly sensitive tool to detect breast cancer. However, though it is a highly sensitive tool (and more sensitive than mammography, ultrasound, and clinical exam combined), it is not a highly specific tool. Many benign, proliferative and inflammatory processes will show increased vascularity on gadolinium-enhanced MRI. This low specificity combined with the higher cost of MRI limits its use as a screening modality for average-risk women. However, the higher sensitivity outweighs the disadvantages of low specificity for screening high-risk women. Women with a National Cancer Institute (NCI) lifetime risk assessment of 20% or greater, those with a known genetic mutation or a first-degree relative with a genetic mutation known to be associated with breast cancer, and those women who have undergone previous chest irradiation, usually for Hodgkin lymphoma, should be counseled on the benefits of supplemental MRI screening. MRI cannot detect the small calcifications that mammography can identify, and therefore, MRI screening is in addition to, not in place of, mammography. Some malignant lesions seen on MRI cannot be seen with any other imaging tool, even in retrospect. Therefore, any institution providing breast MRI services should have MRI-guided biopsy capability or a relationship with an institution that can provide this service.

MRI is indicated in any woman with a new diagnosis of breast cancer. Its primary strength is near 100% sensitivity in the detection of invasive breast cancer. Therefore, it should be used as a tool to define the extent of disease of a known malignancy and to exclude additional sites of disease in the same or opposite breast

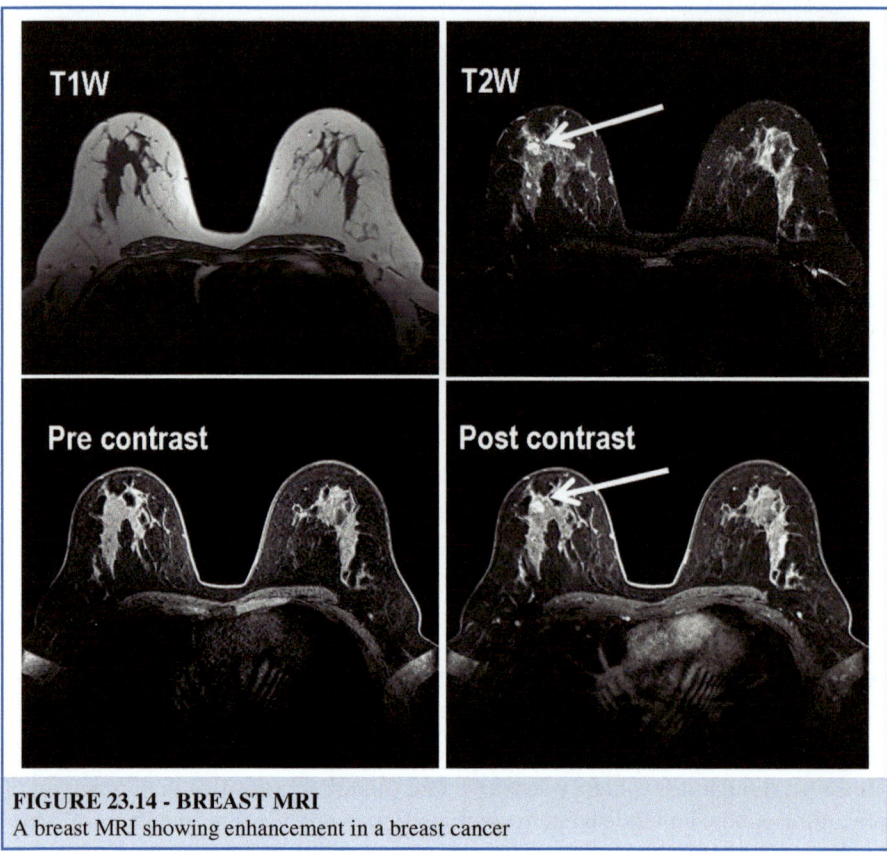

FIGURE 23.14 - BREAST MRI
A breast MRI showing enhancement in a breast cancer

in the preoperative setting. Surgical planning also depends on accurate evaluation of skin, chest wall and locoregional lymph nodes. MRI of the breast is also helpful in assessing tumor response following neoadjuvant chemotherapy, which is initiated prior to surgery to reduce tumor burden and increase the success of breast conservation (Fig. 23.14).

Image-Guided Biopsy

Suspicious findings identified by any imaging modality can be assessed with core needle biopsy under imaging guidance. Mammographic findings such as microcalcifications are best approached with stereotactic mammographic guidance. This method can also be used for the biopsy of mammographically detected masses when there is no ultrasound correlate. Images of the breast are obtained at 15° off center, and this "stereo pair" is used to calculate the x, y, and z coordinates of the location of the abnormality within the breast. After the administration of local anesthesia, a probe is then positioned at these coordinates for sampling. Lesions at the chest wall are difficult to reach with this method and may require other modalities to biopsy.

As mentioned above, ultrasound is often used to evaluate the site of a palpable mass or mammographic abnormality. It is a more comfortable and cost-effective examination for the patient, and lesions in any part of the breast can usually be safely sampled under ultrasound guidance.

BI-RADS®

Table 23.2 shows the BI-RADS® classification used by breast radiologists to communicate findings to other clinicians in a standard and consistent form. BI-RADS stands for Breast Imaging-Reporting and Data System and is a quality assurance tool published by the American College of Radiology. At the end of every mammogram report, one of these numbers is listed.

BI-RADS® is a registered trademark of the American College of Radiology, Reston, VA.

Table 23.2 BI-RADS® classification

Category	Assessment	Explanation
0	Incomplete	Your mammogram or ultrasound did not give the radiologist enough information to make a diagnosis. Follow-up imaging is necessary
1	Negative	There is nothing to comment on; routine screening is recommended
2	Benign finding(s)	A definite benign finding; routine screening is recommended
3	Probably benign findings – initial short-interval follow-up suggested (findings with <2% risk of malignancy)	Findings that have a high probability of being benign (>98%); 6-month short-interval follow-up
4	Suspicious abnormality-biopsy should be considered	Not characteristic of breast cancer, but reasonable probability of being malignant (3–94%); biopsy should be considered
5	Highly suspicious of malignancy-appropriate action should be taken (>95% probability)	Lesion that has a high probability of being malignant (>95%); take appropriate action
6	Known biopsy proven malignancy-appropriate action should be taken	Lesions known to be malignant that are being imaged prior to definitive treatment; assure that treatment is completed

S: The American College of Radiology (ACR) currently recommends annual screening mammography for women at average risk of developing breast cancer starting at age 40. This recommendation factors in the risks and benefits of the relatively low radiation dose associated with the screening test. Recommendations also include ultrasound as the first modality in some instances (e.g., to evaluate palpable abnormalities in younger patients) to avoid unnecessary radiation.

A: The ACR Appropriateness Criteria includes recommendations for imaging for patient symptoms (e.g. nipple discharge and palpable abnormality) and for screen-detected findings using the BI-RADS criteria (Breast Imaging Reporting and Data System).

F: Structured reporting using BI-RADS terminology allows for multiple findings to be accurately categorized and managed concurrently. This allows for potentially malignant findings to not be dismissed in the workup of other findings.

E: BI-RADS allows for screening mammography findings to be categorized using a small number of well-defined terms into clear categories. This allows for a more systematic and efficient workup of breast findings.

References

1. Tabar L, Dean PB, Chen TH, et al. The incidence of fatal breast cancer measures the increased effectiveness of therapy in women participating in mammography screening. Cancer. 2018 (0):1–9.
2. ACR BIRADS Lexicon, American College of Radiology, Reston, VA.
3. Pisano ED, Gatsonis C, Hendrick E, et al. Diagnostic performance of digital versus film mammography for breast-cancer screening – the results of the American College of Radiology Imaging Network (ACRIN) Digital Mammographic Imaging Screening Trial (DMIST). N Engl J Med. 2005;353(17):1773–83. [Published correction appears in N Engl J Med. 2006;355(17):1840.]
4. Ciatto S, Houssami N, Bernardi D, et al. Integration of 3D digital mammography with tomosynthesis for population breast-cancer screening (STORM): a prospective comparison study. Lancet Oncol. 2013;14(7):583–589.
5. Skaane P, Bandos AI, Eben EB, et al. Two-view digital breast tomosynthesis screening with synthetically reconstructed projection images: comparison with digital breast tomosynthesis with full-field digital mammographic images. Radiology. 2014;271(3):655–663.
6. McCormack VA, dos Santos SI. Breast density and parenchymal patterns as markers of breast cancer risk: a meta-analysis. Cancer Epidemiol Biomarkers Prev. 2006;15(6):1159–69.
7. Maniero MB, Lourenco A, Mahoney MC, et al. ACR appropriateness criteria breast cancer screening. J Am Coll Radiol. 2013;10(1):11–4.
8. Wall BF, Hart D. Revised radiation doses for typical x-ray examinations. Brit J Radiol. 1997;70:437–39.
9. Berg WA, Blume JD, Cormack JB, et al. Combined screening with ultrasound and mammography vs mammography alone in women at elevated risk of breast cancer. JAMA. 2008;299(18):2151–63.

PART IV
GENITOURINARY AND ABDOMINAL IMAGING

24 GENITOURINARY ULTRASOUND

Objectives:
1. Understand how ultrasound can be used to evaluate the kidney.
2. Name several causes of abnormal uterine bleeding and appreciate their ultrasound characteristics.
3. Name several masses seen in the ovary and appreciate their ultrasound characteristics.
4. List imaging modalities and applications in the evaluation of fertility and pregnancy.
5. List common causes of scrotal pain.
6. Understand the imaging modalities required to fully evaluate a patient with a malignant testicular mass.

Ultrasound plays the primary role for much of genitourinary imaging with fluoroscopy studies, CT, MRI, and nuclear medicine studies performed to assist in the subsequent evaluation. Ultrasound does not produce ionizing radiation, and examinations rarely require sedation, making it a desirable modality for evaluation of the kidneys, bladder, female pelvic organs, and scrotum in patients of all ages.

Kidneys

Evaluation of the kidneys is frequently performed with ultrasound in patients of all ages. Ultrasound can be used to screen for or monitor the progression of renal disease as the appearance of renal parenchyma becomes brighter, or more echogenic, than a healthy kidney in the setting of chronic renal dysfunction. Common causes of

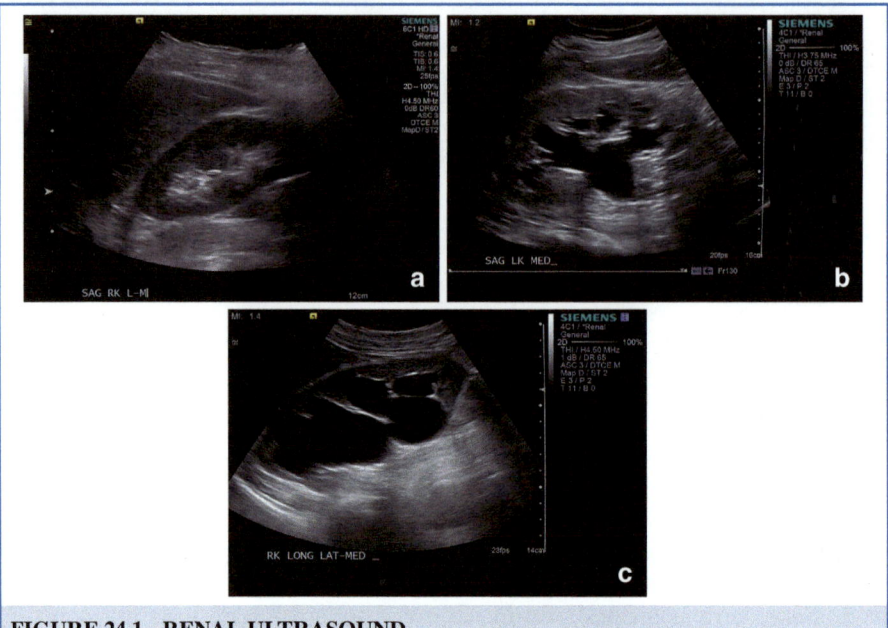

FIGURE 24.1 - RENAL ULTRASOUND
Examples of (**a**) a normal kidney without hydronephrosis, (**b**) a kidney with moderate or grade 2 hydronephrosis, and (**c**) a kidney with severe, grade 4 hydronephrosis

chronic renal disease are diabetes and hypertension. Ultrasound is also used to screen for distention of the renal pelvis with urine, known as hydronephrosis. Hydronephrosis is classified as mild (grade 1) through severe (grade 4) (Fig. 24.1). There are many potential causes of hydronephrosis (vesicoureteral reflux, obstructing ureteral calculi, ureteral stricture, compression from a retroperitoneal mass, etc.), and further imaging with fluoroscopy, nuclear medicine exams, CT, or MRI is required to identify the cause. Similarly, the identification of any renal mass on ultrasound requires further workup with dedicated contrast-enhanced CT or MRI examination to rule out malignancy.

Bladder

Ultrasound of the urinary bladder is frequently used as a point of care tool by nursing staff to evaluate for urinary retention after voiding. In patients suspected of bladder outlet obstruction, diagnostic ultrasound can be utilized to evaluate for causes including prostatic hypertrophy and bladder calculi and to assess for chronicity of obstruction. Findings of chronic bladder outlet obstruction include bladder wall thickening and bladder wall diverticula.

Evaluation of the Uterus and Uterine Bleeding

Abnormal uterine bleeding is bleeding unrelated to normal menstruation and can occur in women of any age. Organic causes of abnormal uterine bleeding include problems related to pregnancy, medication, benign and malignant masses, and systemic disease. Dysfunctional uterine bleeding (DUB) is defined as abnormal bleeding that does not have an organic cause and is commonly related to anovulation and abnormal function of the hypothalamic-pituitary-ovarian axis. Common dysfunctional uterine bleeding terms include menorrhagia (prolonged bleeding), metromenorrhagia (irregular bleeding), and spotting (intermenstrual bleeding).

Ultrasound is commonly used to begin the evaluation of abnormal uterine bleeding. Ultrasound may identify structural causes for abnormal bleeding such as fibroids and polyps that extend into the endometrial cavity. Ultrasound can assess the thickness and contour of the endometrial lining and determine if the bleeding may be the result of a thin atrophic endometrium or a thick endometrium, which may reflect hypertrophy or cancer. Ultrasound may identify structural changes in the endometrium from drugs such as tamoxifen. Pelvic ultrasound can contribute to the evaluation of amenorrhea such as seen with the polycystic ovarian syndrome and pregnancy (Fig. 24.2).

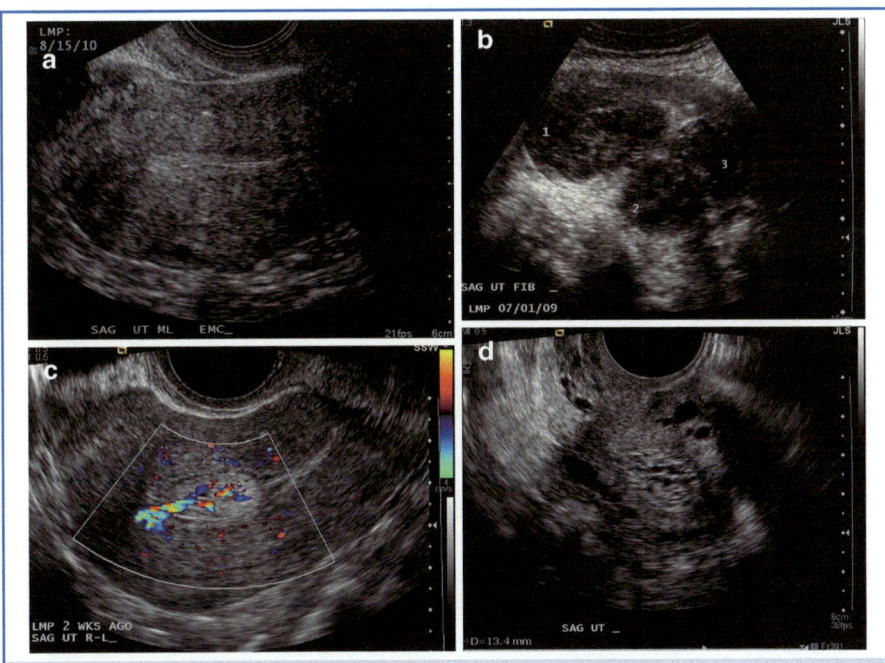

FIGURE 24.2 - TRANSVAGINAL ULTRASOUND
Examples of (**a**) normal endometrium, with bright walls and central cavity delineated by a white line, (**b**) multiple hypoechoic fibroids, (**c**) echogenic polyp with central vascular stalk, and (**d**) cystic changes of endometrium from tamoxifen

Transabdominal ultrasound is commonly performed first to evaluate the pelvis as it provides an "overview" of pelvic structures. The urine-filled urinary bladder is used as an acoustic window to best evaluate pelvic structures. Transvaginal ultrasound is performed with an ultrasound probe that is cleaned and covered with a sterile probe cover and inserted into the vagina. The transvaginal approach provides more detail of the uterus, the endometrium, and the ovaries. Transvaginal pelvic ultrasound evaluation is similar to a speculum pelvic examination, and the patient does not have the discomfort of maintaining a full bladder.

Additional imaging may be prompted by ultrasound findings. MRI may be performed to further evaluate the myometrium and endometrial-myometrial junction. MRI can be used to evaluate for adenomyosis, a process where endometrium is deposited into the endometrial-myometrial junction and myometrium. CT may follow an ultrasound if a pelvic mass is identified and there is a concern for more extensive disease; however, this does involve radiation. Diagnostic imaging does not always explain the cause of abnormal uterine bleeding but may direct the indication and location for biopsy, hysteroscopy, surgery, or follow-up.

Evaluation of the Ovaries

Imaging commonly is an adjunct to physical examination of the adnexa. It may be difficult to tell if a "full" adnexa is merely stool-filled bowel or pathology in the ovaries or in surrounding structures. Ultrasound commonly begins the evaluation. While there are some "classic" ultrasound findings of ovarian structures such as normal functional follicles, hemorrhagic cysts, and endometriomas, many ovarian masses have nonspecific findings (Fig. 24.3).

A complex cystic mass in the adnexa is particularly hard to manage because the differential diagnosis is extensive and includes benign and malignant cystic neoplasm; atypical cyst; endometrioma; dermoid, torsed ovary; abscess, hydro- and pyosalpinx; as well as nongynecologic masses such as mesenteric cysts and nongynecologic processes (Fig. 24.4).

Clinical evaluation is essential to determine if the process needs immediate intervention such as antibiotics or surgery. If a patient is not acutely ill, follow-up ultrasound in two to three menstrual cycles is commonly recommended and performed. If follow-up ultrasound remains concerning, MRI may further characterize the ovarian mass but the patient and her physician may elect to go to laparoscopy for visual and pathologic diagnosis. CT may be performed to determine the extent of disease such as the presence of ascites or peritoneal metastases.

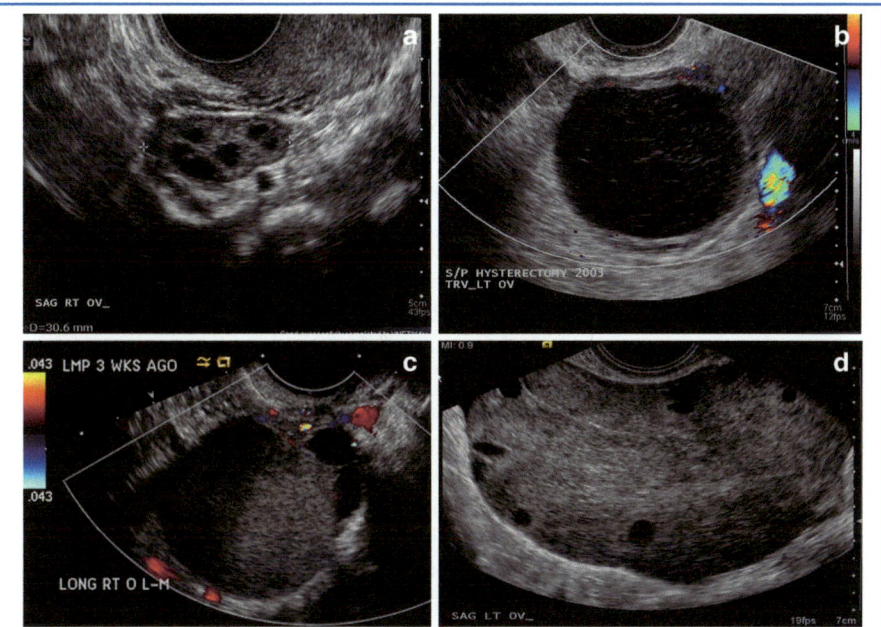

FIGURE 24.3 - TRANSVAGINAL ULTRASOUND
Examples of (**a**) normal ovary, (**b**) hemorrhagic cyst with reticulated mesh-like echoes, (**c**) endometrioma with homogeneous echoes, and (**d**) enlarged torsed ovary with peripheral follicles

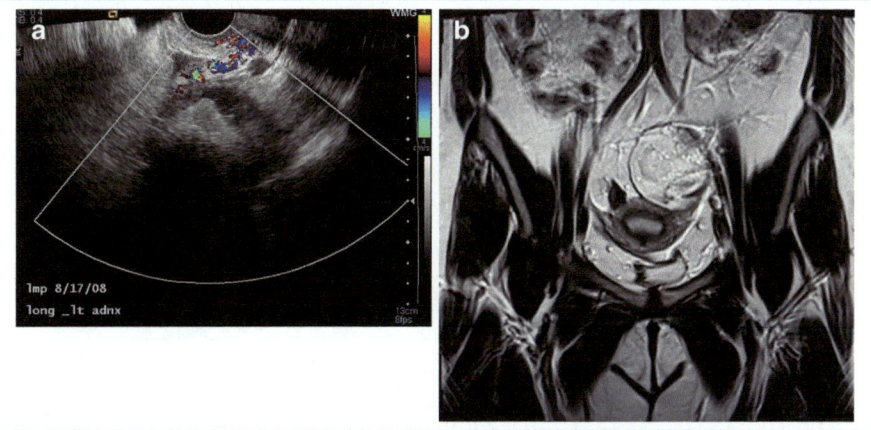

FIGURE 24.4 - OVARIAN DERMOID
"Tip of the iceberg" configuration of an ovarian dermoid (cystic teratoma) is noted on ultrasound: (**a**) the multiple types of tissue that make up a dermoid such as hair, blood, fat, cartilage, and calcifications create an acoustic shadow, which blocks all sound waves, and the mass is essentially obscured. (**b**) The corresponding MRI shows the extent and complex nature of the mass. Fat identified in an ovarian mass on CT or MRI is classic for dermoid

Pregnancy

Evaluation of pregnancy may begin with infertility. Fallopian tube patency can be assessed with hysterosalpingography in which contrast is instilled into the uterine cavity under fluoroscopy. If the fallopian tubes are patent, contrast will spill out of the tubes into the peritoneal cavity. Hysterosalpingography, ultrasound, and MRI can assess the contour of the cavity itself and look for problems that might affect pregnancy such as large fibroids, congenital anomalies, and scarring of the cavity. Fallopian tube blockage and its possible treatment are reviewed in the Genitourinary Interventions chapter. The male partner may be evaluated for problems that may affect fertility such as varicoceles and testicular pathology with a scrotal ultrasound.

Ultrasound is used to assess for the presence of intrauterine pregnancy initially and then for appropriate fetal growth and well-being. Ultrasound is commonly used to assess for ectopic pregnancy when the patient has a positive pregnancy test and may have vaginal bleeding and/or pain. It is important to interpret the ultrasound results in conjunction with the patient's quantitative serum B-HCG levels. That is, sometimes the ultrasound is performed so early that an intrauterine pregnancy cannot be identified and the differential includes very early intrauterine pregnancy, ectopic pregnancy, and early pregnancy loss. Ultrasound is used in the evaluation of retained products of conception and gestational trophoblastic disease (Fig. 24.5).

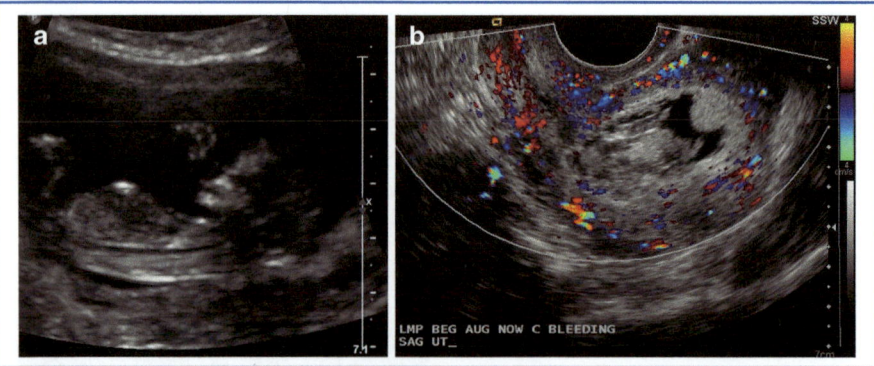

FIGURE 24.5 - EXAMPLES OF (a) INTRAUTERINE FETUS AND (b) IRREGULAR HETEROGENEOUS TISSUE WITH DEGENERATION OF GESTATIONAL TROPHOBLASTIC DISEASE (MOLAR PREGNANCY)

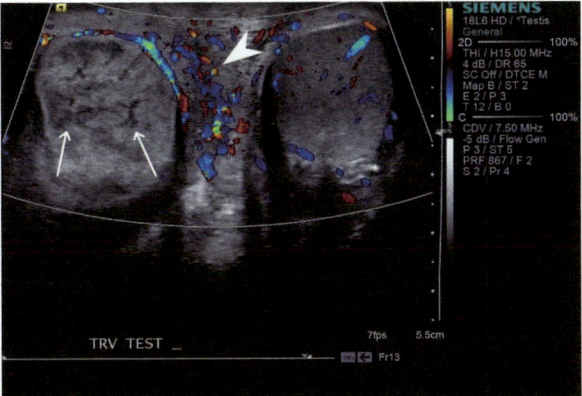

FIGURE 24.6 - TESTICULAR TORSION
Transverse color Doppler ultrasound of the testicles with normal flow seen within the left testi-cle and absent flow in the right testicle due to torsion. Note areas of hypoechoic tissue (*thin white arrows*) within the right testicle indicative of necrosis and increased peripheral vascularity (*white arrowhead*), consistent with reactive hyperemia

Evaluation of the Painful Scrotum

The imaging modality of choice for the evaluation of a patient with a painful scrotum is ultrasound due to its high diagnostic specificity and lack of radiation to gametes. Infection is semi-acute in presentation and can be seen on ultrasound in the epididymis (epididymitis), throughout the epididymis and testicle (epididymo-orchitis), as an abscess within the testicle itself (testicular abscess), or as a collection in the fluid about the testicle (scrotal pyocele). An emergent cause of acute scrotal pain is testicular torsion. This is identified on ultrasound as a decrease or cessation of blood flow in the affected testicle as compared with the unaffected testicle (Fig. 24.6).

Testicular torsion is a surgical emergency, requiring prompt intervention for salvage of the testicle. The most common cause of scrotal pain is from the presence of varicoceles, which are dilated blood vessels in the scrotal sac due to incompetent valves in the gonadal veins. Varicoceles are present in approximately 15% of males and can be a chronic source of pain and an etiology for infertility that can be treated with gonadal vein embolization as described further in the chapter on Genitourinary Interventions (Fig. 24.7).

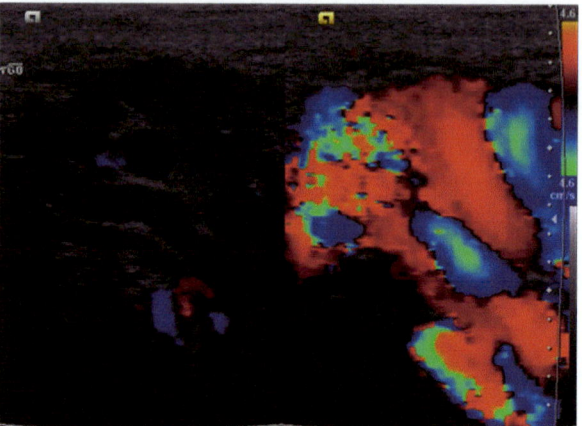

FIGURE 24.7 - VARICOCELE
Ultrasound of the scrotum demonstrating dilated veins (left image) that increases in size and vascularity with Valsalva maneuver (right image), consistent with varicocele

Evaluation of a Painless Testicular Mass

The normal testicle is a 3–5 cm oblong organ which is uniformly homogeneous in echotexture on ultrasound. A discrete mass within the testicle seen on ultrasound is concerning for malignancy. The most common testicular cancer is seminoma (almost 50% of testicular tumors); however, there are many nonseminomatous germ cell tumors as well, such as yolk sac tumor, embryonal cell carcinoma, teratoma, and mixed germ cell tumor to name a few. It is uncommon, however not impossible, to see metastatic disease within the testicles as the testicle is considered a sanctuary site with a tight blood-organ barrier. This makes the transfer of metastatic disease into the testicle unlikely; however, by the same token, it is relatively difficult for chemotherapeutic agents to penetrate the testicle for this same reason. Therefore, diagnosis of testicular cancer on imaging almost always requires orchiectomy and a careful search within the chest, abdomen, and pelvis with CT or MRI for a metastatic disease which would require systemic chemotherapy (Fig. 24.8).

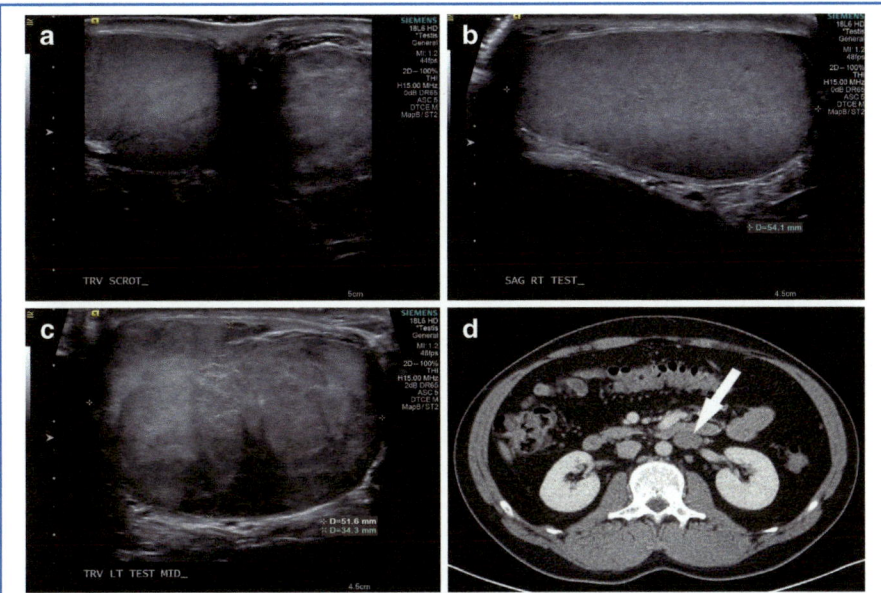

FIGURE 24.8 - TESTICULAR MASS
Transverse ultrasound of the testicles (**a**) with normal appearance of the right testicle and heterogeneous appearance of the left testicle. Longitudinal ultrasound of the right testicle (**b**) with normal homogeneous echotexture compared with the left testicle (**c**) which has been replaced by the tumor which appears as markedly abnormal and heterogeneous echotexture. Axial CT image (**d**) at the level of the kidneys shows metastatic left para-aortic lymphadenopathy (*arrow*)

S: Genitourinary ultrasound is unique in that definitive diagnoses can often be made on ultrasound imaging alone, a modality which is relatively inexpensive, portable, and spares the patient exposure to radiation.

A: Based on the patient's symptoms and physical exam, if a genitourinary pathology is suspected, ultrasound is the appropriate first study in most instances, with MRI the second most appropriate. If ultrasound and MRI do not offer a diagnosis, then consideration can be given to radiation-based modalities such as CT scanning.

F: Ultrasound is the imaging modality most dependent on the ultrasonographer or technologist. Much of the information garnered from an ultrasound exam is "real time" and therefore very dependent on the experience of those obtaining the images.

E: As ultrasound is a real-time modality, decisions about additional imaging and/or treatment can be made during the exam, expediting patient care.

25

ABDOMINAL CALCIFICATIONS

Objectives:
1. Describe the patterns of calcification and their location on radiographs for the following: chronic pancreatitis, vascular structures, uterine fibroids, appendicolith, and renal calculi.
2. State what percentage of renal calculi are normally visible on the plain radiograph.

Chronic Pancreatitis

Calcifications within the pancreas of a patient with chronic pancreatitis (Fig. 25.1) are often multiple, of variable size and shape, and located in the mid-upper abdomen and left upper quadrant at the expected anatomic location of the pancreas.

Vascular Calcifications

Vascular calcifications take on several forms. The most common lower pelvic calcifications are phleboliths (Fig. 25.2), which often appear as numerous, small, round, smoothly marginated calcifications representing calcified thrombi within pelvic veins. They often contain a central lucency that relates to recanalization of the occluded veins.

Vascular structures will often demonstrate peripheral and rim calcifications. Sometimes the calcification is extensive enough to outline the entire vessel or an aneurysm, as can often be seen in the aorta (Fig. 25.3). Pathologic calcifications on

© Springer Nature Switzerland AG 2020
J. Kissane et al. (eds.), *Radiology Fundamentals: Introduction to Imaging & Technology*, https://doi.org/10.1007/978-3-030-22173-7_25

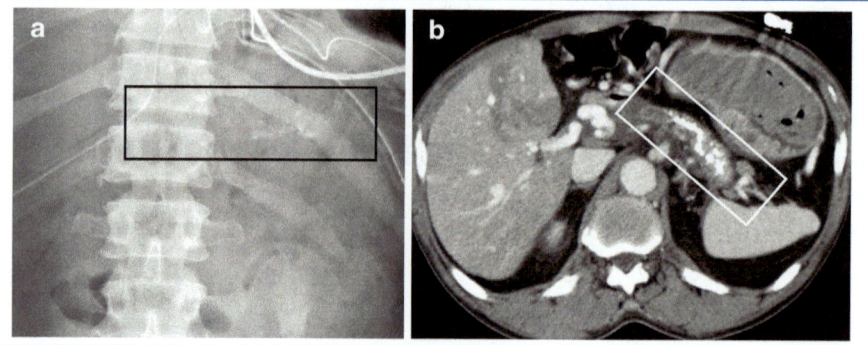

FIGURE 25.1 - CHRONIC PANCREATITIS
Supine radiograph collimated to the pancreatic bed (**a**) and corresponding axial image of contrast-enhanced CT (**b**) show multiple variably sized and shaped pancreatic calcifications (***boxes***)

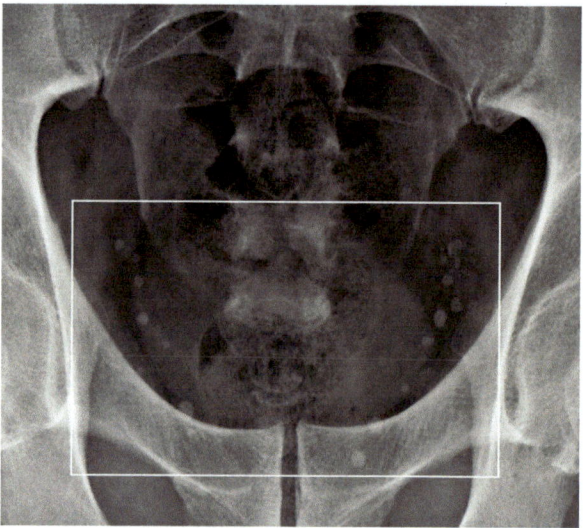

FIGURE 25.2 - PELVIC PHLEBOLITHS
Multiple bilateral rounded calcifications, many with central lucency, located in the lower pelvis with the majority at and below the level of the ischial spine (white arrow)

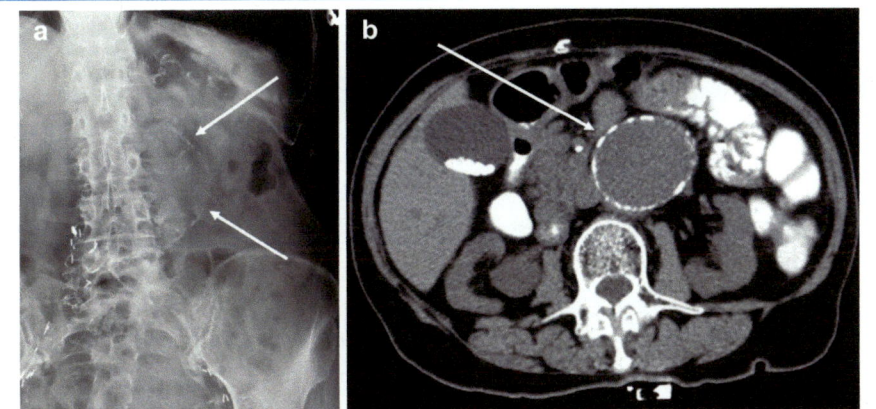

FIGURE 25.3 - AORTIC CALCIFICATION
Supine abdominal radiograph (**a**) and corresponding axial image of a noncontrast CT (**b**) show a rim calcified abdominal aortic aneurysm (***arrows***)

abdominal radiographs should prompt additional evaluation, as an enlarged calcified abdominal aortic aneurysm should be further assessed with alternative imaging modalities such as ultrasound or CT.

Uterine Fibroids

Various tumors, both benign and malignant, may calcify according to different calcification patterns. Popcorn-like calcifications in the pelvis are dystrophic calcifications in uterine fibroids (Fig. 25.4), the most common benign tumor found in the female pelvis.

Appendicolith

An appendicolith is a calcified round or oval stone within the appendix (Fig. 25.5), most commonly found within the right lower quadrant where the appendix is usually located. A calcification is seen in the right lower quadrant of this radiograph (a) of a patient presenting with right lower quadrant pain. When this finding is seen in

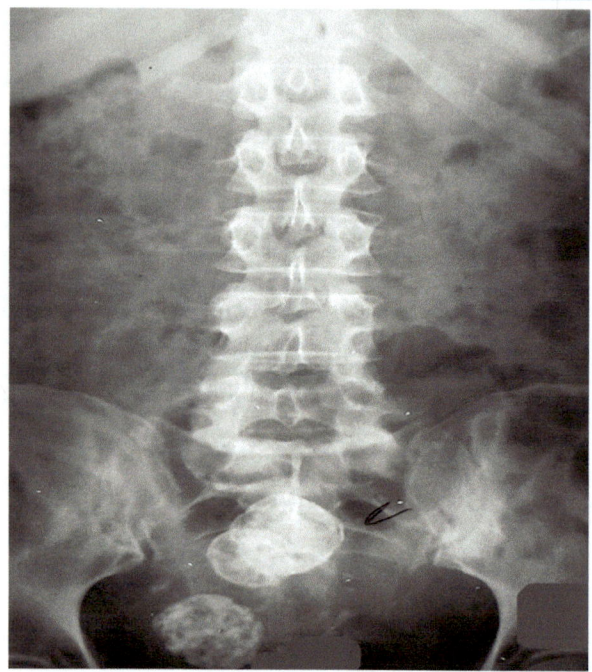

FIGURE 25.4 - CALCIFIED UTERINE FIBROIDS

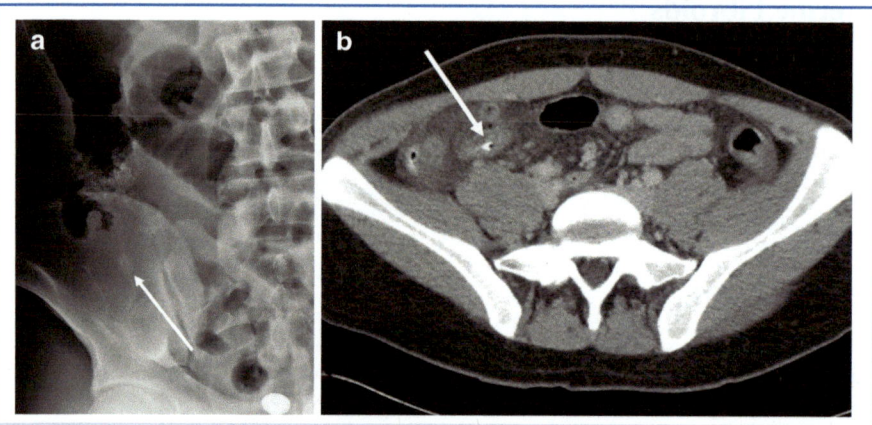

FIGURE 25.5 - APPENDICOLITH
Calcified appendicolith (*arrows*) on AP abdominal radiograph and axial image of a noncontrast CT

association with acute right lower quadrant pain, appendicitis should be strongly considered. The diagnosis and any associated complications including perforation and abscess formation can be confirmed with CT (b) in adults and MRI or US in children.

Urinary Tract Calculi

Approximately, 90% of renal calculi are radiopaque and can be visualized on a radiograph. Urinary tract calculi take on many shapes and can be located anywhere within the collecting system, projecting over the renal outlines and along the expected course of the ureters (Fig. 25.6).

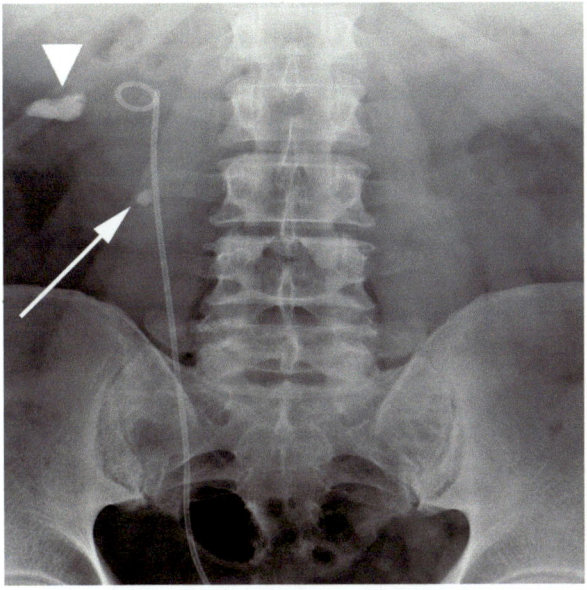

FIGURE 25.6 - URINARY TRACT CALCULI
Large oblong calcified stone in the right kidney (***arrowhead***) and rounded calcified stone within the proximal right ureter (***arrow***) at the level of the third lumbar vertebral body. The right ureteral stent identifies the course of the right ureter

CT is often the first study performed to localize and quantify calcifications in the urinary tract. Calcium-containing stones such as calcium oxalate and calcium phosphate stones are radiopaque and are usually seen on plain radiographs when large or dense enough. Radiolucent stones such as uric acid, indinavir, and pure matrix stones are radiolucent and are not usually visualized on plain radiographs or on CT.

S: In patients who require follow-up imaging with CT to reassess a previously documented urinary tract calculus, low-dose renal stone protocol should be utilized to decrease radiation dose to the patient.

A: Patients with known urinary tract calculi who present with recurrent symptoms may be imaged with an abdominal radiograph if the previously identified calculus was evident on a radiograph or visualized on the CT scout topogram.

F: Differentiation of a phlebolith from a distal ureteral calculus can be made based on the shape and location of the calculus most of the time. Phleboliths have a central umbilicated lucency and are often located at or below the level of the ischial spine.

E: The patient care team is interested in the size of the calculus and its location. Calculi >5 mm are less likely to spontaneously pass. Every effort should be made to accurately measure and report the size of an obstructing calculi.

26 ABDOMINAL HARDWARE AND TUBES

Objectives:
1. Become familiar with common abdominal hardware and tubes.
2. State the desired location of nasogastric and enteric feeding tubes.

Surgical Clips

Different types of clips are used in a variety of procedures performed in abdomino-pelvic surgery. The most common that are encountered radiographically are chole-cystectomy clips. These are readily identified by their appearance and location in the right upper quadrant as seen in Fig. 26.1. Bowel surgery that results in resection and anastomosis will often involve a metal stapler that will leave a chain of small staples similar to those in Fig. 26.1. These staples can be helpful in both fluoroscopy and CT when trying to identify points of obstruction or leakage, though some anastomoses are hand sewn and therefore not readily apparent radiographically. Tubal ligation is a contraceptive procedure which occludes the fallopian tubes and can involve the use of clips located bilaterally within the pelvis.

Gastrointestinal Tubes

It is necessary to become familiar with the appearances and desired positioning of gastrointestinal tubes. Nasogastric, orogastric, and enteric feeding tubes enter the abdomen via the esophagus. Typically, the nasogastric (NG) or orogastric (OG) tube

© Springer Nature Switzerland AG 2020   173
J. Kissane et al. (eds.), *Radiology Fundamentals: Introduction to Imaging & Technology*, https://doi.org/10.1007/978-3-030-22173-7_26

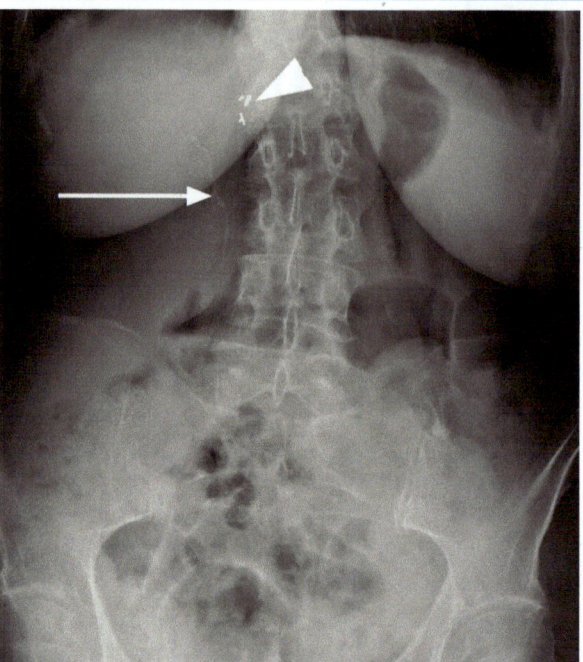

FIGURE 26.1 - TYPICAL POSTSURGICAL CLIPS
Radiograph of the abdomen showing metallic cholecystectomy clips (***arrowhead***) and a bowel resection staple line (***arrow***)

will demonstrate a tip well within the stomach because most tubes have side holes that extend several centimeters back from the tip. In order to effectively decompress the stomach, the side holes should also be located below the diaphragm and not in the esophagus. Enteric feeding tubes are radiographically dense on both sides of the tube (unlike the NG tube) and often have a dense weighted tip. In some clinical settings, it is desirable to have a nasojejunal (NJ) tube with the tip of the feeding tube beyond the ligament of Treitz. Termination past the ampulla of Vater helps to prevent stimulation of biliary and pancreatic secretions. Therefore, the feeding tube should outline the expected course of the duodenum similar to Fig. 26.2. Gastrostomy tubes are another common type of GI tube that are encountered during abdominal imaging. These tubes will have a balloon or flange which maintains their positioning in the gastric lumen.

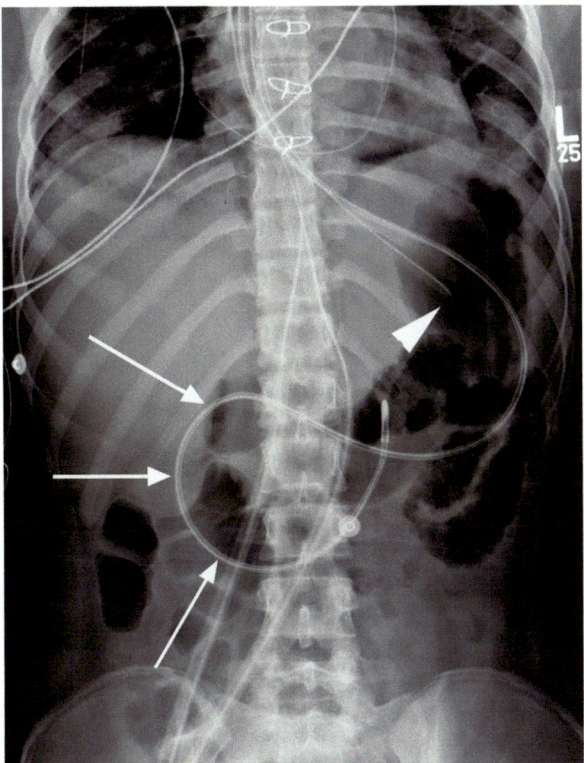

FIGURE 26.2 - UPPER GI TUBES
Radiograph of the abdomen and pelvis demonstrating a weighted-tip NJ tube following the typical course duodenal C loop (***arrows***). The tip of an NG tube is seen near the air bubble of the gastric fundus (***arrowhead***). Additional lines, tubes, and sternotomy clips are seen in the lower chest

Genitourinary Tubes and Hardware

Abdominal radiographs can be used to help verify the location of urinary stents and catheters. Ureteral stents follow the expected course of the ureter from the renal fossa to the bladder and have a loop at each end to help hold them in place as illustrated in Fig. 26.3. Prior to placing a ureteral stent, patients may have a nephrostomy tube placed to decompress an acutely obstructed kidney and afford access for

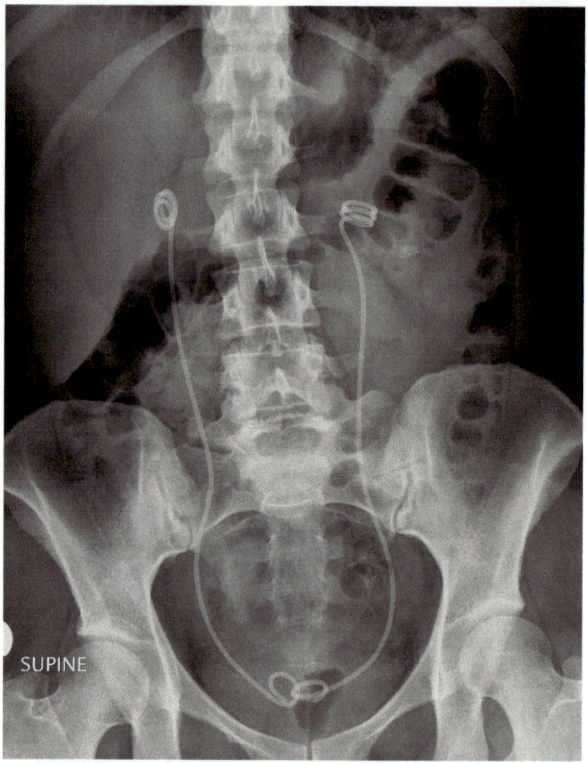

SUPINE

FIGURE 26.3 - URETERAL STENTS
Supine abdominal radiograph showing bilateral internal double-J ureteral stents with ends appropriately positioned in the renal pelvis and bladder

impending stent placement. The nephrostomy tube will have a single looped end located in the renal pelvis and then course externally, where it is connected to a drainage bag. For reference, see Fig. 43.3.

There are additional hardware devices which are utilized for contraception besides tubal ligation clips (Fig. 26.4). An intrauterine device (IUD) is normally seated in the uterine cavity in a characteristic T-shape with the short arms directed toward the cornua of the uterus. The Essure® device comprises two separate flexible inserts that are placed within the lumen of the fallopian tubes to prevent pregnancy (Fig. 26.5). It is imperative to confirm the structural integrity and appropriate positioning of these devices.

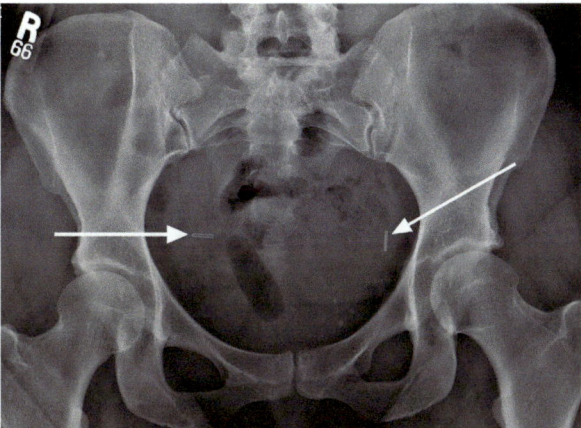

FIGURE 26.4 - TUBAL LIGATION CLIPS
AP view of the pelvis showing metallic bilateral tubal ligation clips (*arrows*) which close the fallopian tubes

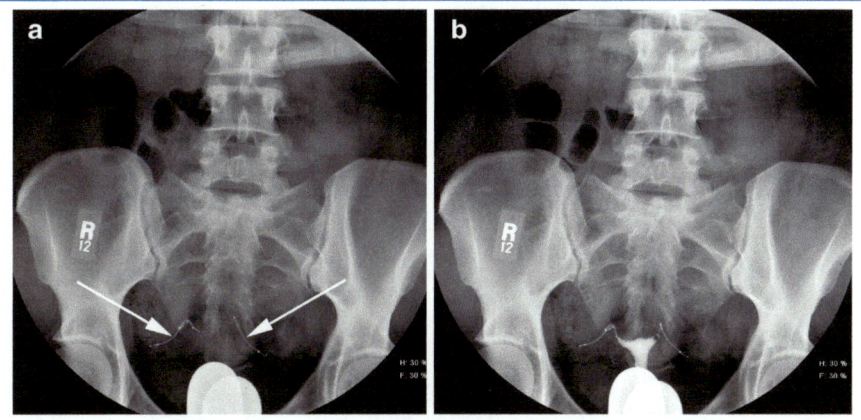

FIGURE 26.5 - ESSURE DEVICE
(**a**) Radiograph prior to hysterosalpingogram showing radiopaque inserts (*arrows*) in both fallopian tubes. Note the vaginal speculum in place along the inferior margin of the image. (**b**) Injection of dye through the cervical os demonstrating the uterine cavity and absence of contrast flow into the peritoneal space, confirming the occlusion of the fallopian tubes. Note a small air bubble in the left cornua

Vascular Hardware

Management of common vascular diseases often includes the use of hardware devices. Abdominal aortic aneurysms can be treated with endovascular stent grafts as seen in Fig. 26.6. Also seen in Fig. 26.6 is an inferior vena cava (IVC) filter, which can be evaluated with radiography for integrity and appropriate position. Arterial embolization sometimes involves the use of metallic coils which are placed endovascularly to impede blood flow and can be readily seen on radiographs. Femoral arterial and venous catheters are placed much less frequently than subclavian or jugular catheters; however they may be encountered on routine abdominal radiographs. In the neonatal population, vascular catheters are frequently seen on abdominal imaging.

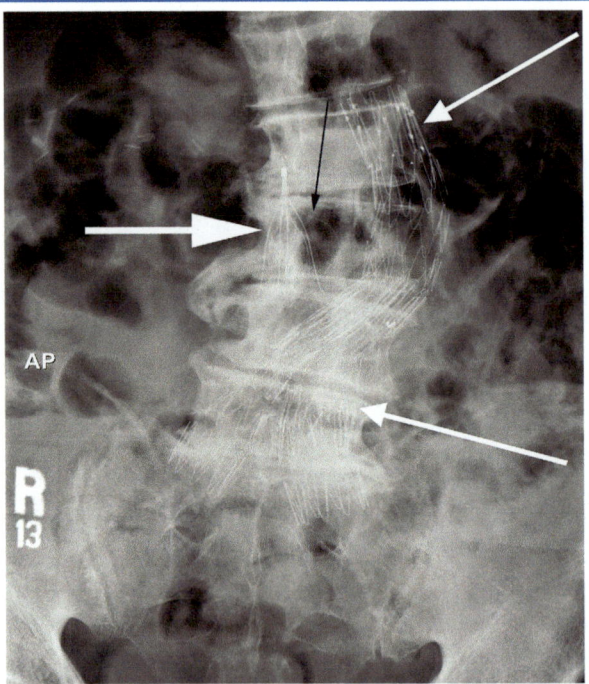

FIGURE 26.6 - TYPICAL VASCULAR HARDWARE
Collimated AP radiograph of an aortoiliac endovascular stent (***thin white arrows***) and an IVC filter (***thick white arrow***). Note that the medial leg of the filter is inappropriately displaced toward midline (***black arrow***)

Miscellaneous Hardware

Numerous other intra-abdominal devices are used and encountered during radiologic examination. Ventricular-peritoneal drainage catheters are designed to alleviate elevated intracranial pressure by draining cerebrospinal fluid (CSF) from the ventricles into the peritoneal space. A "shunt series" includes frontal and lateral radiographs of the skull, a chest x-ray, and an abdominal x-ray so that the entire course of the catheter can be scrutinized. In the abdomen, the catheter will typically coil randomly with the tip shifting its location over time. Surgical drainage catheters can be located anywhere in or around the abdomen and commonly have multiple side holes toward the tip. Multipurpose drainage catheters can be seen in various locations and demonstrate a loop at the end, several side holes, and a radiopaque ring several centimeters from the tip, marking the last side hole. To aid in the assessment of tube patency and position, drains can be assessed fluoroscopically via the injection of water-soluble contrast. Other hardware that may be present includes pancreaticobiliary stents, cyst-gastrostomy tubes or stents, and esophageal stents. Stents may appear as curvilinear radiopaque structures or mesh-like metallic devices.

S: Radiography and fluoroscopy can rapidly and safely aid in the placement and monitoring of abdominal hardware, lines, and tubes while exposing patients to low amounts of ionizing radiation.

A: Radiographs are indicated in the assessment of abdominal hardware and tubes to ensure appropriate positioning and offer a relatively cheap, low risk, and portable means for doing so.

F: An understanding of the anatomy and radiographic appearance of hardware is essential to the safe placement of lines and tubes within the abdomen. For example, successful post-pyloric positioning of nasojejunal feeding tubes can be verified via portable abdominal radiography.

E: It is critical to recognize malpositioned abdominal tubes and devices to avoid patient care delays and adverse outcomes. Incorrectly positioned devices should be reported to the ordering teams without delay, typically via direct or telephone communication.

Suggested Reading

Hunter TB, Taljanovic MS. Medical devices of the abdomen and pelvis. Radiographics. 2005;25(2):503–23.

ABNORMAL AIR COLLECTIONS IN THE ABDOMEN

Objectives:
1. State the difference between an "interface" and a "line."
2. State the expected radiographic findings in pneumoperitoneum in both a supine and upright patient.
3. Discuss the significance of intramural air within the bowel wall.

Pneumoperitoneum

When an air-containing hollow viscus ruptures, air and bowel contents are released into the abdominal cavity, most often into the peritoneal cavity. "Free air," also known as pneumoperitoneum, will collect in the least dependent or highest portion of the peritoneal cavity. Pneumoperitoneum has a broad range of etiologies from benign causes to life-threatening emergencies. Often the investigation of pneumoperitoneum begins with abdominal radiographs. If free air is a concern, CT is performed to confirm and further delineate the extent of free air and determine the source.

In an upright patient, the air outside of the hollow viscus will collect just beneath the diaphragm (Fig. 27.1). In cases where a small amount of air is suspected, an upright chest radiograph, in addition to abdominal radiographs, may also be useful in detecting a pneumoperitoneum. When the patient is not mobile and/or there is a concern for a subtle or loculated collection of air outside of the bowel lumen, CT is recommended.

In cases of pneumoperitoneum, the right hemidiaphragm is abnormally visible as a thin white line. This is a result of an abnormal collection of air under the diaphragm, outlining the diaphragm along with the air superiorly in the lung. Normally,

J. Kissane et al. (eds.), *Radiology Fundamentals: Introduction to Imaging & Technology*, https://doi.org/10.1007/978-3-030-22173-7_27

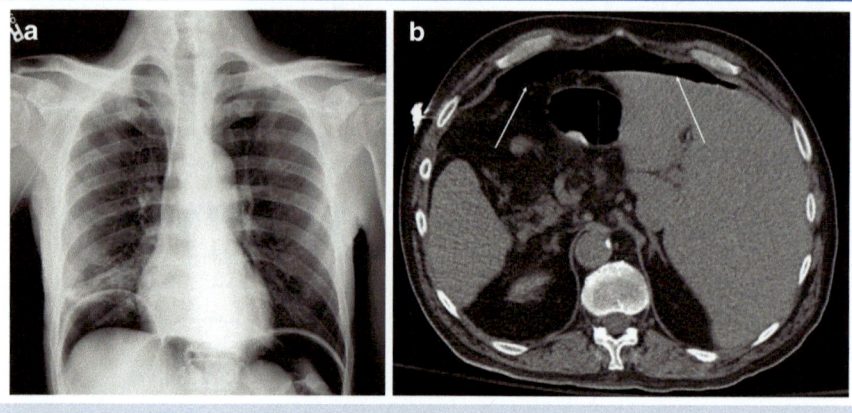

FIGURE 27.1 - PNEUMOPERITONEUM
(a) Note the intraperitoneal free air underneath the diaphragm on the PA chest radiograph. (b) Intraperitoneal free air (*arrows*) in a nondependent position following rupture of a hollow viscus

the diaphragm is not visible as it blends imperceptibly with the adjacent liver, representing an interface (remember the silhouette sign). The change from interface to line is often a useful finding in discerning the presence of abnormal air collections within the abdomen.

Similarly, a change of appearance of the bowel wall from interface to line can also be a helpful finding. Normally, air within the bowel lumen only allows visualization of the inner wall as the outer surface of the bowel wall normally forms an interface with nearby soft tissue structures. When there is free air within the peritoneal cavity, the outer wall of a bowel loop becomes visible as a white line, known as Rigler's sign. Occasionally, intraperitoneal free air can be identified outlining the falciform ligament, known as the falciform ligament sign. Remember patient positioning counts! In the supine patient position, air collects centrally within the abdomen since this, not the subdiaphragmatic region, is the highest point. For this reason, the radiographic presentation of pneumoperitoneum is different in the supine patient versus in the upright patient.

Pneumatosis Intestinalis

Air can also be located within the wall of the bowel itself (Fig. 27.2) as in this case depicting air within the wall of the cecum and ascending colon. This condition is referred to as pneumatosis intestinalis and can be seen in a variety of conditions from benign and idiopathic causes to life-threatening emergency situations such as bowel ischemia. Pneumatosis in infants may reflect the infection necrotizing enterocolitis with complication of bowel wall ischemia.

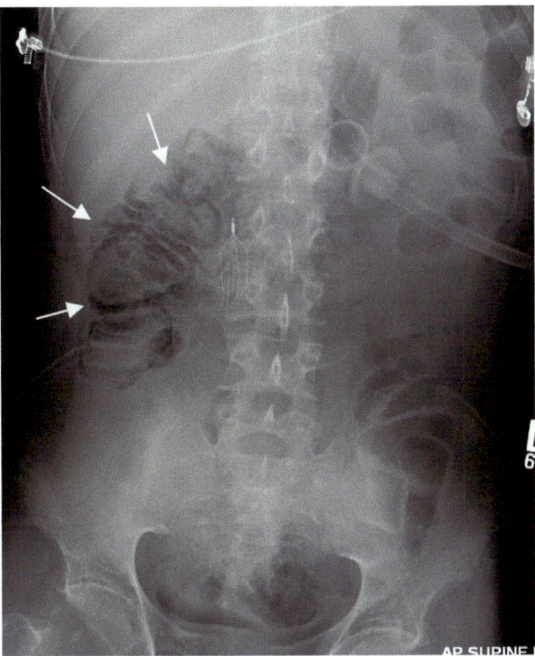

FIGURE 27.2 - PNEUMATOSIS INTESTINALIS

Portal Venous Gas

Portal venous gas is the result of dying or dead bowel and portends imminent patient demise the majority of the time. As the bowel necrosis, gas is absorbed into the draining portal venous system which is comprised of the superior mesenteric, inferior mesenteric, and left gastric veins. From these venous tributaries, the gas is delivered to the liver via the main, left, and right portal veins. When this occurs, air is characteristically seen in the periphery of the liver as portal venous blood flow is hepatopetal (Fig. 27.3). Portal venous air must be differentiated from pneumobilia which is air within the biliary system. Since bile flows out of the liver in the hepatofugal direction, pneumobilia is more centrally located in the liver (Fig. 27.4). Etiologies of pneumobilia are more often benign and related to prior procedures such as papillotomy and surgery such as a Whipple's procedure. When air is peripherally located in the liver, portal venous gas must be suspected and urgently communicated to the clinical team.

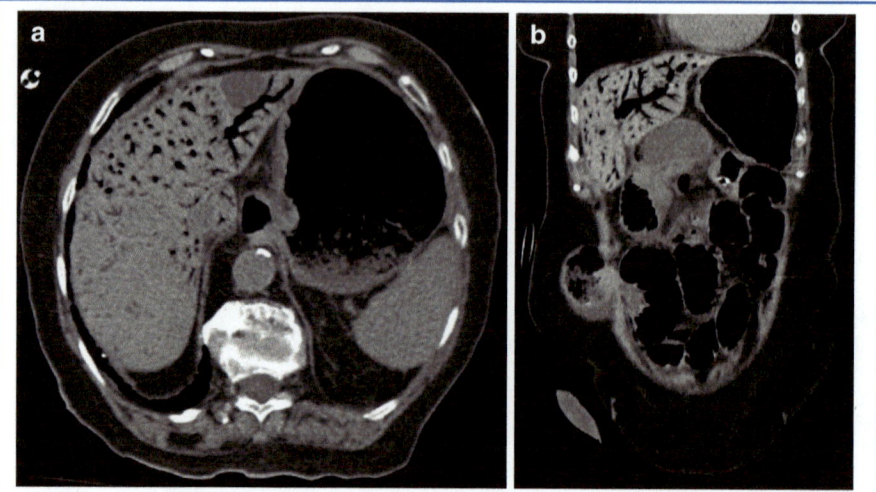

FIGURE 27.3 - PORTAL VENOUS GAS
Axial (**a**) and coronal (**b**) noncontrast CT images demonstrate air within the portal veins in a more peripheral location than pneumobilia

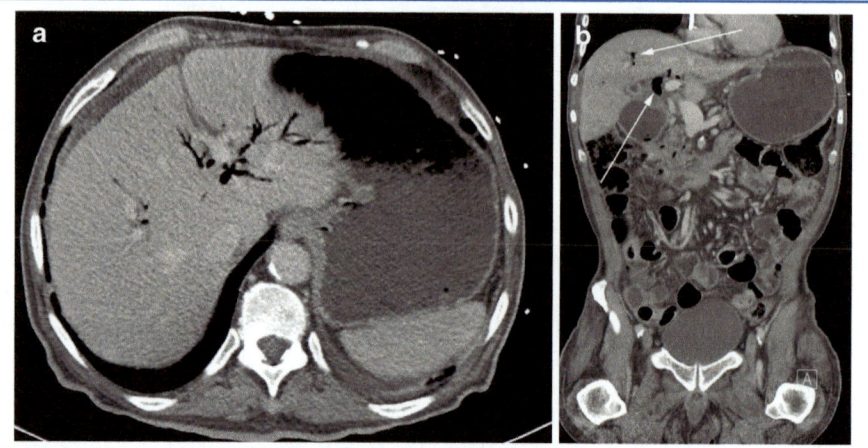

FIGURE 27.4 - PNEUMOBILIA
Axial (**a**) and coronal (**b**) contrast-enhanced CT images show air more centrally located in the liver within the biliary tree (***arrows***)

S: For those patients who are able to sit upright, plain, upright film can help identify free air quickly, without having the patient leave their clinical unit. When there is a concern for free air and the patient is critically ill, not mobile, or has multiple air distended bowel loops, CT is recommended as the initial examination. The CT may offer additional information as to the cause of their clinical status.

A: When a patient is unable to stand, a left lateral decubitus position radiograph obtained with the patient lying on their left side can be helpful in making the radiographic diagnosis of pneumoperitoneum. Free air will rise to outline the nondependent hepatic contour.

F: Utilizing soft tissue interfaces and patient positioning, even small amounts of air can be seen on plain film. Knowing what information is needed, recent surgeries or procedures, and the patient's clinical status will help you choose the most appropriate imaging modality.

E: A positive finding of pneumoperitoneum on imaging warrants a verbal communication to the patient's care team to expedite further management with the recommendation to consider a surgical consultation.

28 | BOWEL OBSTRUCTION

Objectives:
1. Describe the radiographic findings of large and small bowel obstruction.
2. List criteria used to distinguish bowel obstruction from ileus.
3. Define the term "air-fluid level."
4. Understand the advantages and disadvantages of conventional radiography and CT in the evaluation of bowel obstruction.

Gas is normally present in the stomach and colon. Small accumulations of gas may be found in the duodenum and upper portion of the jejunum as well. Scattered collections of gas may be present throughout much of the small intestine in physically inactive patients, patients on narcotics, and those who swallow large amounts of air habitually. Air can be seen as individual accumulations of rounded or ovoid-shaped lucency. If a single loop of normal intestine can be recognized because of gas filling, the shadow is seldom more than 5–8 cm in length. More often, the gas does not form any specific loop pattern. Conventional radiography is a useful and efficient means of evaluating for bowel obstruction. It is readily available, requires little to no patient preparation, is relatively low cost, and exposes the patient to minimal ionizing radiation. Abdominal radiography also serves as means to triage patients for additional (i.e., cross-sectional) imaging.

Small Bowel Obstruction

When individual segments of small intestine are dilated 3–4 cm in transverse diameter, one should consider the possibility that the gas pattern is abnormal. Radiographic findings in small bowel obstruction develop over time as fluid and gas build up proximal to the obstructive process.

J. Kissane et al. (eds.), *Radiology Fundamentals: Introduction to Imaging & Technology*, https://doi.org/10.1007/978-3-030-22173-7_28

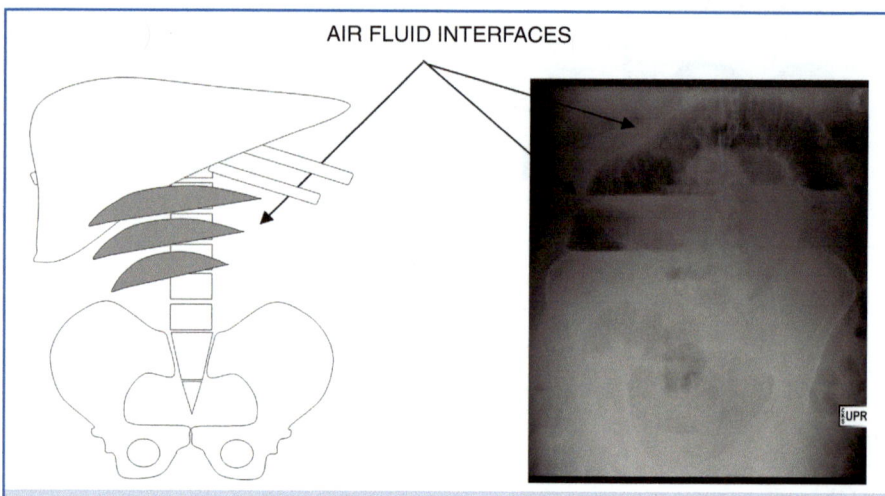

AIR FLUID INTERFACES

FIGURE 28.1 - AIR-FLUID LEVELS
The gas rises above the fluid in the bowel lumen creating gas-fluid interfaces, resulting in "fighting loops of bowel." A gas-fluid interface can be seen normally in the stomach, but not in the small bowel

Gas is visualized readily in supine radiographs, but the presence of fluid can only be confirmed on upright or decubitus views. In the upright view, the gas rises above the fluid, and the interface between gas and fluid forms a straight horizontal margin: an air-fluid level. Figure 28.1 demonstrates an air-fluid level in the small bowel. Air-fluid levels are generally considered to be abnormal in the small intestine. (Note that an air-fluid level is normally observed in the stomach because swallowed air is almost invariably present.) Air-fluid levels may be seen in the first portion of the duodenum where air may be trapped temporarily when the patient assumes the upright position. In the early stage of obstruction, only one or two such gas-distended segments are visualized. With increasing time, more distended loops may become visible. For this reason, serial examinations may be necessary for the diagnosis of small bowel obstruction. As distension increases, more loops become visible, and they tend to lie transversely at different levels, forming so-called fighting loops. Gas-filled loops may be recognized as small intestine rather than colon when they occupy the central portion of the abdomen rather than the periphery. Also, the pattern of mucosal folds in the small bowel, the valvulae conniventes, is finer and closer together than the colonic haustra. Unlike the haustral markings of the colon, these folds traverse the entire width of the bowel loop (Fig. 28.2). This is referred to as the "stack of coins" appearance.

When two gas-filled loops of bowel lie adjacent to one another, the soft tissue density between them represents a double thickness of intestinal wall. Thus, information concerning wall thickness is available. In a simple obstruction, a double thickness of intestine wall seldom amounts to more than a few millimeters in width, since the walls are thinned considerably by the distension. Inflammatory changes in

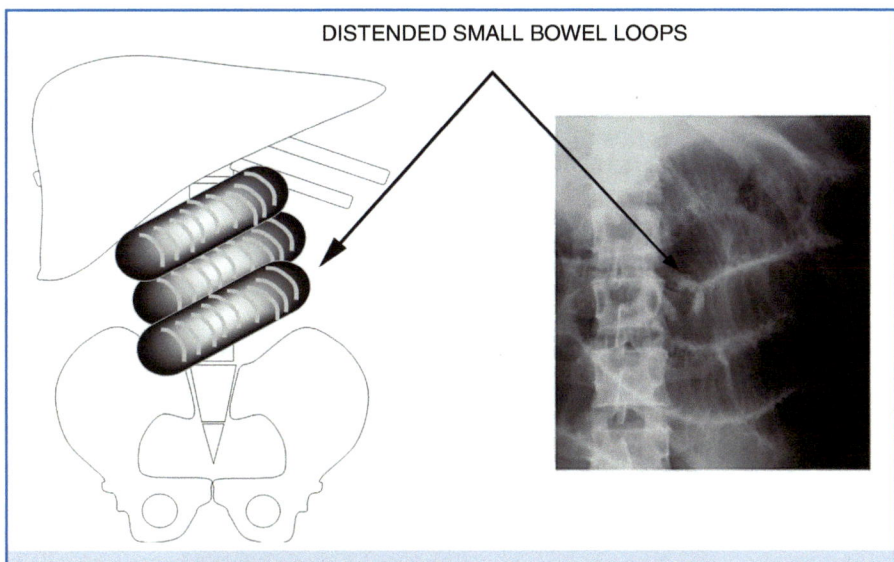

DISTENDED SMALL BOWEL LOOPS

FIGURE 28.2 - DISTENDED BOWEL LOOPS
As the loops of the small bowel distend, they begin to lie on top of each other resembling a stack of coins. The mucosal markings, called valvulae conniventes, cross the small bowel in their entirety

the wall or fluid in the peritoneal cavity interposed between the bowel loops result in a thickening of this soft tissue shadow. Abnormal thickening of the bowel wall indicates a more complex process, such as underlying inflammation, edema, or ascites. If obstruction of the small intestine is complete, little or no gas will be found in the colon, a valuable differentiating point between mechanical obstruction and ileus. However, it is important to note that small bowel obstruction can also present with a conspicuous absence of gas in the abdomen when the small bowel loops are entirely fluid filled.

If the obstruction is very proximal in the small intestine or if the patient has been decompressing the obstruction by vomiting, or if a gastric or biliary tube is in place providing decompression, the gas and fluid which would normally accumulate above an obstruction may not be present, and the typical findings may not be seen on the radiograph.

Large Bowel Obstruction

Gas is normally present in the colon. Because of this, the diagnosis of colonic obstruction (large bowel obstruction) may be made only when the colon is thought to be dilated from the cecum to the level of the lesion. Usually the abnormally

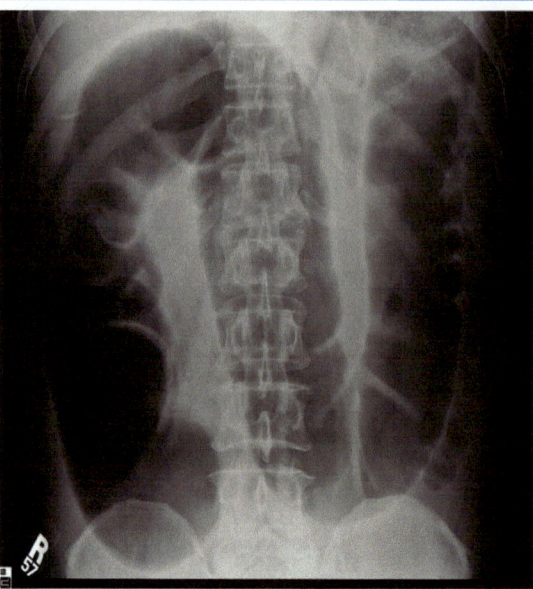

FIGURE 28.3 - TOTAL COLONIC OBSTRUCTION
Note the dilated, air-filled colon from the cecum to the proximal sigmoid. The cecum measures roughly 10 cm transversely

distended colon ends abruptly at the level of the lesion with the colon distal to the lesion free of gas. This is similar to what was previously discussed for the small bowel, and the principle is the same. Namely, distended bowel is found proximal to the obstruction. There is a paucity of gas distal to the obstruction with time. The large bowel is considered pathologically dilated when the diameter is greater than 7 cm in the left colon or greater than 9 cm in the cecum. Figure 28.3 shows the plain abdominal radiograph of a patient with a total colonic obstruction. Can you identify the point of obstruction?

The most likely site for obstruction of the large bowel, as might be expected, is in the rectosigmoid region since this is the most common site for colon carcinoma. The cecum undergoes the greatest distension in colonic obstruction and is the most likely site for perforation even when the obstruction is in the more distal colon. When the ileocecal valve is incompetent and the colon can decompress into the ileum, there is a lower likelihood of perforation. When the cecum distends to ten or more centimeters, perforation becomes a more likely possibility. Fluid levels are of less significance in the diagnosis of colonic obstruction than they are in the small bowel.

Another cause of large bowel obstruction is volvulus. Occurring typically in either the sigmoid colon or the cecum, volvulus refers to a twisting of the bowel around the mesentery, resulting in a closed loop obstruction and proximal bowel dilation. Sigmoid volvulus is most common in elderly patients and on x-ray characteristically demonstrates a large air-filled bowel loop above the transverse colon known as the "northern exposure" sign as seen in Fig. 28.3. Cecal volvulus occurs in younger adults and often demonstrates an air-filled loop of large bowel located in the left upper quadrant.

Evaluation for Obstruction

Computed tomography (CT) is generally considered the study of choice for further evaluation and characterization of obstruction, though at the expense of additional ionizing radiation to the patient. The zone of transition, presence of pneumoperitoneum or free fluid, degree, and etiology of obstruction may all be identified via CT. In addition, CT is readily available, requires minimal patient preparation, and is rapidly performed, allowing for quick triage of the acutely ill patient.

Given the diagnostic yield and ready availability of CT, contrast fluoroscopic evaluation has become less common in the evaluation of obstruction. However, this modality still has significant diagnostic yield as it can be utilized in the simultaneous localization and quantification of obstructive processes. If the location of an obstruction is not known, the colon is studied first, typically with a retrograde (enema) examination. In the setting of suspected obstruction or leak, only water-soluble contrast should be used, as barium-based contrast agents may result in intraluminal barium concretions or peritonitis secondary to peritoneal spillage of contrast.

In evaluating small bowel obstructions, the same principles apply. However, dilute water-soluble contrast is typically administered orally or via an existing gastric tube. Multiple serial radiographs are then taken over the ensuing time period until the contrast can be identified in the colon.

Ileus

There are many conditions which may reduce the motility of the large and small bowel. When this occurs, gas will accumulate within the bowel, giving a distended appearance both clinically and radiographically (Fig. 28.4). Note that the stomach and large and small bowel are all affected in equal proportion suggesting a diffuse rather than focal abnormality. These findings may be useful in distinguishing ileus from bowel obstruction, although certainly this differentiation can be difficult in some patients.

Occasionally, ileus can present focally without diffuse bowel distention. Focal ileus is caused by local inflammation that impairs motility of a small segment of bowel. On plain radiography, this has the appearance of a single dilated bowel loop

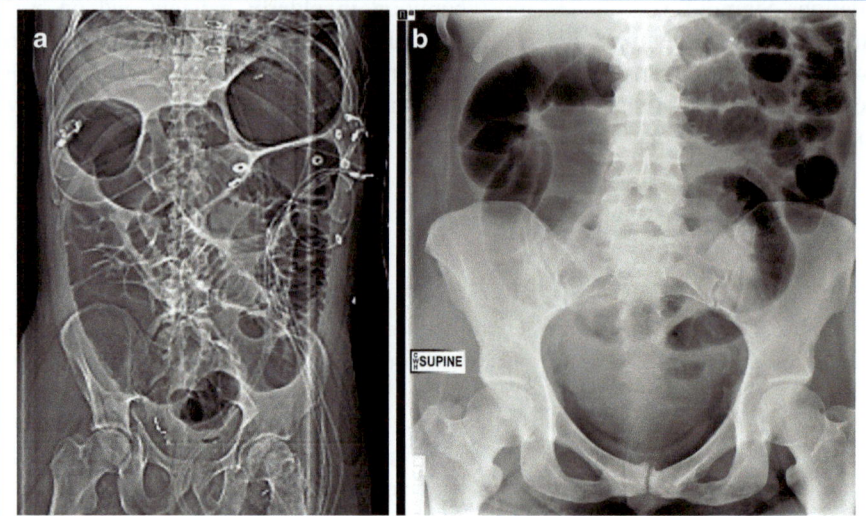

FIGURE 28.4 - ILEUS
Supine scout CT image (**a**) and radiograph (**b**) of two separate patients with ileus. Noted are multiple dilated, gas-filled small and large bowel loops measuring up to 5.5 cm in diameter throughout the abdomen and the upper portion of the pelvis. Equally distended loops of large bowel are seen extending down to the rectum

which can be similar in appearance to bowel obstruction. CT can be used to differentiate ileus from bowel obstruction and to find the etiology for the ileus (e.g., appendicitis, diverticulitis, cholecystitis, etc.). A focal loop of ileus, known as a "sentinel loop," can have the same appearance as an early small bowel obstruction. Serial clinical exams and follow-up radiography may be of use in further differentiation.

Mucosal Edema

Finally, the bowel wall may become edematous either in the presence of or the absence of obstruction. This is characterized by mucosal edema termed "thumbprinting." Bowel edema can be the result of infectious processes (i.e., *C. difficile*), intramural hemorrhage, or ischemia, among other causes.

Figure 28.5 demonstrates a prominent transverse colon with thickened haustra. This usually indicates edema of the bowel wall. The acute development of these findings is concerning, and further diagnostic evaluation with CT is warranted. Conditions which chronically inflame the colon may give a similar appearance. Hence, as in all radiographic interpretations, the clinical history is essential.

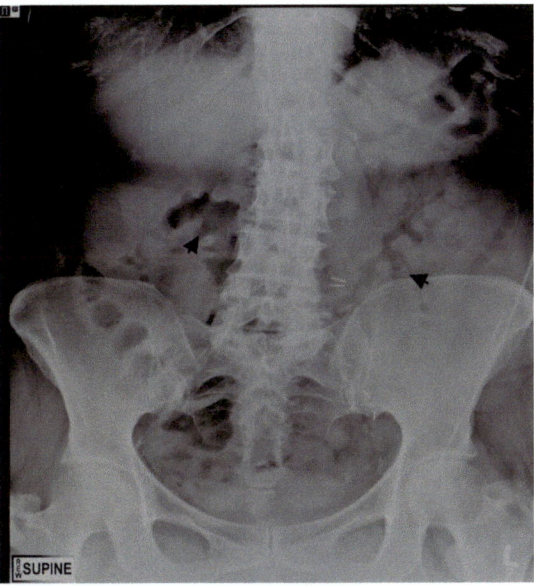

FIGURE 28.5 - LARGE BOWEL THUMBPRINTING
There is the suggestion of bowel wall thickening with thumbprinting of the transverse and descending colon (**arrows**)

S: The rapid assessment and triage of acute bowel abnormalities can be accomplished via conventional radiography, fluoroscopy, and CT, all of which are readily available, quickly performed, and relatively noninvasive. The amount of radiation from each increases from radiography to fluoroscopy and CT.

A: Radiographs and CT are indicated in the initial and follow-up assessment of acute bowel abnormalities, particularly suspected bowel obstruction.

F: An understanding of the anatomy and radiographic appearance of bowel obstruction, ileus, pneumoperitoneum, and other acute bowel abnormalities is necessary for the accurate interpretation of radiographic and CT exams. As an example, recognizing a focal transition point of obstruction on CT examination is invaluable during the ensuing surgical intervention.

E: It is of paramount importance to recognize acute bowel abnormalities, such that appropriate triage and management can occur without increase in morbidity or mortality. Acute abdominal abnormalities, including pneumoperitoneum and obstruction, should be communicated to the ordering service verbally as soon as possible.

29 CONCERNING ABDOMINAL MASSES

Objective:
1. Learn to recognize important masses in the abdomen including abscess, abdominal aortic aneurysm, renal cell cancer, pancreatic mass, and hepatocellular carcinoma.

Abscess

An abscess is a collection of infected fluid and inflammatory debris that has been walled off by the body's immune system. Many infectious or inflammatory processes in the abdomen or pelvis such as appendicitis, diverticulitis, and Crohn's disease can lead to an abscess. Traumatic puncture wounds and foreign bodies can also result in abscess formation. Common locations for an abdominal abscess are the subphrenic and subhepatic spaces. Abscesses can also develop in organs, such as the liver (intrahepatic abscess) or kidney (renal abscess). An abscess must be promptly treated with antibiotics and either percutaneous or surgical drainage to prevent systemic infection or sepsis.

Patients with an abscess clinically present with fever and an increased white cell count on laboratory values. Radiographically, an abscess appears as a loculated fluid collection with a thick, enhancing wall (Fig. 29.1). Free fluid in the body tends to layer dependently, while fluid in an abscess remains loculated. Characteristic features of an abscess include fluid-fluid levels, septations, and most notably air.

Sometimes you will hear the term "phlegmon" used in similar clinical scenarios. A phlegmon is a viscid collection of inflammatory debris. The same disease processes that lead to abscess formation can also cause a phlegmon to develop. On CT, an abscess will demonstrate fluid density (Hounsfield units <20), while a phlegmon often demonstrates higher soft tissue density (Hounsfield units 20–40). A phlegmon requires treatment with antibiotics; however, with little to no fluid component, a

© Springer Nature Switzerland AG 2020
J. Kissane et al. (eds.), *Radiology Fundamentals: Introduction to Imaging & Technology*, https://doi.org/10.1007/978-3-030-22173-7_29

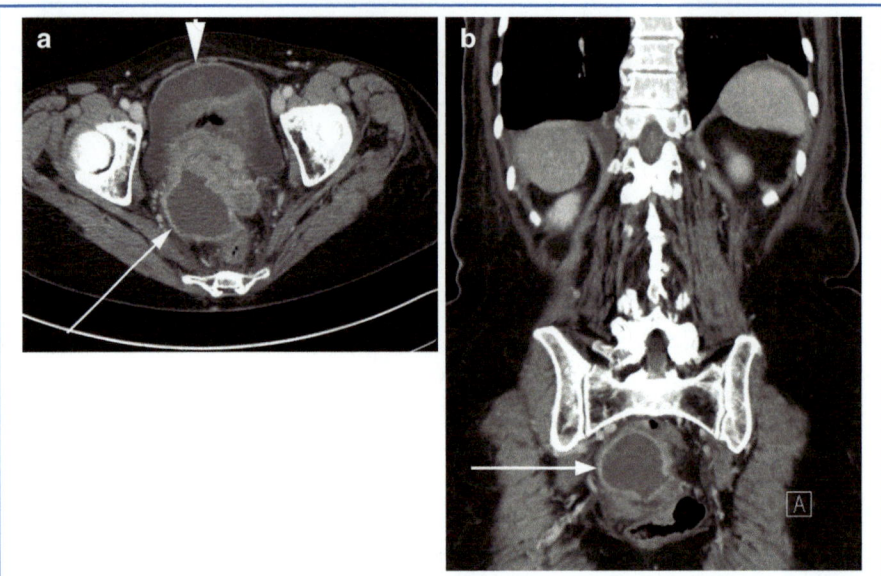

FIGURE 29.1 - ABSCESS
Axial (**a**) and coronal (**b**) contrast-enhanced CT images show a rim-enhancing fluid-filled collection compatible with an abscess (**arrow**). Note the normal appearance of the bladder (**arrowhead**) anteriorly

phlegmon cannot be treated with drainage and generally does not require surgery. A phlegmon and an abscess can be thought of as different points along the spectrum of inflammation.

Abdominal Aortic Aneurysm

Nearly 10% of the population over age 65 has an abdominal aortic aneurysm (AAA). Smoking is a well-known risk factor. Guidelines state that ultrasound screening is indicated in males 65–75 years old with a smoking history. Once the abdominal aorta measures greater than 3 cm, it is considered to be an aneurysm. Ninety percent of AAAs are infrarenal, meaning located below the renal arteries. Location is important for surgical or endovascular planning as repair of an aneurysm above the renal arteries is more complex.

With dissection of an aneurysm, the radiologist may see an intimal flap and the subsequent development of a false lumen. Dissection involving the origin of a branch vessel (e.g., the celiac artery) can lead to ischemia of organs supplied by those branches. Worrisome radiographic findings include the hyperdense

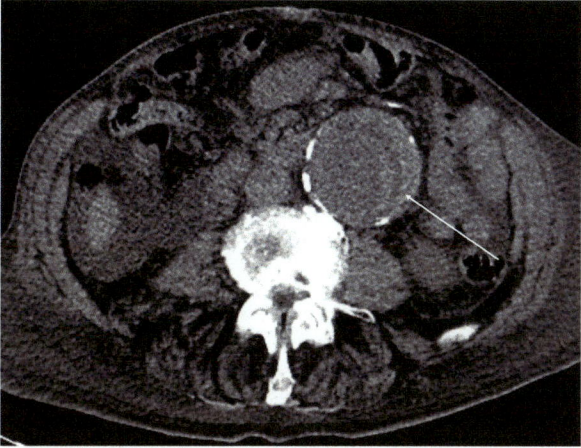

FIGURE 29.2 - ABDOMINAL AORTIC ANEURYSM
Rim-calcified abdominal aortic aneurysm. *Arrow* points out the hyperdense crescent sign, a sign of impending rupture and hemorrhage into the aortic wall

crescent sign which is a sign of impending aortic rupture and represents acute bleeding into the wall of the aneurysm known as an intramural hematoma (Fig. 29.2). Signs of aortic rupture include hemorrhage in the surrounding retroperitoneal tissues or active bleeding which is demonstrated by extravasation of contrast.

Renal Cell Cancer

Renal cell cancer (RCC) is the most common solid renal tumor. Smoking is a known risk factor. Other less common risk factors include Von Hippel–Lindau syndrome and acquired renal cystic disease from chronic hemodialysis. The uncommon, yet classic, clinical triad associated with RCC is a palpable flank mass, flank pain, and hematuria. Other presenting features include fever and weight loss.

Radiographically, RCC tumors are heterogeneous in appearance with brisk enhancement after the administration of intravenous contrast (Fig. 29.3a, b). With every new diagnosis of RCC, the ipsilateral renal vein and the IVC must be examined carefully to look for tumor thrombus involvement, a relatively common occurrence with RCC (Fig. 29.3c). The surrounding renal hilar, pericaval, and periaortic lymph nodes should also be examined for evidence of tumor involvement. Common sites of RCC metastasis include the lungs, bones, liver, brain, and adrenal glands. Renal cell cancer responds poorly to chemotherapy and radiation therapy.

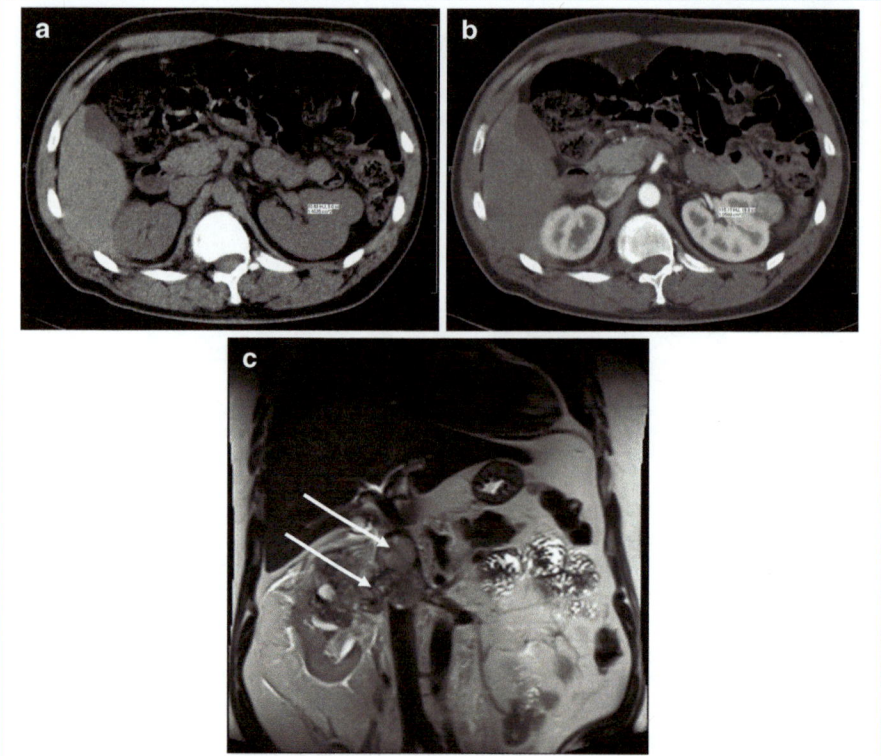

FIGURE 29.3 - LEFT RENAL MASS
(a) Noncontrast axial CT image shows an isodense solid mass arising from the left kidney measuring Hounsfield unit values of 30. (b) Contrast-enhanced CT of the same mass demonstrates rapid arterial enhancement measuring Hounsfield unit values of 115, reflecting enhancement. (c) Coronal MRI image in a different patient demonstrates extensive tumor thrombus in the right renal vein extending into the IVC from a right upper pole RCC

However, it is often curable with surgical resection when found early. Certain patients are candidates for less invasive techniques such as partial nephrectomy or ablation.

Hepatocellular Carcinoma

Hepatocellular carcinoma (HCC) is the most common primary hepatic malignancy in patients with chronic hepatic disease; it is very uncommon in patients without chronic liver disease. Common etiologies of chronic liver disease include chronic alcohol abuse, hepatitis B, hepatitis C and increasingly hepatic steatosis and subsequent development of steatohepatitis. Any solid hepatic mass in a cirrhotic patient is HCC until proven otherwise. HCCs develop along a pathologic continuum from a regenerative nodule to dysplastic nodule to HCC.

Patients often have clinical features of portal hypertension such as ascites, splenomegaly, variceal bleeding, and sometimes encephalopathy. The laboratory test, serum alpha-fetoprotein, can be used to monitor for HCC development or recurrence, in the appropriate clinical population. Radiographically, HCCs may be present as discrete masses but sometimes can be inconspicuous and infiltrating. Classic imaging characteristics of vigorous enhancement and de-enhancement or washout allow for their identification (Fig. 29.4). Like renal cell carcinoma, vascular invasion by tumor thrombus is relatively common. The hepatic and portal veins must be assessed for involvement of tumor thrombus on pretreatment imaging. Definitive treatment is liver transplant. Temporizing treatments include partial hepatectomy, various percutaneous ablations, chemoembolization, and systemic chemotherapy.

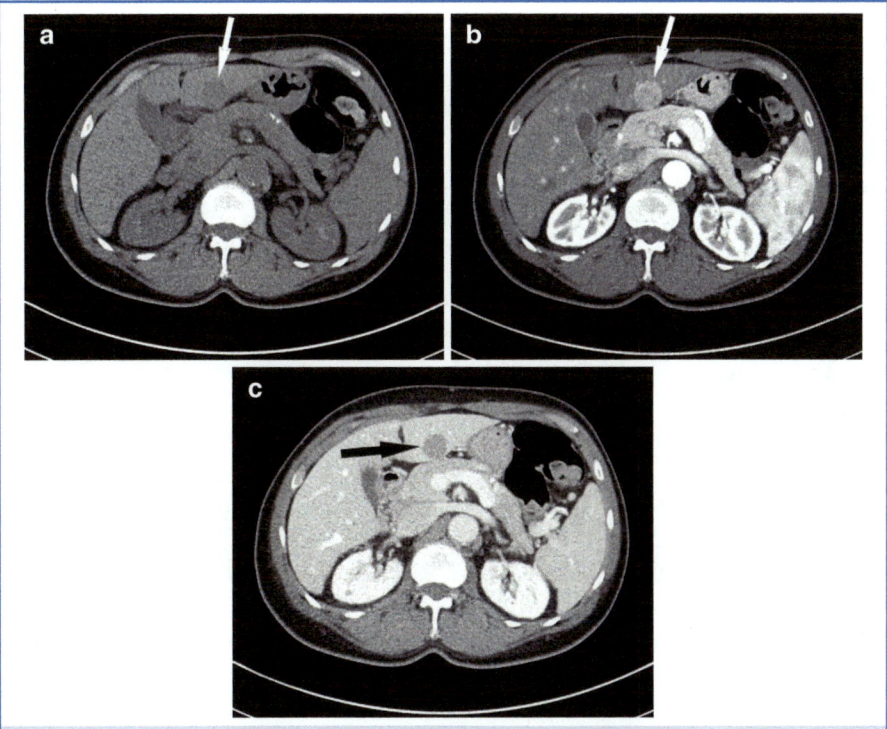

FIGURE 29.4 - HEPATOCELLULAR CARCINOMA ON MULTIPHASIC CT
(a) Noncontrast CT shows a subtle hypodense contour irregularity suggestive of a mass in the periphery of the left lobe of the liver. (b) Contrast-enhanced CT during the arterial phase shows avid enhancement of the mass seen in (a). (c) Contrast-enhanced CT during the venous phase shows that the mass in the left liver has become hypodense consistent with rapid washout of contrast which is characteristic of a hepatocellular carcinoma

Pancreatic Mass

Pancreatic adenocarcinoma is a malignancy with a low five-year survival rate despite aggressive surgical and medical treatment. The poor prognosis is due to the fact that the tumor does not manifest symptoms until late in the course of the disease at which time the tumor is often no longer resectable at time of diagnosis. When clinical symptoms present, they often include abdominal pain, weight loss, and jaundice.

Pancreatic tumors are difficult to detect on standard imaging that has not been tailored to evaluate the pancreas. Often pancreatic adenocarcinoma appears as a hypoenhancing mass located at the site of abrupt main pancreatic duct cutoff with upstream pancreatic gland atrophy. Sixty percent of pancreatic adenocarcinomas are located in the pancreatic head. The best imaging finding to aid in diagnosis of a pancreatic head adenocarcinoma is the double duct sign (Fig. 29.5). This refers to dilation of both the common bile duct and the main pancreatic duct caused by tumor in the pancreatic head compressing both ducts. Evaluation of a pancreatic mass would be incomplete without reporting on features that determine if the tumor is resectable. Radiographic signs of unresectable tumor include vascular involvement (celiac, hepatic, and superior mesenteric artery) and extension beyond the pancreas into other organs.

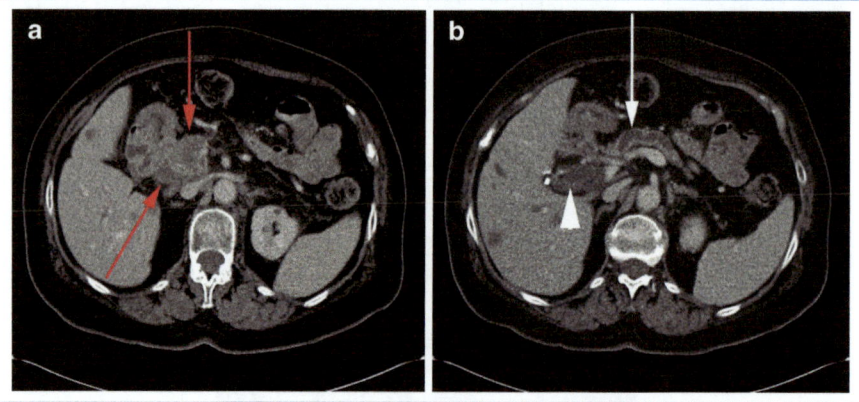

FIGURE 29.5 - PANCREATIC HEAD MASS.
(a) Axial contrast-enhanced CT image of the pancreas shows a heterogeneous hypoenhancing mass in the pancreatic head (***red arrows***). (b) Axial image superior to image (a) demonstrates dilated pancreatic (***white arrow***) and common bile duct (***arrowhead***) known as the "double duct sign"

S: Careful review of clinical risk factors including smoking, prior history of significant alcohol use, etc. helps direct imaging strategies for patients at risk for a variety of intra-abdominal pathology. The risk of radiation exposure in carefully selected patients is outweighed by the risk of a missed diagnosis. Clinical information is critical.

A: The United States Preventive Services Task Force (USPSTF) currently recommends one-time US screening for AAA in men ages 65–75 who have ever smoked.

F: While radiographs may be the first imaging modality to detect calcification along a dilated aorta, radiographs cannot be used as a stand-alone study as it is unable to assess true aneurysm sac size. CTA and MRA are the most appropriate tests for a diagnostic evaluation.

E: Abdominal aortic aneurysm maximum diameter greater than 5.5 cm and rate of enlargement greater than 1 cm per year, as well as periaortic stranding and intramural hematoma, are findings that indicate impending rupture. Positive finding of an aortic aneurysm with impending rupture on imaging warrants a verbal communication to the patient's care team to expedite vascular surgery or cardiovascular interventional radiology consultation.

30 FLUOROSCOPIC EVALUATION OF THE UPPER GI TRACT AND SMALL BOWEL

Objectives:
1. Identify normal anatomy on a "barium swallow" and "upper GI" series.
2. Be able to differentiate mucosal versus extramucosal lesions based on radiographic findings.
3. Describe the radiographic features of malignant esophageal lesions.
4. Know the common locations for esophageal diverticula and their radiographic appearance.
5. Understand the main advantages and disadvantages of the various means of small bowel examination.

Fluoroscopy

GI studies are observed fluoroscopically in real-time imaging to evaluate peristalsis and the rate of flow of contrast. Exposures and limited video captures of key anatomic regions or focal abnormalities are also obtained. Static images covering a large region of the GI tract are acquired at the end of the study for the purpose of giving a geographic perspective of the contrast distribution throughout the GI tract.

Normal Esophageal Motility

Swallowed contrast is propelled by peristaltic waves, which are visible as smooth, segmental, and progressive narrowings of the esophagus. The normal peristaltic wave with swallowing is called the primary peristaltic wave. A secondary wave may occur if the patient swallows quickly after the primary swallow. Figure 30.1 demonstrates a single image from a normal fluoroscopic exam of the esophagus.

© Springer Nature Switzerland AG 2020

J. Kissane et al. (eds.), *Radiology Fundamentals: Introduction to Imaging & Technology*, https://doi.org/10.1007/978-3-030-22173-7_30

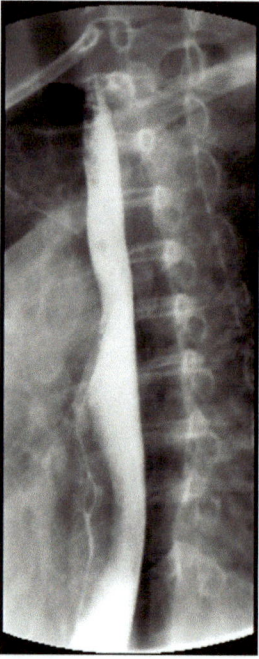

FIGURE 30.1 - NORMAL CONTRAST ESOPHAGRAM
Contrast upper gastrointestinal (UGI) study performed with barium demonstrating a normal esophageal appearance

Abnormal Esophageal Motility

Sometimes abnormalities of esophageal motility may manifest as tertiary
contractions which are seen as multiple small disorganized and transient indentations
of the contrast column within the esophagus. These are generally related to
abnormalities of the neurologic plexus responsible for propagation of the peristaltic
wave. They are commonly seen in older individuals as the plexus and motor function
degenerates with age, but may also be observed in those with underlying
gastrointestinal dysmotility or neurological disorders. Fluoroscopic evaluations
should be correlated with any available manometric examinations.

When the neurologic plexus in the distal esophagus degenerates, spasm without
relaxation of the lower esophageal sphincter may occur, producing a condition
termed achalasia (Fig. 30.2). This results in distension of the proximal esophagus
with collections of ingested food and secretions leading to an increased risk of
aspiration pneumonia. An increasing number of fluoroscopic exams are now being

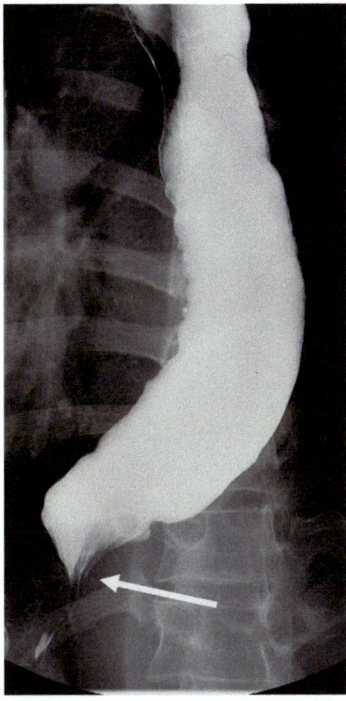

FIGURE 30.2 - ACHALASIA
Malfunction of the neurologic plexus leads to spasm of the lower esophageal sphincter, resulting in a markedly distended esophagus and the classic "birds beak" (***arrow***) narrowing at the level of the lower esophageal sphincter

performed on patients who have undergone peroral endoscopic myotomy (POEM) in which the circular muscles of the esophagus are divided endoscopically for the treatment of achalasia.

Esophageal Carcinoma

Esophageal carcinomata create areas of fixed narrowing, often with mucosal ulceration and overhanging edges that result in "shouldering" of the barium column at the edges of the fixed narrowing. Shouldering of contrast around a narrowing suggests malignancy as compared to smooth margins that occur more frequently about benign lesions as depicted in Fig. 30.3.

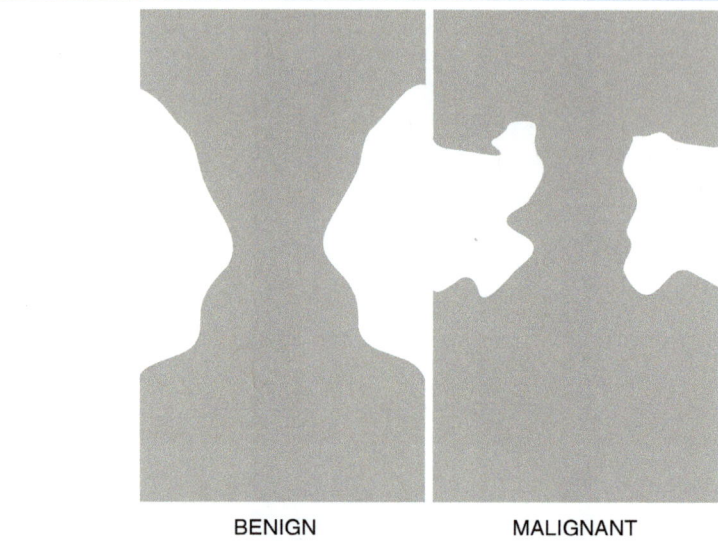

BENIGN   MALIGNANT

FIGURE 30.3 - CONTRAST ESOPHAGRAM
On contrast swallow studies, benign (*left*) and malignant (*right*) lesions have a different appearance. Note the gradual narrowing with smooth margins of the benign lesion versus the overhanging edges and abrupt appearance of the malignant lesion

Esophageal carcinoma occurs most commonly in the mid to lower esophagus (Fig. 30.4). As it is difficult to definitively distinguish a benign esophageal stricture (i.e., caused by gastric reflux) from a carcinoma on fluoroscopy, endoscopic evaluation with biopsy is often necessary.

Esophageal Diverticula

Diverticula of the esophagus take two forms: traction diverticula and pulsion diverticula. Traction diverticula most commonly arise in the region of the carina. They result from retraction of the inflamed subcarinal lymph nodes as they pull on the esophageal mucosa via fibrous adhesions. Pulsion diverticula occur when peristaltic waves exert a positive pressure within the esophageal lumen. Any weakness in the esophageal wall may lead to a "ballooning out" of the mucosa. A common location for esophageal wall weakness is in the upper esophagus posteriorly where the constrictor muscles fail to completely cover the esophageal wall. This region is known as Killian's dehiscence. The pulsion diverticulum formed in this area is termed a Zenker's diverticulum and may be present as a mass in the upper neck. Another common

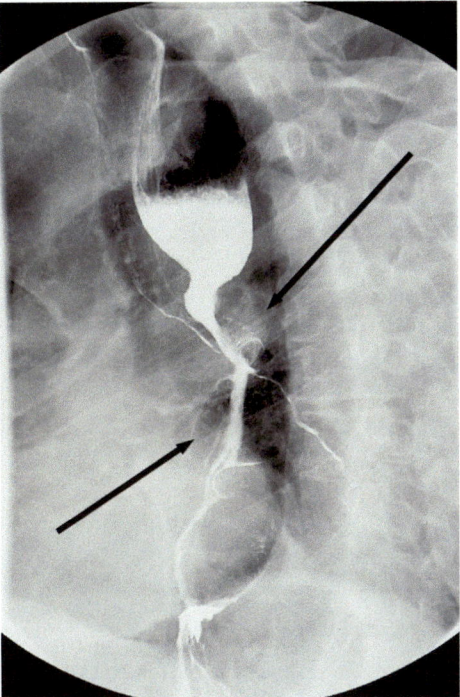

FIGURE 30.4 - ESOPHAGEAL CARCINOMA
Note the irregularity and overhanging edges (***arrows***) resulting in abrupt shouldering of the contrast column above and below the narrowing

location for pulsion diverticula is just above the lower esophageal sphincter. These diverticula are called epiphrenic diverticula and can be associated with achalasia.

Double- and Single-Contrast Upper GI Studies

Standard upper GI studies utilize either a single- or double-contrast evaluation of the esophagus, stomach, and duodenal bulb. In a double-contrast study, barium and air are the two contrast agents. Within the stomach, the barium coats the gastric mucosa, and the air distension allows the mucosal folds of the stomach to be clearly evident (Fig. 30.5).

In a single-contrast upper GI series, barium is the only contrast agent. The stomach is nearly filled with barium, and the mucosal detail is not as evident. Single-contrast studies are faster to perform and result in less radiation exposure; however, mucosal information is expectedly more limited.

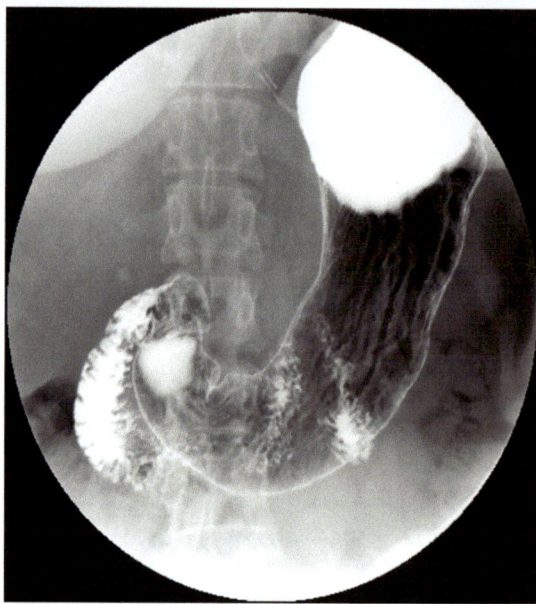

FIGURE 30.5 - DOUBLE-CONTRAST GASTRIC STUDY
Note the detail of the gastric and duodenal mucosa

Filling of ulcer craters with barium produces small collections of contrast within the gastric wall. Gastric folds may radiate toward the ulcer as a result of inflammation. Ulcers may be malignant or benign, and endoscopic evaluation is often required for differentiation. Adenocarcinoma is the most common gastric malignancy and can present as an irregular solitary filling defect or as a diffuse infiltrative lesion that rigidly narrows the gastric body and antrum in a pattern termed "linitis plastica."

After evaluation of the stomach, static images are obtained of the duodenal bulb and proximal "C" loop of the duodenum as it curves around the head of the pancreas. The duodenal bulb and post-bulbar portion of the duodenum are common places for ulceration and diverticula formation. The duodenum ends anatomically at the ligament of Treitz which should be at the same craniocaudal level as the duodenal bulb and lies to the left of the midline.

Small Bowel Follow-Through

A single-contrast study of the contrast column may be followed through the small bowel as it passes distally through the GI tract, termed "a small bowel follow-through" (Fig. 30.6). This will reveal gross abnormalities such as mucosal masses,

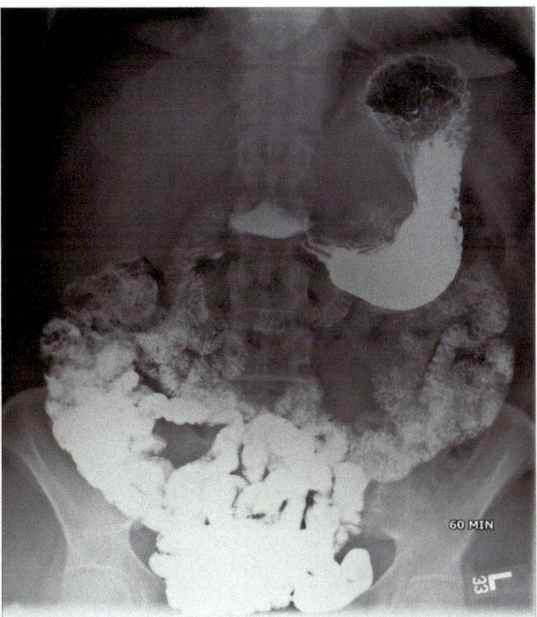

FIGURE 30.6 - SMALL BOWEL FOLLOW-THROUGH
Detail of the mucosal lining is visible as barium passes through the small bowel

strictures, and mass effect displacing the small bowel loops, in addition to serving as a rough indicator of overall small bowel transit time and motility. The small bowel follow-through terminates when contrast is seen within the cecum of the colon, having passed through the terminal ileum and the ileocecal valve.

Conventional Enteroclysis

A double-contrast study of the small bowel, termed an "enteroclysis," may be performed for the purpose of further elucidating small bowel anatomy. By placing an enteric tube distal to the ligament of Treitz, occluding the jejunal lumen with a balloon and slowly injecting soluble barium and methylcellulose as a "solid column," a double-contrast effect is achieved. Multiple single exposure images of the small bowel are obtained with fluoroscopy. The study is concluded once contrast reaches the cecum.

Small bowel malignancies may be either primary or metastatic and usually will appear as focal narrowing or strictures of the small bowel and/or nodular filling defects. Given the dynamic nature of the exam, this study can be useful for detecting low-grade small bowel obstruction secondary to Crohn's disease and postoperative

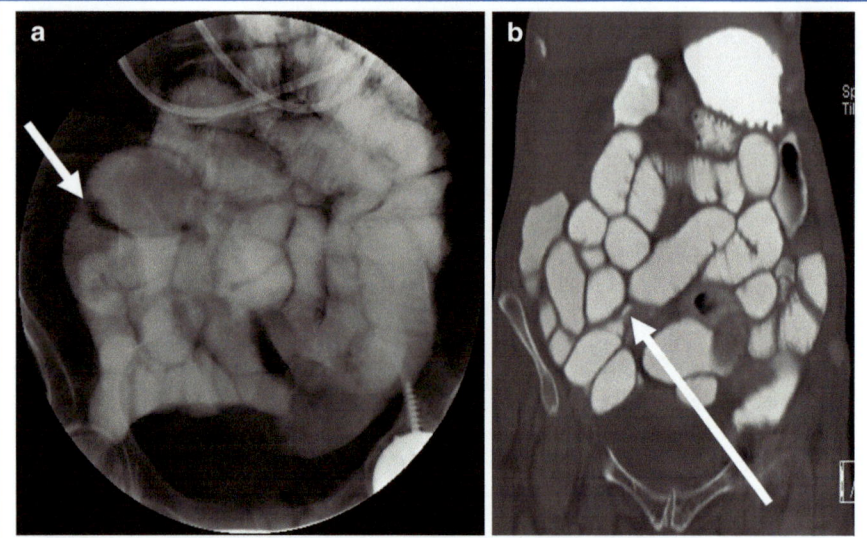

FIGURE 30.7 - CONVENTIONAL VERSUS CT ENTEROCLYSIS
(**a**) Conventional enteroclysis demonstrates a focal area of narrowing in the distal ileum (***arrow***).
(**b**) Coronal image from a CT enteroclysis of the same patient demonstrates the focal area of narrowing in the distal ileum in the same location as the narrowing seen on conventional enteroclysis (***arrow***). CT enteroclysis had the added advantage of being able to demonstrate multiple different areas of narrowing in this patient (not shown) as well as evaluating bowel wall thickness and extraluminal pathology

adhesions (Fig. 30.7). Active Crohn's disease may also be detected with this type of examination, although the diagnostic modality of choice for evaluation of Crohn's disease is CT or MR enterography.

This study is more difficult for the radiologist to perform and for the patient to tolerate. Therefore, it is used only in select situations, as when cross-sectional and endoscopic evaluations have proven unrevealing.

CT Enteroclysis

This type of study evaluates the small bowel in a similar manner to conventional enteroclysis. However, barium and methylcellulose are not used as contrast agents. The patient receives either positive (radiopaque) contrast, such as barium or diluted water-soluble contrast, or negative (radiolucent) contrast, such as water, prior to being taken to the CT scanner. Typically, the scan is performed once contrast has reached the cecum. CT enteroclysis is more sensitive for the detection of small strictures and mucosal inflammation such as in Crohn's disease.

Postoperative Imaging

Conventional fluoroscopic evaluation has become less frequently utilized in the day-to-day evaluation of gastrointestinal complaints owing to the expanding role of cross-sectional imaging and endoscopy. In the postoperative setting, however, fluoroscopy has gained a larger role as a low-risk (as compared to a return to surgery) evaluation of anatomy, leaks, or fistulae in patients post gastric bypass, esophagectomy, and stent placement. Of note, barium is contraindicated when a leak is suspected as it can stimulate an inflammatory response and peritonitis. Therefore, fluoroscopy with a water-soluble contrast agent is commonly performed to identify anastomotic leakage or stenosis.

S: Contrast fluoroscopy exams provide readily accessible anatomic and physiologic data. However, care should be taken to minimize the risks of ionizing radiation both to examiners and patients alike. Consultation with health physics personnel should be considered particularly in children. In addition, barium should not be used in the setting of suspected obstruction or perforation. Care should be taken to avoid the use of water-soluble contrast in the setting of possible aspiration.

A: While radiographs and CT play roles in evaluation of the upper gastrointestinal tract and small bowel, contrast fluoroscopy examination allows for real-time evaluation of physiology, anatomic delineation, and localization of focal abnormalities, such as leaks. This modality is of particular use in the postoperative setting, in which complications and variant anatomy are frequently of clinical concern.

F: An understanding of upper gastrointestinal and small bowel physiology, normal and postoperative anatomy is essential in the interpretation of fluoroscopic GI exams. As an example, it is key to recognize the presence of a gastro-gastric fistula in the patient who is status post Roux-en-Y gastric bypass or to localize an esophageal leak status post intervention.

E: Fluoroscopic examination of the upper GI tract and small bowel can be used in elective and emergent settings and allow for the relatively rapid detection of potentially acute but correctable findings. Actionable findings require immediate communication to the appropriate providers.

31 IMAGING OF THE COLON

Objectives:
1. Explain the difference between a single- and double-contrast barium enema.
2. List the typical findings seen in colonic malignancies.
3. Describe the radiographic appearance of colonic diverticula and polyps.
4. Develop a basic understanding of the principles of CT colonography (virtual colonoscopy).

As with the upper GI series, fluoroscopic colonography can be performed in either a single or double-contrast fashion. In single-contrast studies, the colon is filled only with opaque contrast such as barium or water-soluble contrast. This study can demonstrate extrinsic displacement of the colon, strictures, and large intraluminal filling defects (Fig. 31.1). Double-contrast studies involve partially filling the colon with barium followed by insufflation with a gas (air or carbon dioxide) via a rectal tube placed in the rectum for the purpose of elucidating polyps, early carcinomas, or inflammatory bowel disease. If there is a concern of obstruction or perforation, single-contrast water-soluble enema may be used (Fig. 31.2a).

An important part of fluoroscopic colonography is thorough bowel preparation, including a clear liquid diet and laxatives for a day or two prior to the exam for the purpose of clearing the GI tract of stool. This may be difficult for some patients; however, without adequate preparation, the diagnostic yield of the exam is limited.

Figure 31.2b is a single image from a normal double-contrast barium enema study. On the normal barium enema study, you should be able to identify the rectal ampulla, the sigmoid colon, descending colon, transverse colon, ascending colon, and cecum. Filling of the appendix is variable, even when normal and present. Note that the barium column is impinged upon by regularly occurring mucosal folds called haustra. These haustra are somewhat less prominent in the rectosigmoid region; however, loss of normal haustral markings may indicate pathology.

© Springer Nature Switzerland AG 2020
J. Kissane et al. (eds.), *Radiology Fundamentals: Introduction to Imaging & Technology*, https://doi.org/10.1007/978-3-030-22173-7_31

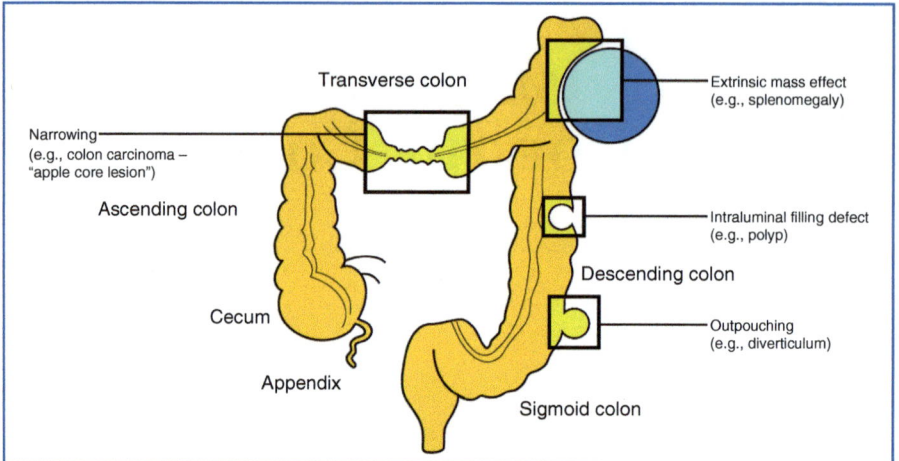

FIGURE 31.1 - FLUOROSCOPY OF THE COLON
Note the different segments of the colon and the resulting appearance of the large bowel in the setting of narrowing or stricture, extrinsic or mural mass, filling defect (i.e., intraluminal lesion), and outpouching of the contrast column (i.e., diverticula)

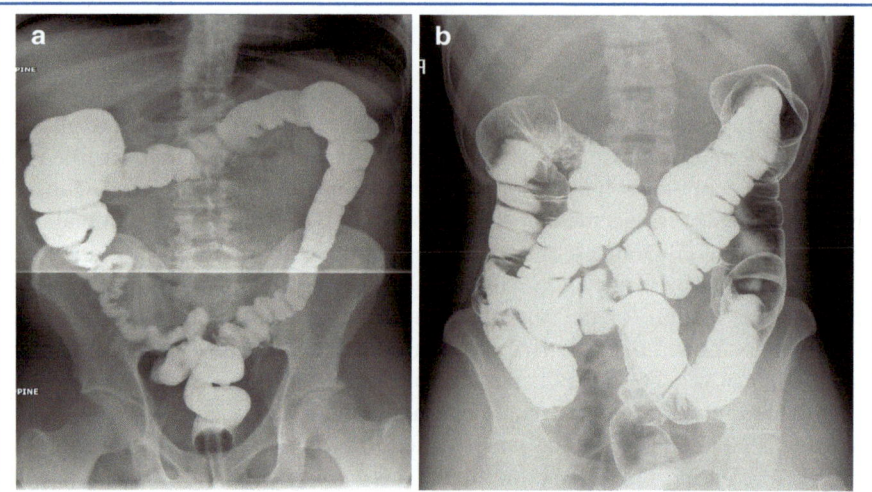

FIGURE 31.2 - (a) SINGLE-CONTRAST AND (b) DOUBLE-CONTRAST ENEMA
Although a single-contrast study may be easier to perform, mucosal detail is better seen on the double-contrast study

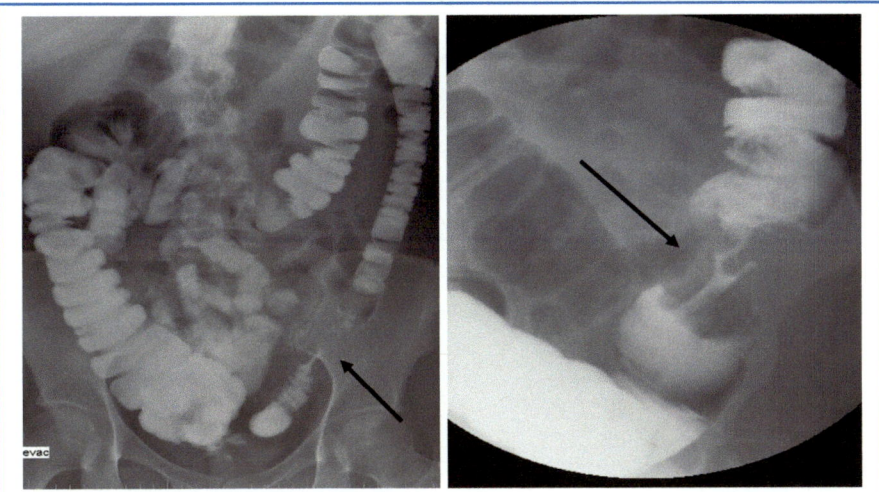

FIGURE 31.3 - APPLE CORE LESION OF THE SIGMOID COLON
Again, note the abrupt caliber change and the irregular margins (*arrows*)

Colon cancer demonstrates the same fluoroscopic abnormalities that are seen with other GI tract malignancies including loss of normal peristalsis, disruption of the normal mucosal pattern, and overhanging edges or "shouldering" of the contrast column about a narrowed segment as seen in the typical "apple core" lesion in Fig. 31.3. The rectosigmoid region is the most common site of colonic carcinoma.

Colonic Diverticula and Polyps

Diverticula are outpouchings of mucosa between weak taenia coli muscles. They are more common with age, and while they can involve any part of the gastrointestinal tract, diverticula more commonly involve the colon as seen in Fig. 31.4 which demonstrates numerous outpouchings of the sigmoid colon.

Polyps can be either benign or premalignant. Adenomatous polyps are on the spectrum of premalignant lesions that with time progress to adenocarcinoma. Barium enema, especially a double-contrast barium enema, is a relatively low-cost, low-risk procedure for the detection of these polyps. It is important to note that double-contrast barium enema is less sensitive than optical or virtual colonoscopy in the detection of small polyps. Colonoscopy has largely replaced barium enemas; however, colonoscopy is more expensive, invasive, and requires a moderate level of conscious sedation which is contraindicated in some patients.

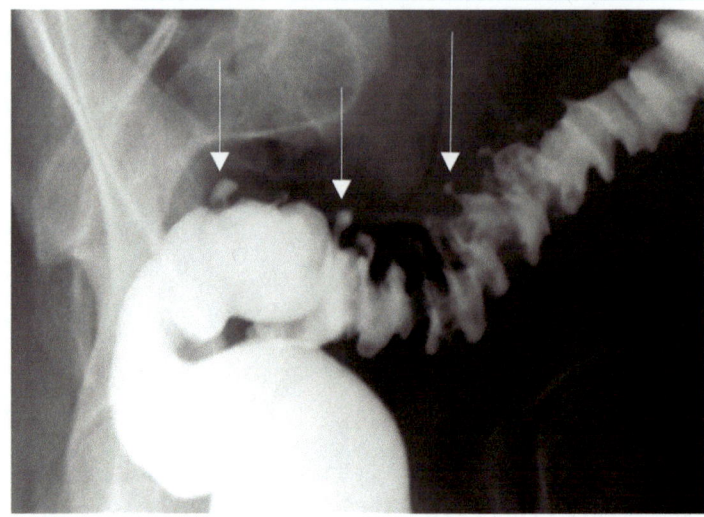

FIGURE 31.4 - SIGMOID DIVERTICULA
Multiple outpouchings along the sigmoid colon consistent with colonic diverticulosis

CT Colonography (Virtual Colonoscopy)

Computed tomography colonography (CTC) or "virtual colonoscopy" has been shown by several multicenter studies to be as effective in the detection of polyps greater than 5 mm as optical colonoscopy which has led to increased utilization of CT colonography for both screening and diagnostic exams.

For this type of study, the patient undergoes the same thorough bowel preparation required for an optical colonoscopy. The patient is then placed in the CT scanner, a rectal tube is inserted, and the colon is distended with carbon dioxide via a special insufflation pump. The CT scanner is used to obtain very thin slices through the abdomen and pelvis, and images are reconstructed in axial, coronal, and sagittal planes. The patient is then rescanned in the prone and sometimes lateral decubitus positions (Figs. 31.5, 31.6, and 31.7).

The CT images are then reviewed using special software in 2-D (axial, coronal, or sagittal) and 3-D modes (virtual colonoscopy fly through images). Colonic polyps are considered significant if they measure >5 mm from the base of the stalk to the top of the polyp. In general, polyps ≤5 mm on CTC are not reported, or if they are reported, a recommendation of follow-up colonoscopy (optical or CT) in 5–7 years can be made. Polypectomy is recommended for any patient with >3 polyps or any polyp >10 mm, regardless of patient age.

There is some controversy over how polyps measuring between 6 and 9 mm should be managed. Current recommendations suggest polypectomy for 1–2 polyps

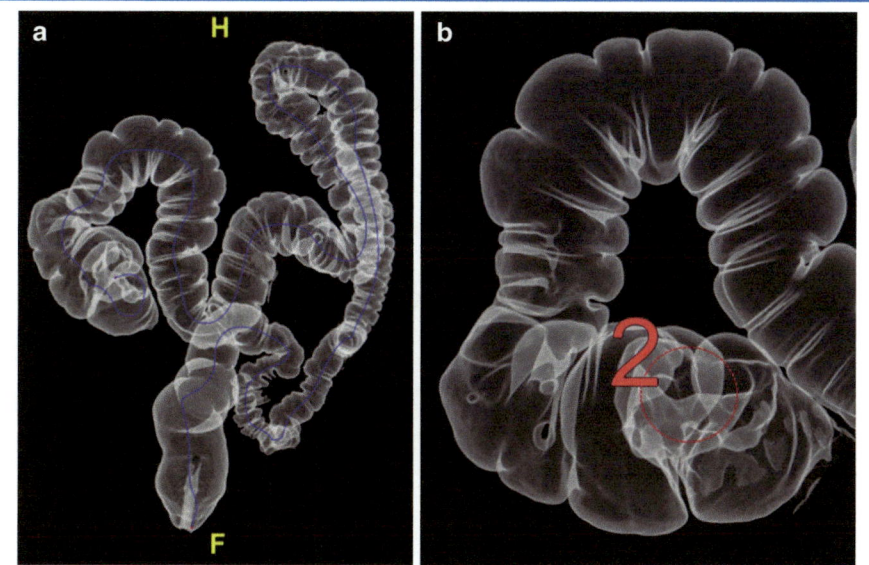

FIGURE 31.5 - CT COLONOGRAPHY
(**a**) This demonstrates a "double-contrast" image obtained by the CT scanner and is used as a "road map" during the virtual colonoscopy portion of the study. (**b**) This is a magnified "double-contrast" view of the cecum. There is a large filling defect in the cecum

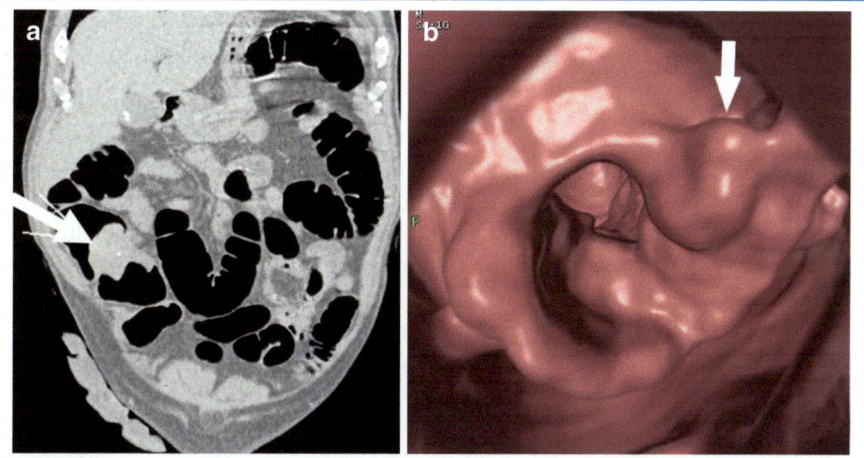

FIGURE 31.6 - CT COLONOGRAPHY
(**a**) Coronal 2-D CT image of the colon demonstrates a large irregular filling defect in the cecum (*arrow*). (**b**) This is a 3-D CT image of a "virtual colonoscopy" study demonstrating the same large mass in the cecum (*arrow*) as seen in (**a**). Biopsy specimen of this large mass came back as invasive adenocarcinoma, T4

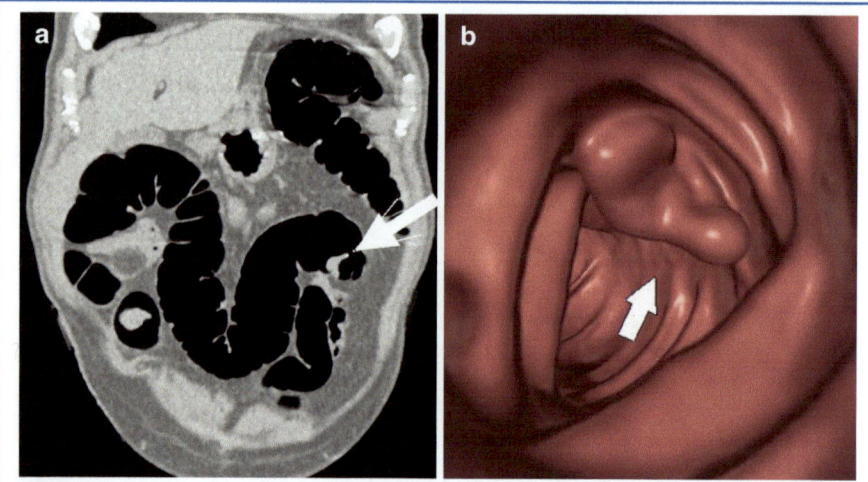

FIGURE 31.7 - CT COLONOGRAPHY
(a) Coronal 2-D CT image of the colon also shows a polyp in the transverse colon in the same patient (*arrow*). (b) This is a 3-D CT image of a "virtual colonoscopy" study in the same patient, demonstrating the polyp in the transverse colon (*arrow*). Biopsy specimen of this polyp came back as benign adenoma

measuring 8–9 mm if the patient is healthy enough to undergo optical colonoscopy and intervention. Three-year follow-up with colonoscopy is recommended for 1–2 polyps measuring 6–7 mm. Ultimately, however, it is a shared decision-making process between the patient and their healthcare team based on patient comorbid conditions when polyps measure between 6 and 9 mm.

S: Recommendations from the United States Preventive Services Task Force (USPSTF) for average-risk individuals over the age 50 include either optical colonoscopy every 10 years, computed tomographic colonography (CTC) every 5 years, or a stool-based test every 1 to 3 years, depending on the sensitivity of the stool-based test. The potential findings must be weighed against the use of radiation.

A: CT colonography colorectal cancer screening in high-risk individuals such as hereditary nonpolyposis colorectal cancer, ulcerative colitis, or Crohn colitis is usually not appropriate. Optical colonography should be performed in this patient population as this allows for biopsy.

F: Incidental extracolonic malignancies and aortic aneurysms are detected in approximately 2–3% of patients during CTC. Structured reporting may facilitate accurate identification of these findings.

E: Verbal communication and discussion of any relevant study limitations during CTC or barium enema is important in order to assess the sensitivity of the examination performed and need for any further diagnostic workup.

32 IMAGING OF THE GALLBLADDER

Objectives:
1. State the strengths and weaknesses of each of the following radiographic tests used for evaluation of the gallbladder and related structures: ultrasound, IDA scan, percutaneous transhepatic cholangiogram, ERCP, and CT scan.
2. Understand the typical imaging findings of acute cholecystitis on ultrasound.

Right upper quadrant pain is one of the most common clinical presentations, and the gallbladder is one of the most frequently imaged organs in this setting. There are numerous available imaging examinations for evaluation of the gallbladder. This chapter discusses each of these briefly but is certainly not complete in its coverage of the various limitations and sequencing of these tests. Of note, radiology is not the only specialty to image the gallbladder as emergency department physicians and surgeons commonly image this organ at the bedside using ultrasound.

The Gallbladder on Plain Radiograph

Figure 32.1 shows discreet radiopacities in the right upper quadrant of the abdomen, each measuring approximately 1 cm in size. Based on the radiographic density compared to the ribs, one can easily surmise that these are densely calcified. They represent calcified gallstones within the gallbladder. Gallstones are composed primarily of cholesterol, and therefore most are lucent on abdominal radiographs. Only 10–15% of gallstones calcify sufficiently for visualization on a plain radiograph.

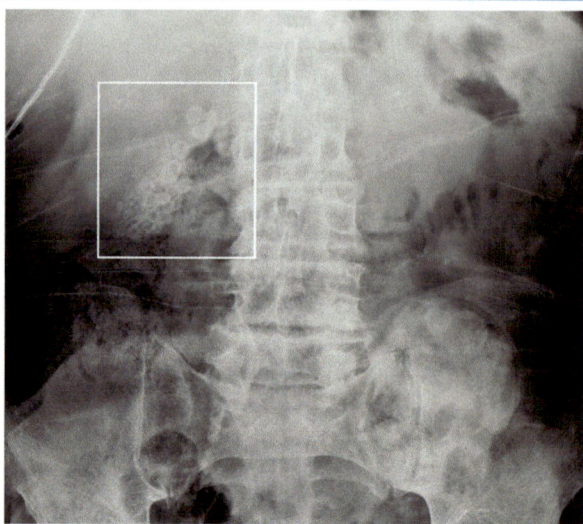

FIGURE 32.1 - GALLBLADDER STONES
The appearance and location of these calcifications are typical of gallstones

Visible gallstones are seen as lamellated calcific densities in the right upper quadrant of the abdomen, which are usually clustered in groups. They range in size from several millimeters to several centimeters.

A uniformly dense calcification of the entire gallbladder wall, termed "porcelain gallbladder," is associated with chronic gallbladder inflammation. Porcelain gallbladder may be considered a premalignant condition that can be associated with gallbladder carcinoma in approximately 10% of cases.

Gallbladder on Ultrasound

Ultrasound is the preferred method for detecting the presence of gallstones. It is advantageous in that it utilizes no ionizing radiation, though it is operator and patient dependent.

Gallstones within the gallbladder are seen as bright echoes within the anechoic, bile-filled gallbladder (Fig. 32.2). Distal to the bright echoes representing the gallstones, there is "shadowing" because of non-transmission of sound through the stones. This is seen as dark bands without any echoes similar in configuration to the beams of a car's headlights and is sometimes called the "headlight sign." Ultrasound is made more difficult in patients with copious bowel gas since sound is poorly

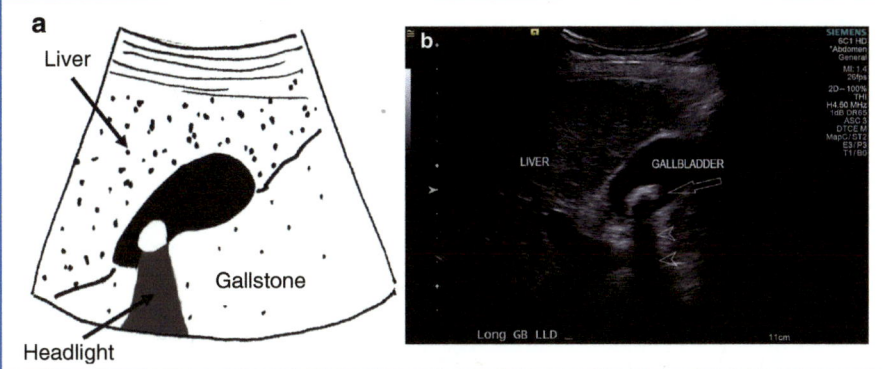

FIGURE 32.2 - GALLSTONES ON ULTRASOUND
In the above diagram (**a**) representing an ultrasound image (**b**), the gallstone (*white-lined arrow*) in the gallbladder has an acoustic shadow (*white-lined arrowheads*) behind it called the "head-light sign"

transmitted through air. Moreover, ultrasound is also difficult in very obese patients since the sound is greatly attenuated by the thick body wall.

Characteristic findings on ultrasound in acute cholecystitis include gallbladder distention, wall thickening (>3 mm), pericholecystic fluid, nonmobile stone in the gallbladder neck or common bile duct (CBD), and sonographic Murphy's sign. In the case of choledocholithiasis (stones in the CBD), the CBD may be dilated to 7 mm diameter or greater. Note that the CBD may be prominent even in the absence of an obstructing CBD stone if there is history of cholecystectomy.

Hepatobiliary Scintigraphy

Nuclear medicine studies may also be used in evaluating possible gallbladder dysfunction (see Chap. 37). These studies are often performed when other imaging is equivocal and additional evaluation is needed. A group of compounds in the iminodiacetic acid (IDA) group are employed. Each of these is labeled to a radioactive compound and injected intravenously. The compound is then selectively extracted from the blood pool by the hepatocytes and excreted through the bile ducts with subsequent filling of the gallbladder and spillage into the duodenum. This occurs according to a predictable time course.

Failure to visualize the gallbladder at the appropriate time may indicate a cystic duct obstruction (e.g., from gallstones) or some degree of dysfunction (such as is seen in chronic cholecystitis). An example of acute cholecystitis is given in Fig. 32.3.

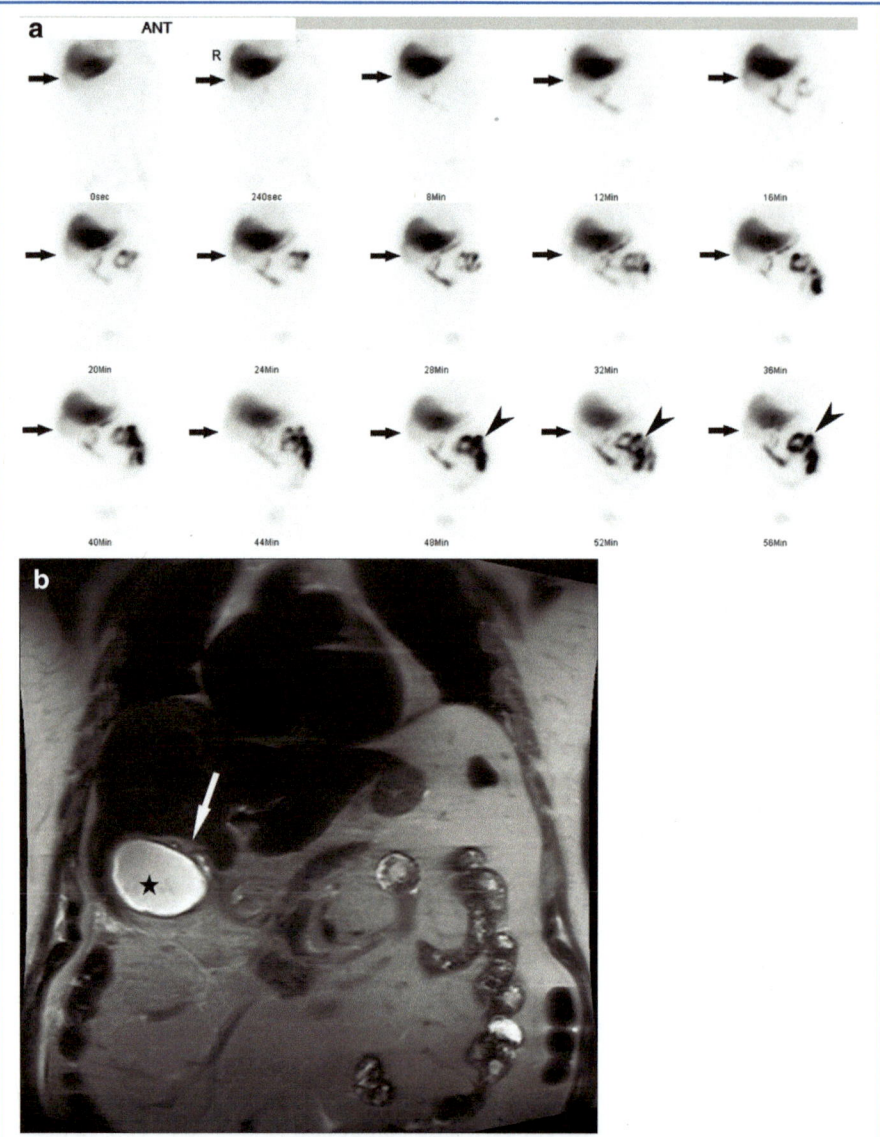

FIGURE 32.3 - ACUTE CHOLECYSTITIS ON HIDA SCAN
There is normal hepatic extraction of radiotracer and excretion/clearance into the biliary system
and eventually the small bowel (*black arrowheads*); however, there is nonvisualization of the
gallbladder in the gallbladder fossa (*black arrows*) on HIDA scan (**a**) consistent with acute
cholecystitis. For comparison, coronal T2 MRI of the abdomen from the same patient (**b**) demonstrates the location of the gallbladder (*star*) with associated pericholecystic inflammation
(*white arrow*)

Visualizing the Biliary Tree

Contrast may be used to directly opacify the biliary tree (Fig. 32.4). This can be done from one of three approaches (Fig. 32.5). A percutaneous transhepatic cholangiogram (PTC) is performed by placing a needle through the abdominal wall

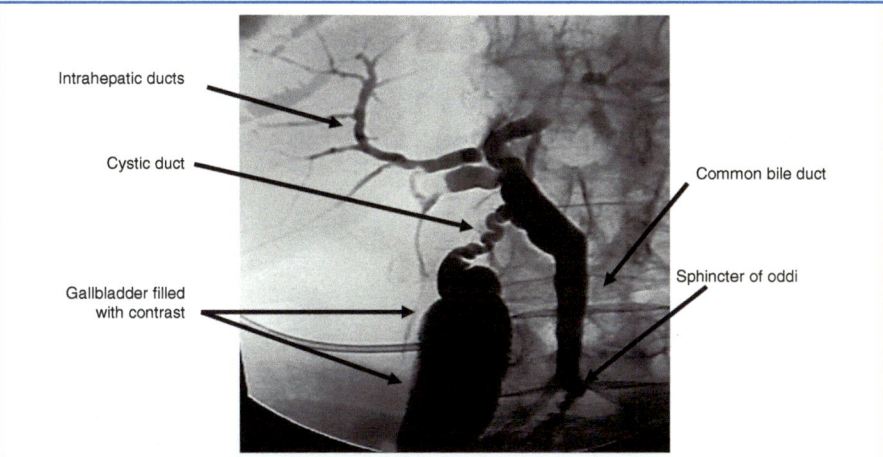

FIGURE 32.4 - GALLBLADDER AND ADJACENT STRUCTURES
On this cholecystostomy study, contrast is injected via the indwelling gallbladder drain. Note the contrast-opacified gallbladder and the cystic duct as well as the adjacent biliary structures

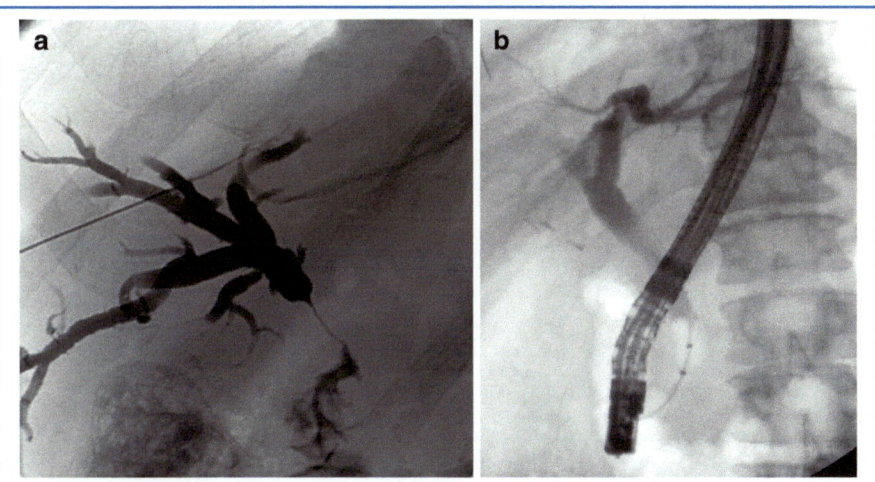

FIGURE 32.5 - PTC (A) AND ERCP (B)
In the PTC (**a**), contrast is introduced transhepatically. In the ERCP (**b**), contrast is introduced in a retrograde fashion

directly into one of the intrahepatic bile ducts. Contrast is then injected through the biliary tree and flows distally toward the point of obstruction. This is performed by interventional radiologists. Alternatively, gastroenterologists can cannulate the ampulla of Vater and inject contrast into the biliary tree in a retrograde manner through the endoscope in a procedure called endoscopic retrograde cholangiopancreatography (ERCP). This will likewise opacify the biliary tree and point out any filling defects or focal narrowing. An additional advantage of ERCP is that the pancreatic duct can also be visualized. Intraoperative cholangiograms are also performed by surgeons via direct cannulation of the biliary tree, typically the cystic duct.

Often, following gallbladder removal, a "T-tube" is left in place to serve as a stent and prevent bile duct obstruction immediately following surgery. When the question of a retained gallstone within the biliary tree or obstruction to biliary flow due to postsurgical stricture or edema is raised, contrast may be infused through the T-tube, opacifying the biliary tree and demonstrating whether or not an abnormality is present (Fig. 32.6).

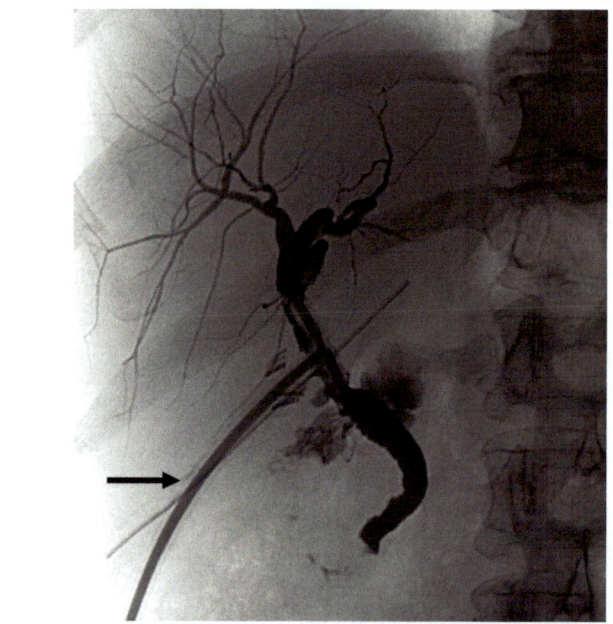

FIGURE 32.6 - CHOLANGIOGRAM
Contrast is injected through the T-tube (*arrow*) to opacify the biliary tree

Gallstones on CT

Finally, in the course of performing an abdominal CT for other reasons, gallstones may often be demonstrated as radiographically dense foci within the fluid-filled gallbladder (Fig. 32.7). Gallstones may not be seen on CT scan if they are composed mostly of cholesterol and not calcium.

Remember that the diagnosis of gallbladder disease and its complications remains complex and challenging. The use of a radiologist as a consultant to recommend and perform one or more of the appropriate studies described above will help to find the accurate diagnosis.

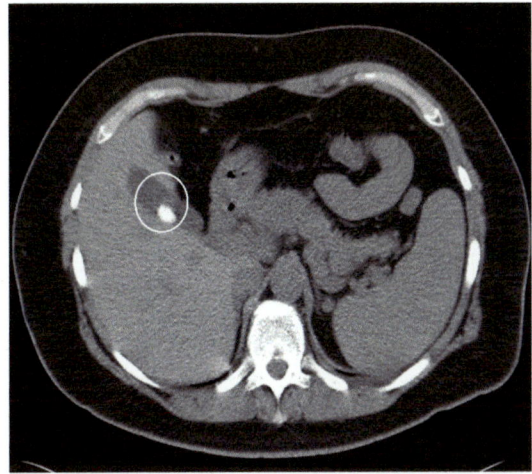

FIGURE 32.7 - GALLSTONE ON CT
Appearance of a gallstone with significant amounts of calcium on CT

S: Imaging evaluation of the hepatobiliary disease patient is a multimodality and multidisciplinary process and may include CT, MR, ultrasound, fluoroscopy, and nuclear imaging. Attention should be directed to aggregate radiation risk, contrast risks, and MR compatibility throughout the evaluation.

A: Initial evaluation of biliary disease is typically via sonography, with MR and nuclear biliary imaging reserved for more complicated cases or those requiring assessment of biliary tree anatomy and physiology, respectively.

F: Interpretation of biliary imaging requires knowledge of normal and variant biliary anatomy and physiology, as well as an understanding of complications and postoperative changes.

E: While many hepatobiliary findings may be non-emergent, acute findings such as cholecystitis, posttransplant ductal leak, or suspected biloma should be communicated to the clinical team without delay.

<table>
<tr><td>

33

</td><td>

INCIDENTAL ABDOMINAL LESIONS

</td></tr>
</table>

Objective:
1. Become familiar with the most common routinely detected incident lesions on CT scans.
2. Recognize standard of care management algorithms for incidental lesions.

Introduction

High-quality cross-sectional imaging has revolutionized medical and surgical diagnosis and aided in patient management; however, it has also led to imaging overutilization as well as the discovery of a large number of incidental findings that may require further evaluation to determine whether they may be safely dismissed or if further clinical care is required.

This chapter discusses several of the most common incidental findings and offers evidence-based management recommendations based upon the *Journal of the American College of Radiology* article on this subject [1]. The guidelines listed below assume a relatively healthy population with reasonable life expectancy. In patients with multiple or severe comorbidities or with limited life expectancy, these guidelines may not be appropriate, and decisions should be tailored on an individual basis.

Incidental Cystic Renal Lesion

Renal cysts are some of the most commonly encountered incidental findings. The Bosniak criteria are a well-studied evidence-based approach to the management of renal cysts. The Bosniak criteria describe five (I, II, IIF, III, IV) categories of renal

© Springer Nature Switzerland AG 2020
J. Kissane et al. (eds.), *Radiology Fundamentals: Introduction to Imaging & Technology*, https://doi.org/10.1007/978-3-030-22173-7_33

cystic lesions based upon distinct imaging characteristics. The concept is that the more purely cystic a lesion is, the more likely it is benign. The more calcification, solid components, enhancement, or thickened walls a lesion has, the more likely it is to be malignant.

Categories I and II do not require follow-up and include simple cysts, cysts with fine calcifications and/or thin internal septa, and non-enhancing hyperdense cysts. Category IIF (F stands for "follow-up") has indeterminate features and should be followed up at 6 and 12 months and then yearly for 5 years to assure stability. Categories III and IV should be referred for surgical consideration at the time of diagnosis (Fig. 33.1).

Size is not a determinant in renal cystic lesions. Interval growth or stability of a lesion may delineate benign from malignant renal cystic lesions.

Incidental Solid Renal Lesion

Renal lesions which are greater than water density may be solid, proteinaceous, or hemorrhagic. Lesions less than 1 cm are too small to definitively characterize with most imaging modalities. Also, it is important to thoroughly search for macroscopic fat within a solid renal lesion. If gross fat is identified in the lesion, then the lesion can almost always be diagnosed as an angiomyolipoma, a benign lesion composed of vascular, muscular, and fatty elements. Of course there are always exceptions,

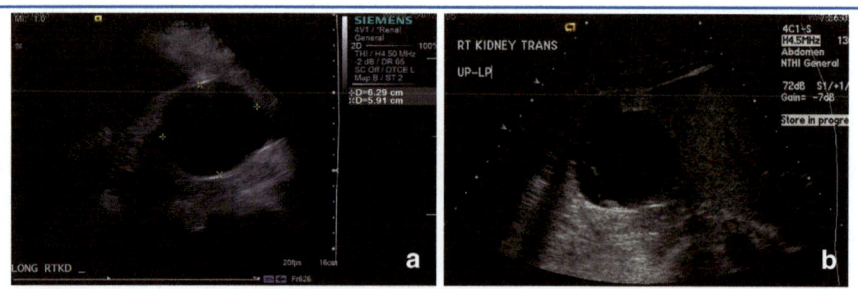

FIGURE 33.1 - (A) ULTRASOUND IMAGE OF A SIMPLE RENAL CYST
Features include well-circumscribed lesion, anechoic (black), thin imperceptible wall, and posterior acoustic enhancement (whiter area behind the cyst) consistent with a Bosniak I lesion. (**b**) Ultrasound image of a more complicated renal cyst. In comparison to image (**a**), this cyst has a thickened internal septation with nodularity along the wall posteriorly, rendering this a Bosniak III lesion at minimum

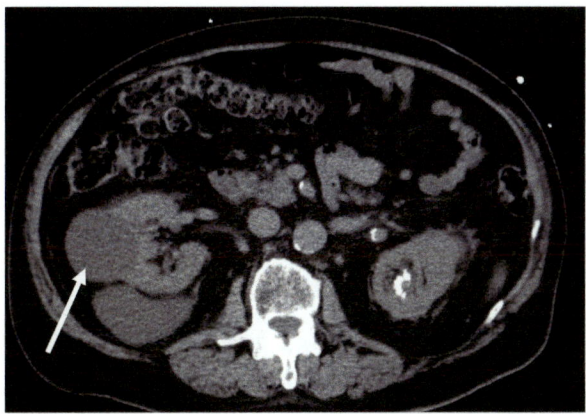

FIGURE 33.2 - LARGE SOLID RENAL LESION ARISING IN THE RIGHT KIDNEY
Given the intermediate density of the lesion, it is indeterminately characterized and warrants
further imaging evaluation

and rarely renal cell carcinoma can incorporate fat within it by enveloping the adjacent perirenal or central sinus fat.

Solid renal lesions have the potential to be malignant and need to be evaluated with an enhanced dedicated imaging study such as renal protocol CT or MRI (Fig. 33.2). Lesions that demonstrate any area of significant post-contrast enhancement are worrisome and should be referred for surgical evaluation.

Historically, biopsy of a renal lesion prior to surgical resection has not been routinely performed; however, a recent paradigm shift in urology has now led to an increased number of renal mass biopsies for lesions measuring under 4 cm to avoid the unnecessary resection of small benign renal masses.

Incidental Hepatic Lesion

Incidental hepatic lesions are common. In fact, nearly half of patients without malignancy have benign hepatic lesions at autopsy. Any hepatic lesion in an oncology patient must be evaluated to exclude malignancy. The recommended approach for evaluating incidental hepatic lesions involves assessing lesion size and patient risk. Despite a complex algorithm based upon these factors and imaging characteristics, the crux of the approach is that any size of a lesion in a high-risk patient needs further evaluation with advanced imaging (CT or MRI) and potential biopsy. The majority of benign lesions are hepatic cysts or biliary hamartomas (which do not

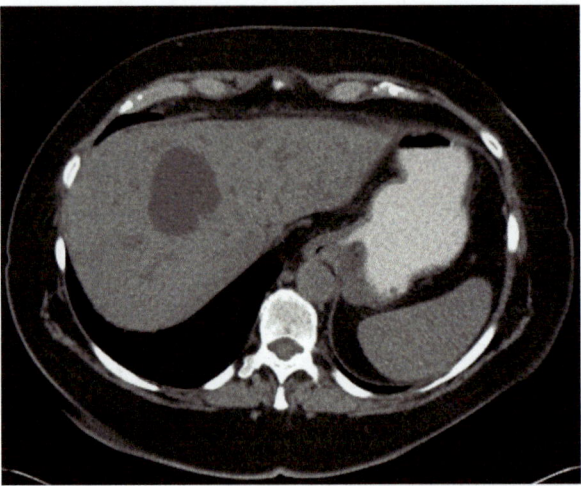

FIGURE 33.3 - LARGE HYPODENSITY IN THE CENTER OF THE LIVER
In a patient with a known malignancy, this would be concerning for metastasis. However, without that history, it most likely represents a large hepatic cyst

enhance) and hemangiomas (which can have a characteristic enhancement pattern) (Fig. 33.3). High-risk patients are those with known malignancy or cirrhosis or patients with risk factors predisposing to the development of cirrhosis (hepatitis, sclerosing cholangitis, etc.). In all other patients, the decision to dismiss or follow up is based upon size and specific imaging characteristics.

Incidental Adrenal Lesion

It is estimated that 3–7% of the population has an incidental adrenal lesion. Studies indicate that the overwhelming majority are benign nonfunctioning adenomas. Therefore, it is important to definitively characterize these lesions on imaging.

The assessment of incidental adrenal lesions is primarily based upon imaging features. If an incidental adrenal lesion has Hounsfield units (HU) of less than 10 on a non-contrast CT exam, it can be definitively diagnosed as a benign adrenal adenoma (Fig. 33.4). For lesions 1–4 cm in size that are greater than 10 HU, it is recommended that the patient be rescanned using a specific CT adrenal protocol. This protocol scans the patient at different time points after intravenous contrast administration to calculate a value termed "adrenal washout." The concept is that a benign adrenal adenoma will enhance and then quickly wash out the contrast, whereas an adrenal metastasis (and presumably adrenal carcinoma) will enhance and retain the

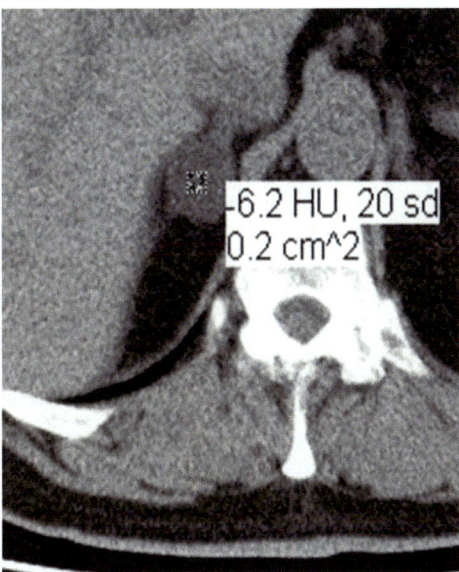

FIGURE 33.4 - NOTE THE ROUND LESION ARISING FROM THE RIGHT ADRE-NAL GLAND
The Hounsfield units measured −6.2 which is diagnostic of a benign lipid-rich adrenal adenoma

contrast (showing delayed washout). Biopsy should be recommended for a lesion with delayed washout. Lesion size and patient history of malignancy are also important factors. Lesions larger than 4 cm are likely malignant and are referred for possible surgical excision. Certain tumors such as functioning adrenal cortical tumors and pheochromocytomas are almost always associated with clinical symptoms and elevated biochemical markers in the patient's blood or urine.

Incidental Pancreatic Lesion

Incidental pancreatic cysts in patients without clinical or laboratory findings of pancreatic disease are relatively common findings. The most common cystic lesion found in the pancreas is a pseudocyst, which is a low-density collection typically developing as a consequence of pancreatitis 4–6 weeks after onset. Cystic pancreatic neoplasms are generally benign or low-grade malignancies. There are three main categories of cystic pancreatic neoplasms: mucinous neoplasm, serous neoplasm, and intraductal papillary mucinous neoplasm (IPMN) (Fig. 33.5). Serous tumors are benign but can enlarge. Mucinous tumors and IPMNs have a malignant potential.

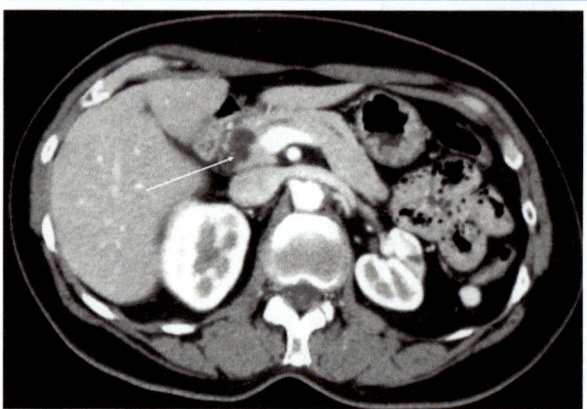

FIGURE 33.5 - AXIAL CT IMAGE AT THE LEVEL OF THE PANCREAS SHOWING A MULTICYSTIC LESION OF THE PANCREATIC HEAD

Table 33.1 Pancreatic cystic lesion follow-up

Lesion type	Follow-up
Cystic lesions, 2 cm or less	F/U MRI or CT at 1 year
Cystic lesions, 2–3 cm	MRI with MRCP
Serous lesions	Follow q 2 years
Lesion without classic radiology findings	Follow q 6 months for at least 2 years
IPMN	Follow q 6 months for at least 2 years

Size is the predominant variable used in the evaluation of incidental pancreatic lesions. In the absence of a recent pancreatitis, pancreatic cystic lesions less than 2 cm should be followed up with CT or MRI in 1 year. If the lesion is unchanged in size and appearance, no further follow-up is needed. If the lesion grows or changes on follow-up or if the initial lesion is 2–3 cm in size, MRI with MRCP (MR cholangiopancreatography) is generally recommended. If a serous lesion is diagnosed, then it should be followed up every 2 years. If an IPMN is diagnosed, follow-up is recommended every 6 months for at least 2 years. If the lesion does not have classic radiology characteristics, then annual follow-up is recommended. If the initial lesion is greater than 3 cm and serous neoplasm cannot be definitively diagnosed, then cyst aspiration using endoscopic ultrasound guidance should be attempted. See Table 33.1.

S: Contrast-enhanced CT can be safely performed when patient GFR is >45 mL/min. In the setting of moderately impaired renal function (GFR between 30 and 45 mL/min), a lower dose of IV contrast can be safely given along with IV hydration before and after the exam for most patients. Severe renal impairment with GFR <30 mL/min is often a contraindication for CT and MRI contrast.

A: Patients with mild IV contrast reactions can be pretreated according to various regimens, usually using a combination of steroids and Benadryl and then safely undergoing a contrast-enhanced examination.

F: Specialized imaging protocols are tailored for dedicated evaluation of specific pathology within organs including MRCP, adrenal protocol CT, renal protocol MRI, and various liver protocols for CT and MRI. It is important to specify the clinical question to be addressed in order to acquire the study appropriately.

E: Positive finding of an unexpected malignancy warrants a verbal communication to the ordering healthcare provider to expedite further clinical management. Frequently, the radiologist can help advice the clinician on the next appropriate imaging study.

Reference

1. Berland L, Silverman S, Gore R, et al. Managing incidental findings on abdominal CT: white paper of the ACR Incidental Findings Committee. J Am Coll Radiol. 2010;7(10):754–73.

34 INFLAMMATORY AND INFECTIOUS BOWEL DISEASE

Objectives:
1. Know the radiographic manifestations of bowel inflammation and the three general etiologies.
2. Know the radiographic manifestations of Crohn's disease (CD) and ulcerative colitis on radiographic, fluoroscopic, and cross-sectional studies.
3. Realize that there is considerable overlap in the radiographic findings found in these processes and that biopsy may be necessary for definitive diagnosis.
4. Understand the significance of toxic megacolon.
5. Understand the major advantages and disadvantages of fluoroscopy and cross-sectional techniques with respect to inflammatory and infectious disease of the bowel.

Colitis

Colitis is defined radiographically as colonic wall thickening of 3 mm or more when the bowel is distended (Fig. 34.1). Often the bowel wall in colitis will enhance after intravenous contrast administration. There are three chief etiologies in the differential diagnosis of colitis: infection, inflammation, and ischemia.

Numerous types of infections can cause colitis. Two of the most severe forms are pseudomembranous colitis and typhlitis. Pseudomembranous colitis is often a pancolitis. The toxin of the *Clostridium difficile* bacteria causes colonic mucosal ulceration which leads to the formation of pseudomembranes composed of mucin, fibrin, and inflammatory cells. Typhlitis is a neutropenic colitis that is classically seen in leukemic patients. It involves the cecum and/or ascending colon. Both of these forms of colitis may be severe and cause marked wall thickening and pericolonic inflammation and can result in colonic perforation.

© Springer Nature Switzerland AG 2020
J. Kissane et al. (eds.), *Radiology Fundamentals: Introduction to Imaging & Technology*, https://doi.org/10.1007/978-3-030-22173-7_34

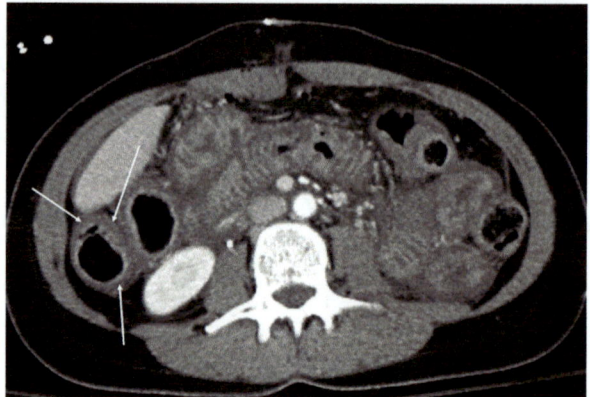

FIGURE 34.1 - COLITIS
Wall thickening of the ascending colon (*arrows*) related to a nonspecific colitis

Ischemia causes a segmental colitis. Segmental refers to the fact that only portions of the colon supplied by the vessel in question are affected. Ischemic colitis tends to occur at the watershed areas of vascular distribution: the splenic flexure and rectosigmoid regions. Figure 34.2 demonstrates ischemic colitis involving the cecum and ascending colon in a patient with atherosclerotic disease. When ischemic colitis occurs, it can progress to bowel necrosis with air in the bowel wall (pneumatosis intestinalis).

There are two common types of inflammatory colitis, ulcerative colitis and Crohn's disease (Fig. 34.3), though these are not mutually exclusive and there may be overlapping features.

Crohn's Disease (CD)

In Crohn's disease, also termed regional enteritis, bowel inflammation is transmural (involving the entire thickness of the bowel wall), may be discontinuous (with intervening skip areas of normal bowel between affected segments), and involves the entire GI system, anywhere from the mouth to the anus. The distal ileum and colon are most commonly involved. Though rarely performed anymore due to the prevalence of CT and MR enterography (MRE), the earliest radiographic findings on double contrast examinations of the colon are tiny aphthous ulcers which appear as white "pinpricks" in the mucosa as barium fills the tiny ulcers. These are very difficult to visualize with single contrast technique, though a single contrast exam is useful in quantification of disease-related strictures. CT scan does not show the mucosal abnormalities as well as fluoroscopic examination, but can demonstrate distribution and extent of disease.

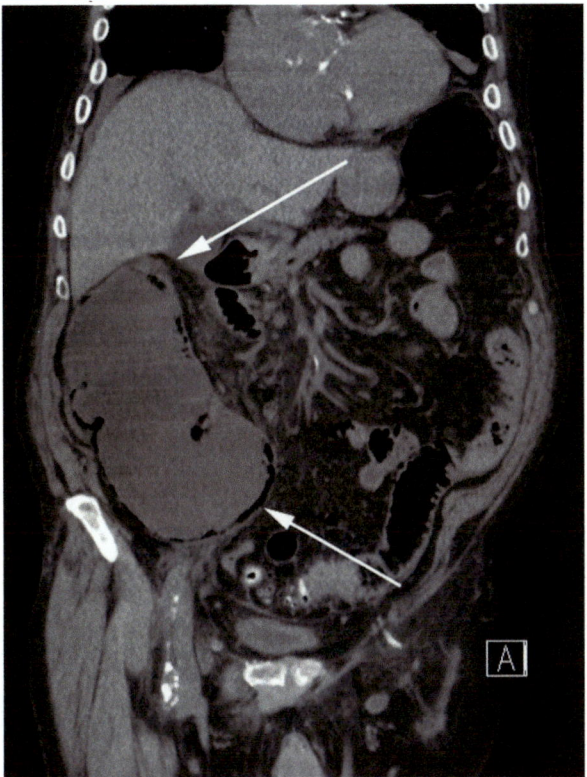

FIGURE 34.2 - ISCHEMIC COLITIS
Coronal CT image demonstrating ischemic changes in the cecum and ascending colon. Note the pneumatosis in the bowel wall (*arrows*) and inflammatory stranding in the pericolonic fat. Vascular calcifications are present in the right common femoral artery indicative of long-standing atherosclerotic disease

Crohn's Cobblestoning

Deep linear ulcers may form in Crohn's disease creating an intersecting network of ulceration which results in a characteristic appearance called cobblestoning (Fig. 34.4). Note how the ulcers are larger and deeper, not aphthous any longer. Cobblestoning may also occur in advanced ulcerative colitis, an example of the radiographic overlap in appearance between ulcerative colitis and Crohn's disease. Notice that patches of ulceration are often separated by completely normal mucosa commonly referred to as "skip" areas. With advanced disease, the bowel wall thickens and becomes fibrotic, sometimes with stricture formation. Again, strictures may form in either ulcerative colitis or Crohn's disease, another example of the radiographic similarity which may be present in these two processes.

CROHN'S DISEASE	ULCERATIVE COLITIS
Skip Lesions, Entire GI Tract	Confined to Colon
Eccentric	Concentric
Fistulae Common	Fistulae Rare
Pseudopolyps Seen	Pseudopolyps, 20%
Toxic Dilatation Very Uncommon	Toxic Dilatation, Uncommon
Rectal Involvement 50%	Rectal Involvement 95%
Perianal Fistulae and Fissures	Anus Normal
Terminal Ileum Strictured and Irregular	Terminal Ileum Dilated and Wide Open

FIGURE 34.3 - CD VERSUS ULCERATIVE COLITIS (GENERAL RULES)
There are several distinguishing characteristics separating the two entities, helping to distinguish them radiographically

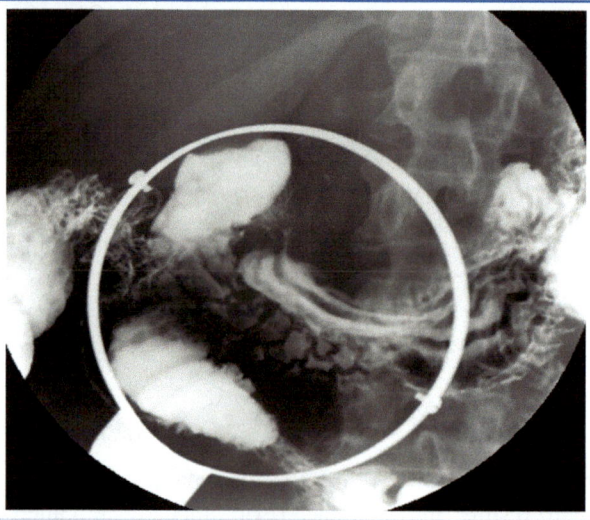

FIGURE 34.4 - CROHN'S COBBLESTONING
Cobblestone appearance of the second and third portion of the duodenum in a patient with known Crohn's disease. The ulcers fill with white barium and show up as white cobblestones

"String Sign" and "Lead Pipe" Appearance

Narrowing of the terminal ileum, often referred to as the "string sign," also occurs in Crohn's disease and is related to both spasm and stricture formation. Fistulas are a frequent complication of Crohn's disease and may extend from the cecum and ascending colon to the terminal ileum or the sigmoid colon. There is also a significant increase in the frequency of ileoileal fistula. Fistulas are optimally defined by single-contrast fluoroscopic examination (small bowel follow through) or cross-sectional enterography (typically CT enterography). Other complications of Crohn's disease include perforation, hemorrhage, and colonic malignancy.

At a more chronic stage, CD may cause diffuse fibrosis and spasm of the longitudinal muscles of the wall of the affected colon, giving a characteristic "lead pipe" appearance (Fig. 34.5) due to obliteration of the normal colonic haustral folds and typically involving the descending colon. Complications of CD include not only small and large bowel fistulas but also enterocutaneous fistulas, abdominal abscess formation, small bowel strictures, bowel obstruction, and perforation.

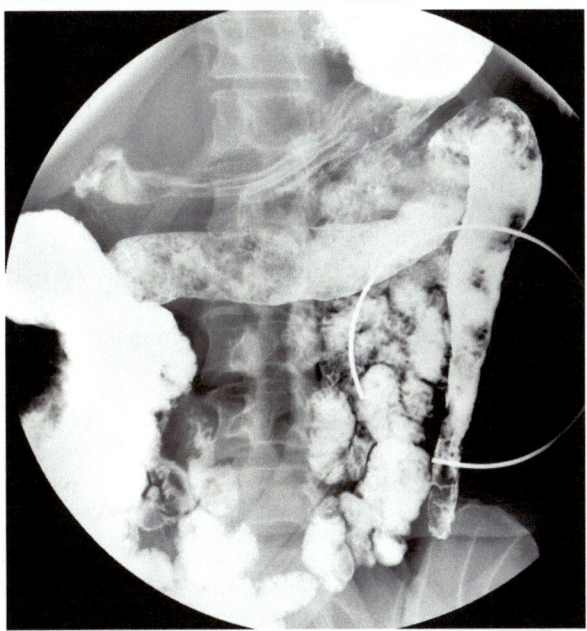

FIGURE 34.5 - LEAD PIPE APPEARANCE
Single-contrast enema in a patient with a long history of Crohn's disease shows the "lead pipe" appearance of the transverse and descending colon

Ulcerative Colitis

Ulcerative colitis begins in the rectum and progresses proximally. The rectum is spared in about 5% of patients. The colonic involvement is relatively uniform and symmetric. During the early stages of ulcerative colitis, the mucosa loses its normal even texture and demonstrates a finely stippled appearance through the barium coating of the mucosa. This is related to multiple shallow ulcerations with surrounding edema, which provide a granular appearance. In ulcerative colitis, inflammation involves the mucosa only and does not extend throughout the bowel wall. For this reason, fistula formation is much less common in ulcerative colitis than in Crohn's disease.

Polypoid Changes in Inflammatory Bowel Disease

Three types of polypoid changes may be seen in both ulcerative colitis and Crohn's disease:

1. Pseudopolyps are islands of inflamed edematous mucosa seen between denuded and ulcerated areas of the bowel wall.
2. Inflammatory polyps are areas of inflamed mucosa resulting in polypoid elevation.
3. Post-inflammatory polyps are seen in the quiescent phase of ulcerative colitis and may be composed of normal or inflamed mucosa.

All of these "polyps" are thought to originate from ulcerations of the mucosa with severe undermining. Long fingerlike outgrowths, called filiform polyps, are thought to be related to a reparative process. With healing, the colon may regain a normal appearance or may lose its haustra and shorten, resulting in the "lead pipe" colon, a sign of "burnt-out colitis."

Ulcerative Colitis and Colon Cancer

Patients with extensive, long-standing ulcerative colitis are at an increased risk of developing colorectal carcinoma. The incidence begins to rise steeply after 10 years of active disease. The risk is greatest when total colitis is present. Carcinoma in patients with ulcerative colitis is more likely to occur in multiple sites.

Rather than producing an intraluminal mass, colon carcinoma associated with inflammatory bowel disease may infiltrate and spread along the bowel wall, giving rise to deceptively benign-appearing strictures. Colon cancer is also more difficult to diagnose in patients with chronic ulcerative colitis because it is associated with symptoms related to or mimicked by the underlying disease. Colonoscopy and biopsy are used for long-term follow-up in patients with chronic pancolitis. In some patients, prophylactic colectomy may be performed.

Toxic Megacolon

Figure 34.6 shows a patient with toxic megacolon. Toxic megacolon is an acute nonobstructive dilation of the colon which is seen in different kinds of inflammatory bowel disease. This patient with a diagnosis of ulcerative colitis presented with fever, bloody diarrhea, and abdominal distension.

The diagnosis of toxic megacolon is manifested here by a dilated transverse colon, paucity of haustral markings, and some thickening of the bowel wall. Attempts should be made to identify this condition on plain radiograph because of the high risk of perforation. One of the most dramatic and ominous signs that may develop in the course of ulcerative colitis is this rapid development of extensive colonic dilatation and edema. Note that since the underlying colon is diseased, the chance of perforation is extremely high.

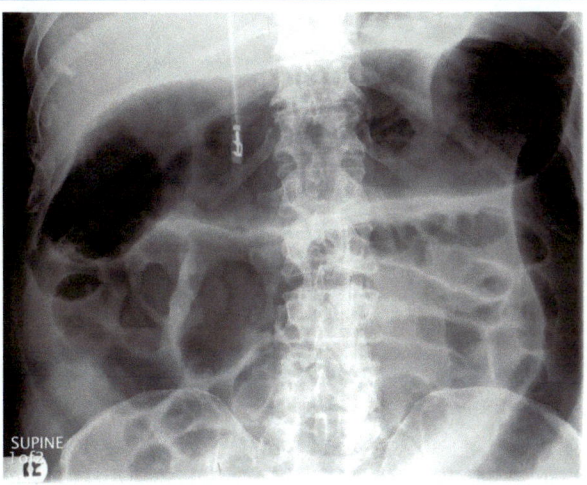

FIGURE 34.6 - TOXIC MEGACOLON
Megacolon appearance with a dilated transverse colon

Enterography and Advanced Imaging

Small bowel enterography can be used to evaluate for active or chronic changes of Crohn's disease. When traditionally performed with CT, the patient is instructed to drink dilute oral contrast and also receives intravenous contrast in an effort to demonstrate mucosal enhancement often seen with inflammation from Crohn's disease. In addition to mucosal enhancement, bowel wall thickening will be appreciated due to the inflammatory change and distention with oral contrast.

MRI is increasingly being utilized in the setting of inflammatory bowel disease, particularly Crohn's disease. Given the importance of minimizing ionizing radiation exposure in the setting of long term surveillance, MR enterography (MRE) is a particularly useful alternative to CT enterography and fluoroscopy in the young IBD population. MRI is also superior to CT in the evaluation of perianal disease and fistulae. Recent advances in MR technology allow faster acquisition times which decrease the effects of bowel motion which had previously degraded image quality. Before the exam the patient will drink oral contrast to provide bowel distention as they would with CT enterography. Bowel wall enhancement is assessed with intravenous gadolinium administration (Fig. 34.7). MRI findings in the setting of inflammatory bowel disease again will include bowel wall thickening, luminal narrowing,

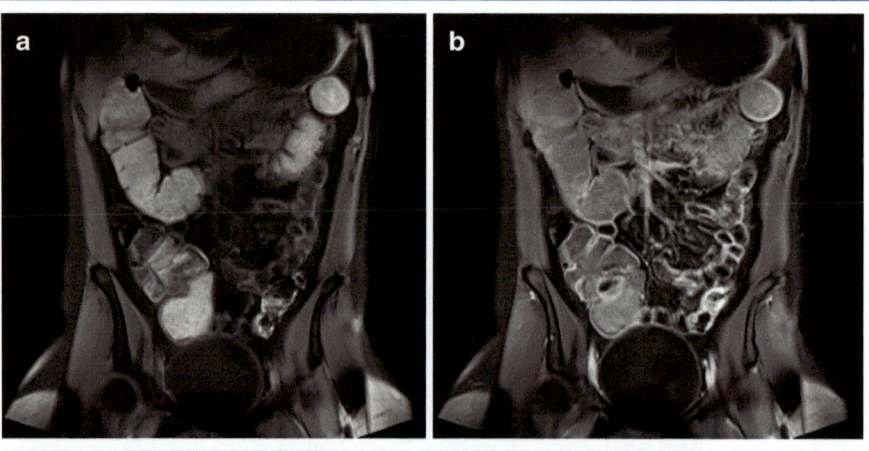

FIGURE 34.7 - MRI ENTEROGRAPHY
(**a**) T1-weighted image with fat saturation showing a normal image from MRI enterography. Note the PO contrast within the loops of large and small bowel. (**b**) T1-weighted post-contrast image with fat saturation demonstrating typical bowel wall enhancement and no focal inflammatory change

and avid enhancement in the setting of active disease. MR enterography has the added advantage of differentiating a fibrotic lesion from an inflammatory stricture and therefore helps determine surgical versus medical management.

S: Imaging of the patient with suspected inflammatory or infectious bowel disease should take into account risks of radiation, MR compatibility, and contrast exposure.

A: In the absence of an endoscopic exam, initial evaluation of these processes may include CT or MR enterography, the latter of which is preferred to mitigate radiation risk in patients who will likely require lifelong surveillance imaging. Once more common, small bowel follow-through exams and enteroclysis have become less utilized following the advent of CT and MR enterography.

F: An understanding of the pathologic processes and their CT and MR manifestations is necessary for useful interpretation of these exams. For example, it is important to understand that acute disease changes may manifest with increased mural enhancement, but that interpretation should also take into account the possibility of abscesses, strictures, or other sequelae of diseases.

E: The evaluation of infectious and inflammatory bowel disease is a multidisciplinary and multimodality endeavor. However, radiologists may be the first to detect early signs of inflammatory or infectious disease of the bowel, and these findings should be relayed to the ordering providers without delay, such that appropriate intervention can occur in a timely fashion. For example, the expedient identification of a pancolitis could suggest *C. difficile* infection, which is amenable to antimicrobial treatment.

35 INTRA-ABDOMINAL LYMPHADENOPATHY

Objectives:
1. List the various radiographic modalities which may be employed for the purpose of detecting abdominal and pelvic lymphadenopathy.
2. List two limitations of computerized tomography in the evaluation of abdominal lymphadenopathy.
3. Identify the following structures on a normal abdominal CT scan: aorta, inferior vena cava, kidneys, liver, pancreas, and spleen.
4. State the indications for intravenous and/or gastrointestinal contrast prior to an abdominal CT scan.

Lymphadenopathy

Lymph node enlargement, also known as lymphadenopathy, may be found in many conditions, both benign and malignant. Benign lymph node enlargement can occur in response to different infections such as tuberculosis and fungal disease. Malignant lymphadenopathy can occur in primary lymphatic diseases such as Hodgkin's disease and non-Hodgkin's lymphoma as well as other malignancies that metastasize to regional lymph nodes.

Computerized Tomography (CT) Scanning

CT scanning is an extremely useful method for detecting intra-abdominal lymph node enlargement. Lymph nodes appear as round or ovoid soft tissue structures many times surrounded by fat (Fig. 35.1).

© Springer Nature Switzerland AG 2020
J. Kissane et al. (eds.), *Radiology Fundamentals: Introduction to Imaging & Technology*, https://doi.org/10.1007/978-3-030-22173-7_35

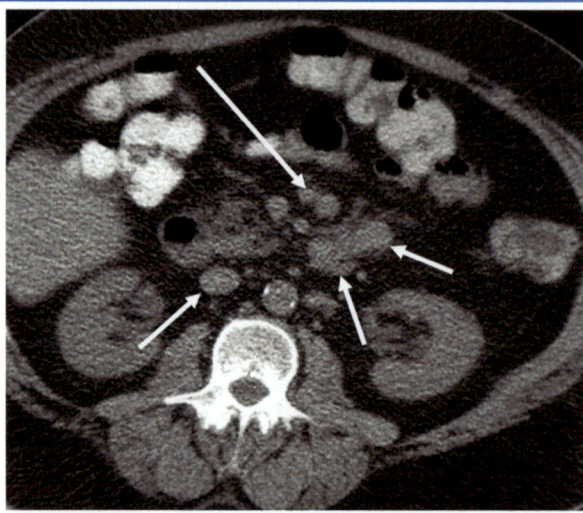

FIGURE 35.1 - ABDOMINAL LYMPH NODES
Mesenteric lymph nodes and para-aortic lymph nodes can be seen as abnormal soft tissue densities on CT scan

Lymph nodes are considered abnormal on CT when they are enlarged. Normal size criteria for a lymph node depend on the location within the body. One of the limitations of CT is that some lymph nodes may be replaced with tumor but not enlarged. Hence, there will be some false negatives where disease has replaced nodal tissue but has not enlarged the nodes. Similarly, not all enlarged nodes herald a malignancy; thus, false-positive cases may be encountered. Another limitation of CT scanning relates to the presence or absence of intra-abdominal fat. Since fat has a very low density on CT scan, it serves to separate and define the normal abdominal structures. In patients who are very thin or have a paucity of intra-abdominal fat, it may be difficult to distinguish the borders of normal anatomic structures from enlarged lymph nodes, thus limiting the study. The injection of intravenous contrast or the placement of contrast within the GI tract either orally or by rectum may help to define bowel loops and normal anatomic structures from abnormal masses. For this reason, patients may be asked to drink a low-density barium mixture; normal barium as used in an upper GI series would be too dense and create artifacts on CT, inhibiting the detection of abnormal lymph nodes. Other water-soluble contrast agents may also be used.

Intrinsic to the detection of abnormal lymph nodes in the abdomen is the ability to define normal anatomic structures (Fig. 35.2). Small blood vessels in the abdomen and pelvis can be confused with lymph nodes on single axial images. However, with the ability to electronically scroll through the examination on a PACS workstation, ovoid/round lymph nodes can easily be differentiated from linear vessels by following these anatomic structures over several images. Because of its capacity to distinguish different tissue densities such as soft tissue, air, fat, and bone, CT is the primary modality of choice in patients in whom an abdominal mass lesion or lymphadenopathy is suspected.

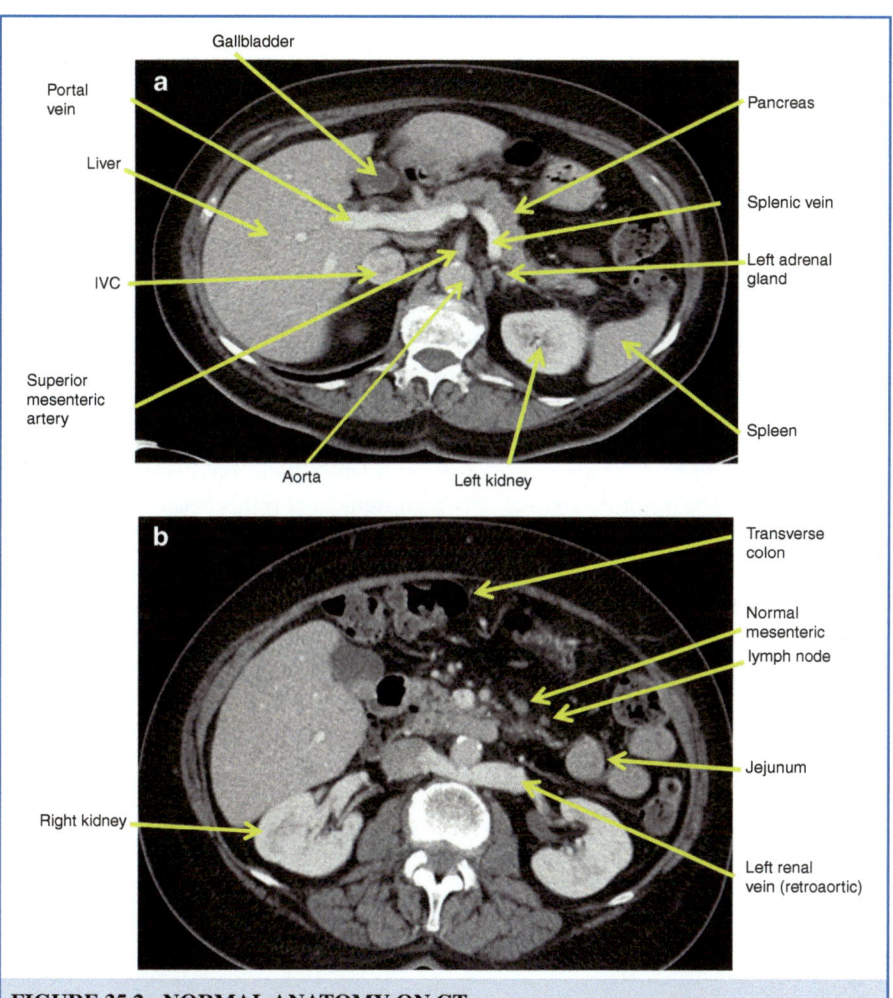

FIGURE 35.2 - NORMAL ANATOMY ON CT
Familiarity with normal cross-sectional anatomy is helpful in order to identify abnormalities such as lymphadenopathy on CT

In the case of malignant neoplasm spread to the lymphatic system, tumors can have typical or preferred nodal groups that will be involved in the earlier stages of the disease prior to diffuse metastasis. Organs often have a regional nodal chain that is responsible for lymph drainage and subsequently can be seeded with tumor causing enlargement. Malignancy of the esophagus and stomach characteristically involves the celiac, perisplenic, and gastrohepatic nodes. Hepatic and biliary cancer will spread to the portal and pancreaticoduodenal nodes. Lymphadenopathy of mesenteric nodes is associated with small bowel cancer. Right-sided colon carcinoma involves the superior mesenteric nodes, while left-sided cancers spread to the inferior mesenteric nodes. Classically testicular cancers will spread to the periaortic retroperitoneal lymph nodes due to their embryologic origin. For this reason, findings of periaortic lymphadenopathy in an otherwise young healthy male should prompt further investigation with testicular ultrasound.

S: Ultrasound is able to identify changes in lymph node morphology and echotexture in addition to size abnormalities with no radiation exposure to the patient.

A: Patients having undergone thyroidectomy for papillary thyroid cancer and neck lymphadenectomy for melanoma undergo surveillance imaging with neck ultrasound as standard of care imaging to evaluate for lymphadenopathy.

F: Enlargement of a lymph node is assessed by short axis in many anatomic locations, for example, at the porta hepatis, and axilla however is also assessed by long axis dimension in other anatomic locations, for example, in head and neck stations.

E: Imaging findings suspicious for primary or metastatic involvement of lymph nodes should be reported and verbally communicated if this is unexpected for the patient encounter. Management recommendations may include consideration of short-interval follow-up repeat exam, additional extent of disease evaluation with another modality such as PET/CT, or direct tissue sampling with biopsy depending on the patient factors including presenting history and location of the abnormality.

PART V
NUCLEAR MEDICINE

36 NUCLEAR MEDICINE CARDIAC IMAGING

Objectives:
1. List advantages of radionuclide imaging for calculation of the left ventricular ejection fraction (LVEF) over cardiac catheterization and echocardiography.
2. Describe principles of "electrocardiogram-gated" (ECG-gated) imaging.
3. Describe the physiologic rationale for myocardial perfusion imaging (MPI) of the myocardium.
4. Identify which type of stress is better for MPI.
5. List common radiopharmaceuticals used in MPI.
6. Define redistribution and which MPI radiotracer has this property.
7. Define normal, ischemic, and infarction patterns on MPI.
8. Define myocardial viability and list imaging approaches.

Multigated Acquisition (MUGA) Scan

The radionuclide ventriculography (also known as multigated acquisition (MUGA) scan, gated blood pool imaging, and radionuclide angiography) is performed by "labeling" a patient's red blood cells with ^{99m}Tc pertechnetate. Imaging of the blood in the heart is then performed, focused on the cardiac chambers and synchronized to the beating heart. The camera starts imaging each beat when triggered by the Q-wave on the electrocardiogram (ECG) – this type of acquisition is called *ECG-gated*, and it takes 10–15 min to obtain one planar projection.

Usually, three planar views are obtained (Fig. 36.1) – anterior, left anterior oblique (LAO), and left lateral views. The projection that provides the optimal angle for differentiating the activity of both ventricles is the LAO view, as the apex of the

J. Kissane et al. (eds.), *Radiology Fundamentals: Introduction to Imaging & Technology*, https://doi.org/10.1007/978-3-030-22173-7_36

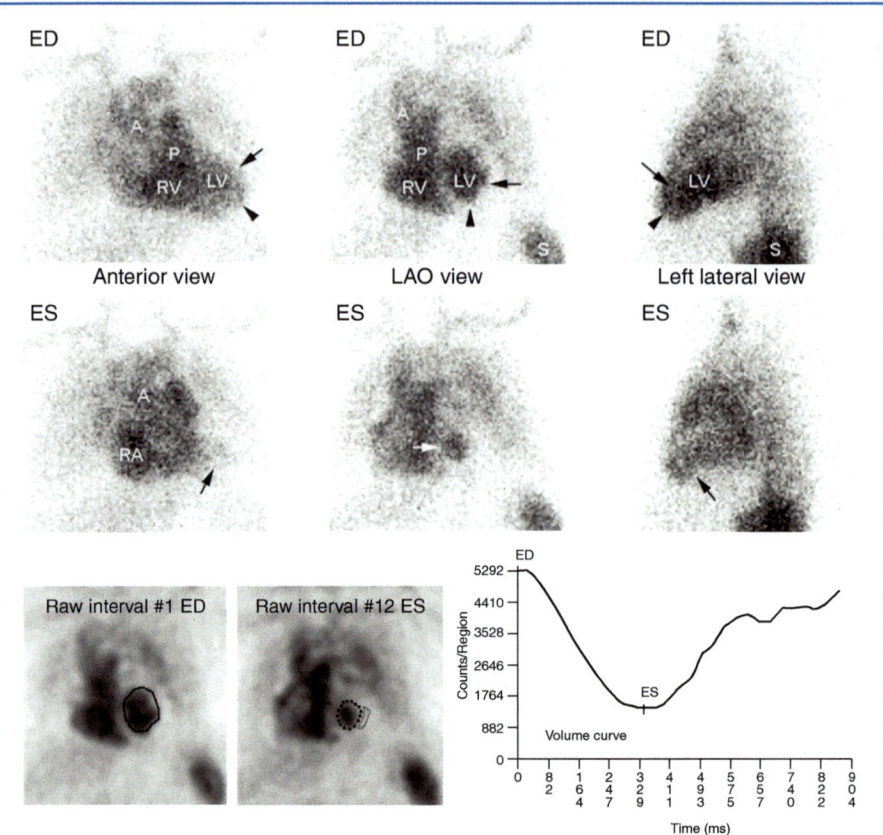

FIGURE 36.1 - MUGA SCAN
The acquisitions were obtained in anterior, left anterior oblique (*LAO*), and left lateral views for 29 intervals each. Activity in the left ventricle (*LV*), right ventricle (*RV*), pulmonary outflow conus (*P*), anterolateral wall (*arrow*), and apex (*arrow head*) is seen on anterior ED frame, while ES frame shows activity in the right atrium (RA), aorta, and inferior septal segment (*arrow*). LAO view depicts normal activity in the spleen (*S*) and the location of lateral (*black arrow*) and inferior apical (*arrow head*) segments on ED frame, while the septal segment is pointed out (*white arrow*) on ES frame. The anterior (*arrow*) and apical (*arrowhead*) segments are annotated on ED frame, while the inferior segment (*arrow*) is annotated on ES frame. Lower panel shows the ED and ES intervals with the LV regions of interest automatically identified by computer edge-detection algorithm. The same is done on every frame of 29 intervals, and those LV counts are plotted as the volume curve shown to the *right*

heart is angled toward the left side of the body. This allows the camera to look down the barrel of the ventricles, clearly separated by the septum. Some also refer to this as the "best septal view."

The MUGA calculation of left ventricular ejection fraction (LVEF) is volume based as follows:

$$LVEF = \frac{LV\,activity\,at\,end\,diastole - LV\,activity\,at\,end\,systole}{LV\,activity\,at\,end\,diastole} \times 100$$

LVEF can also be calculated using cardiac catheterization and echocardiography; however, the volume is estimated in these exams by a geometrical formula that does not account for variations in LV shape. Currently, the main indication for MUGA is the determination and monitoring of systolic function (LVEF) in patients with cardiac disease or at risk for developing drug cardiotoxicity, particularly from certain chemotherapy agents (e.g., doxorubicin, trade name Adriamycin). Normal LVEF is equal to or greater than 50%. The images can also provide information on chamber size and volume, qualitative regional wall motion, chambers' contractile synchrony, and diastolic function.

Myocardial Perfusion Imaging (MPI)

Myocardial perfusion imaging (MPI) is a technique that primarily depicts coronary blood flow at the level of myocardial tissue perfusion. It was initially imaged using planar scintigraphy, but single-photon emission computed tomography (SPECT) is now most commonly used because of its improved accuracy. Based on many of the same principles as computed tomography (CT), SPECT is a three-dimensional volume-based acquisition that can be reformatted into axial, coronal, sagittal, and oblique slices for complex image analysis and interpretation. This is ideal for the obliquely positioned left ventricle, as reformatted slices can be made to conform to the standard cardiac axes. This imaging can also be obtained with ECG gating, which allows not only for assessment of wall perfusion patterns but also assessment of three-dimensional wall motion and estimation of volume-based LVEF. While there is evidence that combined SPECT/CT may provide the best accuracy, it is rarely used because of the additional radiation exposure acquired from CT. Currently used gamma-emitting nuclear cardiology imaging agents include thallium-201 chloride (^{201}Tl) and ^{99m}Tc-labeled agents, such as sestamibi and tetrofosmin [1]. ^{82}Rubidium chloride (^{82}Rb) is a positron emitter used for MPI with PET or PET/CT.

^{201}Tl is a potassium cation analogue, transported in and out of the myocardium by Na$^+$/K$^+$ cellular pumps. ^{201}Tl uptake therefore reflects perfusion and myocardial cell viability. ^{201}Tl is injected intravenously at peak stress, and images are obtained in 10–15 min. Areas of ischemia and infarction are seen as decreased activity on the image, as neither narrowed or occluded vessels are able to dilate appropriately during stress. The patient is then allowed to rest, and *delayed* (*redistribution*) images are obtained 4 h later, at which time segments supplied by narrowed arteries will show similar flow as compared to adjacent healthy arteries, while areas supplied by occluded vessels will continue to show decreased activity. The study is usually completed in about 5 h.

The ^{99m}Tc-labeled agents localize in the myocardium by passive diffusion rather than active uptake and thus not as avidly as ^{201}Tl. These agents bind to intracellular structures such as mitochondria and remain bound without any significant washout (no redistribution). Therefore, the imaging approach is different from that of ^{201}Tl. Typically, a smaller amount of activity will be injected at rest and imaged first. Then, at peak stress (either peak exercise or with vasodilator administration), a larger amount of activity is injected and imaged in order to override the residual activity initially injected at rest. With these agents, the study is usually completed in 2–3 h.

The best form of stress during cardiac imaging is physical exercise performed on a treadmill. Exercise increases coronary blood flow and is also helpful in assessing exercise tolerance (symptoms and ECG changes that develop with increasing exercise), as well as the patent's hemodynamic response (blood pressure and heart rate changes). All of these findings are important for diagnostic and prognostic purposes, as well as clinical management.

A normal study should demonstrate homogeneous tracer distribution (Fig. 36.2). A perfectly normal study is rare in SPECT imaging, as there are commonly attenuation artifacts. "Attenuation" refers to blocking of photons from reaching the camera surface, commonly due to superficial soft tissue structures such as breast tissue. This can frequently cause areas of decreased activity, even in patients with normal perfusion. Considerable skill and experience are required to distinguish those artifacts from real perfusion defects.

Ischemic myocardium will appear as a perfusion defect on stress imaging that appears normal at rest (Fig. 36.3). If a defect on stress imaging does not demonstrate normal activity at rest, the defect is called *fixed*. This implies an area of infarction (fibrosis). There is a spectrum of defect severity, from slightly reduced activity to completely absent activity. The likelihood of coronary artery disease and risk of cardiac events and cardiac death increases with increasing severity and size of ischemic perfusion defects.

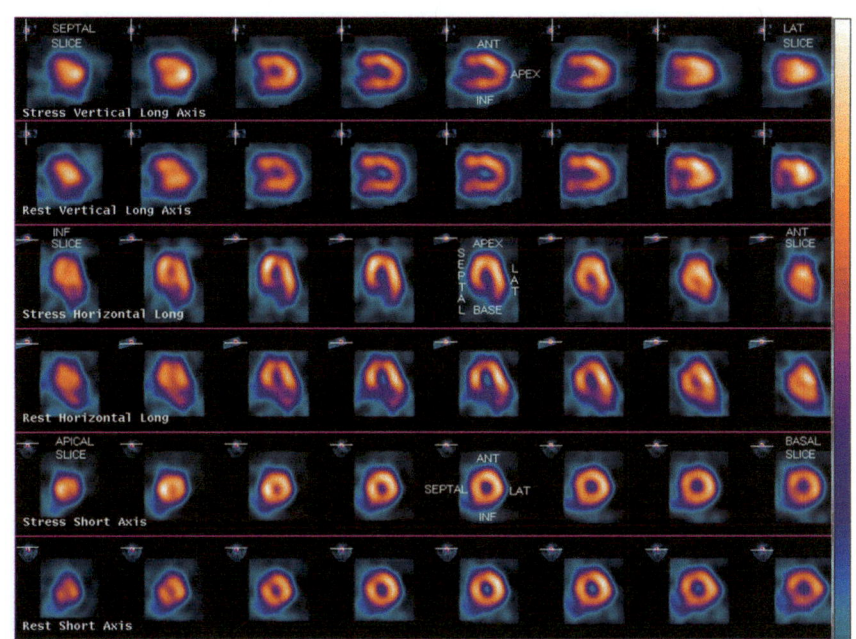

FIGURE 36.2 - NORMAL THALLIUM MYOCARDIAL PERFUSION SCAN
Normal thallium-201 SPECT slices are shown in three standard axes, post-stress on the top, and resting (or redistribution) slices on the lower row of each pair. The ventricle is displayed in relationship to the long axis of the left ventricle rather than the standard body axes. The major left ventricular segments are anterior (*ANT*) wall, inferior (*INF*) wall, lateral (*LAT*) wall, septal wall, and the apex. The opposite end of the left ventricle from the apex is called the base. The beginning and ending slices of each post-stress row are labeled according to their anatomic location. Notice the *color bar* at the right that shows relative color coding of activity, from lowest at the bottom to highest (presumably normal) at the top

Myocardial Viability Imaging (MVI)

Myocardial viability imaging (MVI) is indicated for characterization of myocardial cells in dysfunctional segments as either viable (alive and amenable to recovery of function) or nonviable (irreversibly damaged and replaced by fibrosis). This information is critical in some patients with coronary disease prior to bypass surgery. Since ^{201}Tl can characterize both perfusion and cellular metabolism (Na$^+$/K$^+$ pump function), it is used for assessment of viability in clinical practice. ^{201}Tl can be injected at rest with images obtained at 30 min and 4 h later for characterization of

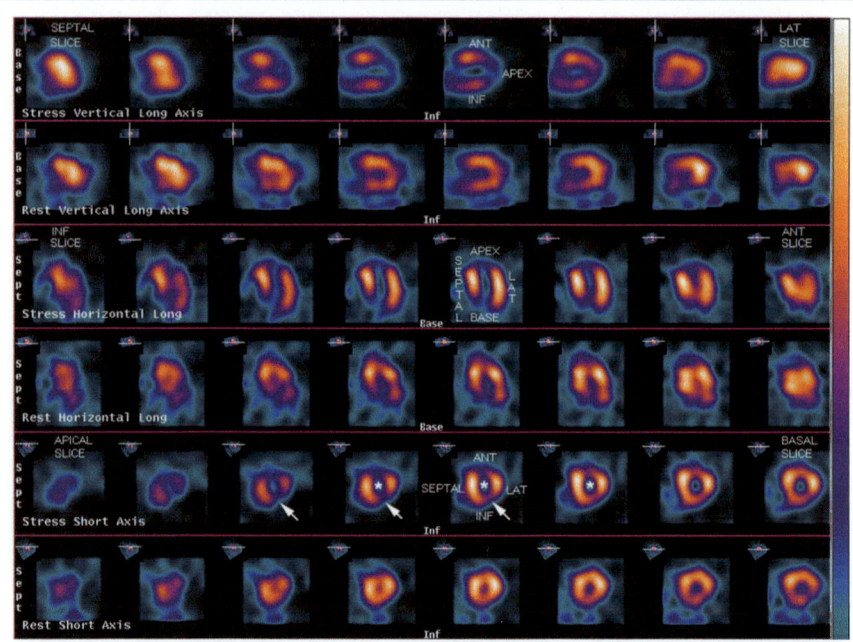

FIGURE 36.3 - ABNORMAL THALLIUM MYOCARDIAL PERFUSION SCAN
Thallium-201 chloride SPECT showing a severe perfusion defect on post-stress images involving the distal anterior wall, extending to the apex and periapical region. The 4-h-delay images show complete redistribution, consistent with severe ischemia in the left anterior descending (*LAD*) coronary artery distribution. The lesion is likely in the mid- to distal LAD, distal to the major septal branches takeoff, based on spared septal activity. Compare the inner cavity size on the post-stress, mid-ventricular short axis slices (annotated by asterisks) to the cavity size on the resting images. This is an example of transient ischemic dilation (*TID*), which is a sign that suggests significant stress-induced ischemia that involves more than one vessel. Indeed, there is also a moderate-to-severe inferolateral perfusion defect (*arrows*) that redistributes, consistent with ischemia in the left circumflex coronary artery

viability. Some patients may require another image at 24 h to demonstrate redistribution of activity into viable myocardial cells. Regions of the left ventricular wall with greater than 50% of normal segment uptake on any of the imaging sequences are considered viable.

S: In the investigation of myocardial ischemia, SPECT myocardial perfusion imaging (MPI) with ^{99m}Tc-labeled agents is an important first-line test in a patient with chronic chest pain and a high likelihood of coronary artery disease. Note that any modality in which cardiac stress is induced carries a risk of an acute cardiac event. It is important to closely monitor patients throughout the stress process, including a concurrent EKG and the presence of trained personnel to institute ACLS protocols if required.

A: ^{99m}Tc SPECT MPI is listed among the most appropriate tests for chronic chest pain in the presence of a high probability of coronary artery disease (ACR AC 9). Alternatives at this same level of appropriateness include chest radiograph, cardiac MRI, and coronary arteriography. SPECT MPI carries the highest radiation dose of these tests but provides much more detailed cardiac information than a chest radiograph, is much less expensive than an MRI, and does not require an arterial puncture in comparison to arteriography. Note that chest radiographs are often performed alongside other appropriate modalities to exclude other etiologies of chest pain. Stress echocardiography provides no radiation exposure but may provide less information if optimal views of LV are limited by a transthoracic approach (ACR AC 8).

F: ^{99m}Tc SPECT MPI is performed at stress and at rest. Stress may take the form of treadmill exercise or pharmacologic vasodilation. A diagnosis of ischemia is made when defects in myocardial perfusion are visualized on stress images but are not visualized on rest images, suggesting a flow-limiting stenosis in the corresponding coronary artery distribution. A myocardial infarction is diagnosed when a perfusion defect is seen in the same region on both rest and stress images, with decreased (or absent) regional wall motion on dynamic images.

E: A SPECT MPI examination that is positive for ischemia often leads to coronary arteriography for further characterization of the stenosis and immediate intervention with balloon angioplasty and possibly coronary stenting. Small areas of ischemia may be managed medically, while larger areas (or the presence of multivessel disease) may require coronary artery bypass graft (CABG) surgery.

Reference

1. Baggish AL, Boucher CA. Radiopharmaceutical agents for myocardial perfusion imaging. Circulation. 2008;118(16):1668–74.

37 GASTROINTESTINAL NUCLEAR MEDICINE

Objectives:
1. Define hepatobiliary scintigraphy.
2. Understand common indications for HBS.
3. List essential diagnostic criteria for HBS indications.
4. Define the gastric emptying test (GET).
5. List the indications for GET.
6. Understand the essentials about gastrointestinal (GI) bleeding scan test.
7. List the appropriate indications for GI bleeding scan.
8. Understand the critical plans that should be optimally made prior to GI bleeding scan.
9. Define the Meckel's scan and its indication.

Hepatobiliary Scintigraphy

Hepatobiliary scintigraphy (HBS) is a nuclear medicine test that uses a radiotracer that is extracted from the blood by hepatocytes due to its bilirubin-like structure. Thus, this tracer allows dynamic visualization of hepatocyte function (clearance of radiotracer from the blood by the liver) and bile flow (radiotracer passage through the bile ducts and into the bowel). The most common radiotracer used is ^{99m}Tc-mebrofenin. The most common indications for this test include acute cholecystitis (AC), chronic abdominal pain due to functional gallbladder disorders (also known as "gallbladder dyskinesia" and other terms), and postsurgical biliary leak. The imaging is usually carried out in dynamic 2D planar mode (Fig. 37.1a), but static 2D planar imaging and occasionally SPECT or SPECT/CT may be helpful to clarify or resolve uncertain findings.

© Springer Nature Switzerland AG 2020

J. Kissane et al. (eds.), *Radiology Fundamentals: Introduction to Imaging & Technology*, https://doi.org/10.1007/978-3-030-22173-7_37

The pathophysiological cause of acute cholecystitis is obstruction of the cystic duct. Nonvisualization of gallbladder (GB) activity on HBS functionally demonstrates cystic duct obstruction, which cannot be directly imaged by any other noninvasive test. Hence, HBS has the advantage of the highest specificity over other modalities such as ultrasound, CT, and MRI (which only show indirect signs of GB inflammation) and is indicated when other tests render equivocal results. The key to obtaining reliable HBS results is in careful patient preparation. For example, if the test is done shortly after a meal (which stimulates GB contraction and emptying), radioactive bile will not be able to enter the contracted gallbladder during the test and could cause a false-positive result. Treating a patient's pain with morphine for over 24 h before the test is conducted results in constriction of the sphincter of Oddi, forcing bile back into the GB due to the resulting back pressure, preventing flow of radioactive bile into the gallbladder and leading to a false-positive result. As such, avoiding morphine or other narcotic medications is essential prior to the test. In a properly prepared patient without recent narcotic use, however, administering morphine *during* the test would expedite GB filling by the same back pressure, expediting the results and enhancing specificity of the test.

The essential finding in functional gallbladder disorder is abnormal gallbladder emptying, tested on HBS by calculating ejection fraction (EF) following stimulated gallbladder contraction. Cholecystokinin (CCK) is a compound released by the stomach in response to a fatty meal, causing gallbladder contraction and release of bile into the small bowel to aid in the emulsification of fats for adequate digestion. In the HBS setting, this is imitated though the infusion of sincalide, a synthetic form of CCK. When stimulated, the amount of bile ejected from the gallbladder can be calculated as a percentage to measure the gallbladder ejection fraction (GB EF) (Fig. 37.1). The normal GB EF is 38% or greater (Fig. 37.1b) when 0.02 µg of sincalide is infused over 60 min. The slow infusion rate is critical, as infusion too

FIGURE 37.1 - HEPATOBILIARY SCINTIGRAPHY (HBS) AND GALLBLADDER EJECTION FRACTION (GBEF)

HBS of a patient with chronic abdominal pain (a) with normal hepatocellular function in the first 4 min as all radiotracer has cleared from the cardiac blood pool (*C*) and is concentrated in the liver (*L*). There is further normal biliary function seen in the top two panels: at 12–16 min, tracer is seen in the gallbladder (*GB*) and common bile duct (*CBD*); at 16–20 min, tracer is seen at the ampulla of Vater (*AOV*); at 20–24 min, tracer has reached the duodenum (*arrow*) and jejunum (*arrowheads*); at 56–60 min, there is further filling of the GB via the cystic duct (*CD*) and minimal tracer remains in the liver. Below the black line are images taken poststimulation with sincalide (synthetic CCK), demonstrating rapid, vigorous emptying of the GB which are used to measure GB EF as seen in (b). Post-sincalide composite image shows the GB region of interest (*ROI, black dotted outline*) which is corrected by the background activity in the liver (*gray broken outline*) as plotted on the graph over time (*white squares* connected by *dotted white line* representing GB activity; *gray dashed* line representing background liver activity on graph). The calculated GB EF of 88% is normal

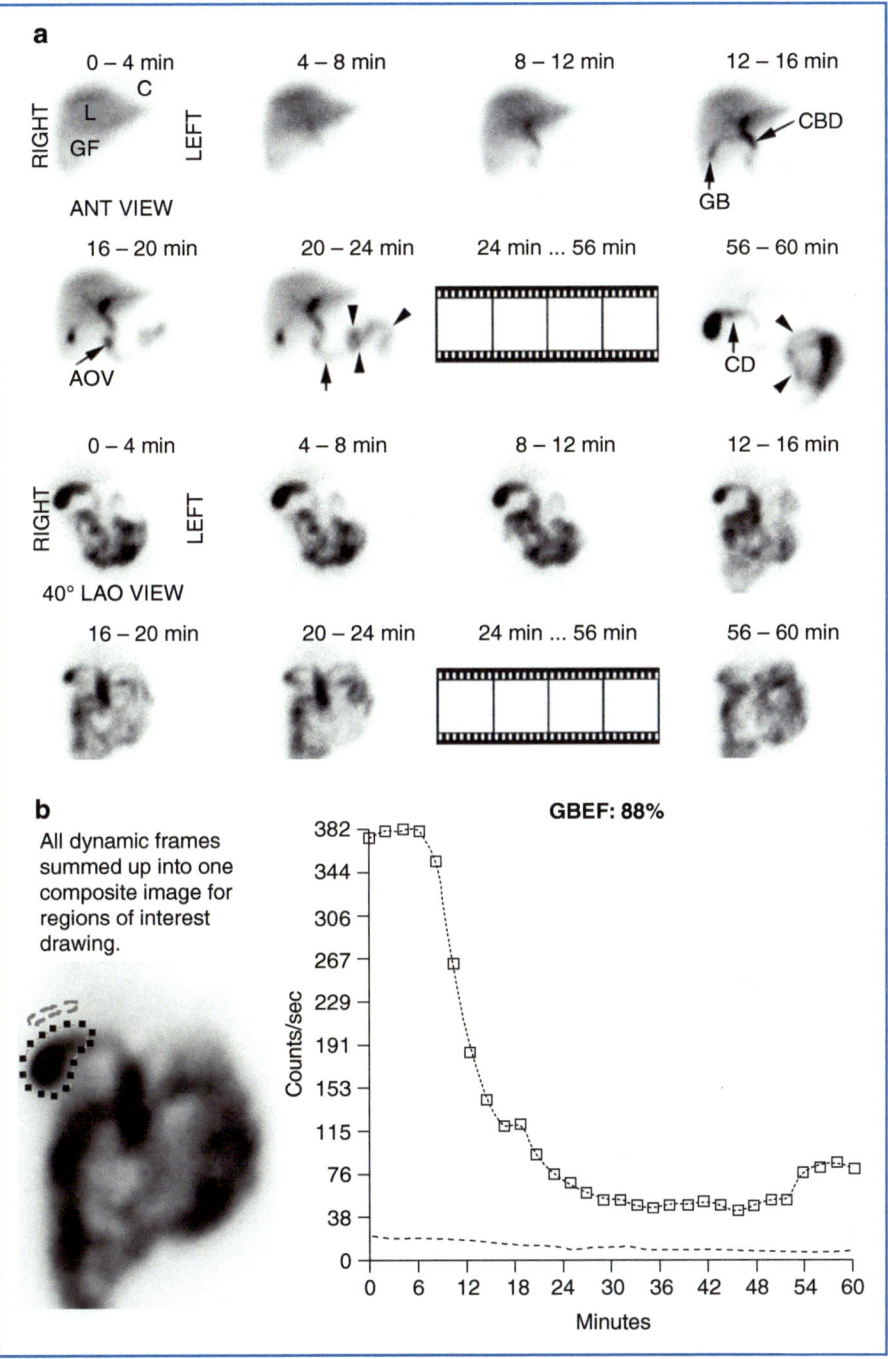

a

0 – 4 min   4 – 8 min   8 – 12 min   12 – 16 min

RIGHT   C   LEFT

L

GF

CBD

GB

ANT VIEW

16 – 20 min   20 – 24 min   24 min ... 56 min   56 – 60 min

AOV

CD

0 – 4 min   4 – 8 min   8 – 12 min   12 – 16 min

RIGHT   LEFT

40° LAO VIEW

16 – 20 min   20 – 24 min   24 min ... 56 min   56 – 60 min

b

All dynamic frames summed up into one composite image for regions of interest drawing.

GBEF: 88%

Counts/sec

382
344
306
267
229
191
153
115
76
38
0

0   6   12   18   24   30   36   42   48   54   60

Minutes

quickly may cause the patient to experience abdominal pain due to gallbladder spasm. Patients with abnormal GB EF often undergo laparoscopic cholecystectomy, which relieves their pain.

When cholecystectomy is complicated by an incompletely closed cystic duct or from injury to other parts of the biliary tree, HBS can also be used to investigate for a *bile leak*. A positive scan will show radiolabeled bile as it escapes (*leaks*) outside the biliary system or bowel lumen, showing its spread along extraluminal surfaces and the formation of discrete collections.

Gastric Emptying Test

The gastric emptying test (GET) quantifies and depicts the process of the emptying of a radioactively labeled meal from the stomach lumen. The international standard solid meal for this examination consists of egg whites (equal to two eggs) fried with ^{99m}Tc-sulfur colloid, two slices of bread, strawberry jam, and 120 mL of water. Indications for GET include functional dyspepsia, diabetic gastroparesis, and assessment of emptying before gastric surgery (e.g., fundoplication, etc.). Static images are obtained in the anterior and posterior projections at time 0 (immediately following food consumption) and at 1, 2, and 4 h after ingestion. The normal ranges for the percentage of meal emptied from the stomach are $\geq 10\%$, $\geq 40\%$, and $\geq 90\%$ at 1, 2, and 4 h, respectively. Emptying of >70% at 1 h is considered rapid gastric emptying (i.e., dumping syndrome).

If a solid meal cannot be used, 300–500 mL of water labeled with radiotracer can be used as an alternative. Of note, solid meals empty in a linear fashion, while liquid meals empty exponentially. Whole milk or baby formula labeled with ^{99m}Tc-sulfur colloid can be used for gastric emptying in small children and is called a "milk scan." Note that due to curdling of the milk when it interacts with stomach acid, it effectively becomes a solid meal when consumed. In addition to gastric emptying, the study also evaluates gastroesophageal reflux, which is another common problem in small children and neonates who have failure to thrive.

Gastrointestinal Bleeding Scintigraphy

Gastrointestinal (GI) bleeding scintigraphy scans dynamically depict blood pool distribution and can identify active extravasation of blood into the intestinal lumen. ^{99m}Tc-labeled autologous red blood cells (^{99m}Tc-RBCs) are used for this study, and labeling can be performed in any nuclear medicine facility using a commercial kit. It requires 1–3 mL of whole blood, and the entire labeling process is completed within 20 min. Once started, the scan protocol can continuously and/or intermittently monitor for bleeding over the ensuing 24 h. GI bleeding is typically intermittent, and active blood loss is difficult to evaluate clinically. Given this, GI bleeding scintigraphy is the most sensitive modality for detection of occult GI bleeding, as it can detect as little as 0.04 mL/min of blood loss.

Figure 37.2 demonstrates a normal distribution of ^{99m}Tc-RBCs first, followed by the appearance of a small bowel bleed. This demonstrates the location of active bleeding and will help other services, such as interventional radiology, identify and embolize the culprit vessel more quickly. It should be noted that the longer the time elapsed following visualization of an active bleed on GI bleeding scan, the less likely it will still be present on angiography as GI bleeding is typically intermittent. Therefore, it is critical to have a clear plan in place with involved services (angiography and/or surgery) to intervene before a patient arrives for the scan. If the next step in clinical management is not considered until after active bleeding has been found on the scan, the time needed for decision making and action will often cause a lengthy delay and may allow the bleeding to stop and render subsequent angiography futile.

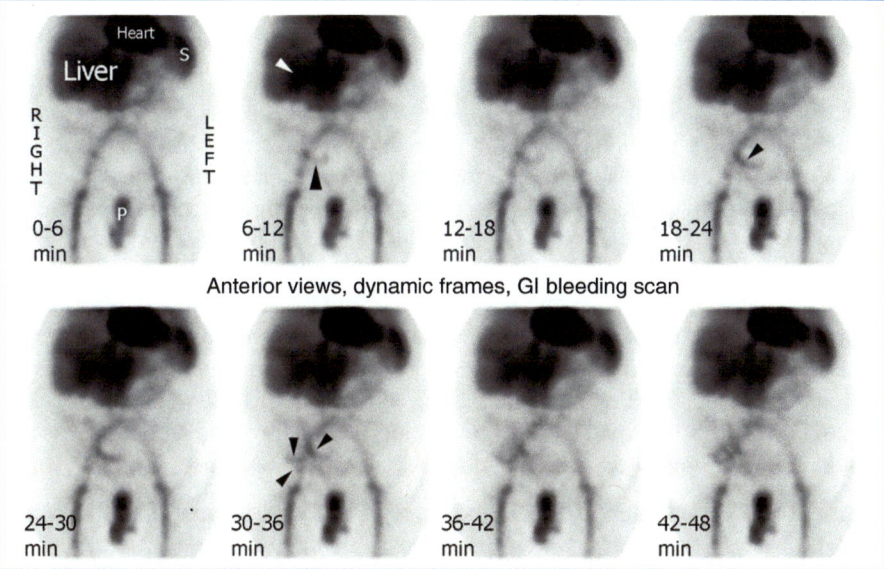

Anterior views, dynamic frames, GI bleeding scan

FIGURE 37.2 - GASTROINTESTINAL BLEEDING SCAN
Gastrointestinal bleeding scan with initial normal tracer activity in the blood pool: heart, aorta, vena cava, iliac vessels, liver, spleen (*S*), and cavernous body of the penis (*P*). The subtle curvilinear activity along the liver (*white arrowhead*) is normal tracer in the porto-hepatic vessels. On the 6–12 min frame, there is a new subtle curvilinear area of activity (*black arrowhead*) to the right of the abdominal midline. Its central position suggests small bowel. However, diagnostic definition of active GI bleeding requires two additional criteria: change in intensity and movement. The intensity of this activity grows with time, as seen on 18–24 min frame and at 30–36 min, the activity moves in a loopy zigzag pattern, typical for the small bowel. Of note, the activity in the penis can be confused with rectal bleeding. While this activity also becomes more intense, it doesn't move, therefore not fulfilling the bleeding criteria

Although a GI bleeding study can diagnose upper GI bleeding (above the ligament of Treitz) with high sensitivity, it is not indicated as the initial workup. If gastric aspirates through nasogastric tube and/or endoscopy are negative, then it becomes reasonable to pursue a GI bleeding scan. In contrast, a GI bleeding scan *is* indicated in the initial workup of acute lower GI bleeding. Colonoscopy is of limited value because intraluminal blood makes visual identification of the bleeding source difficult. Angiography can be used to both diagnose and treat a lower GI bleed. To detect bleeding during angiography, however, the patient must be actively bleeding at approximately 1 mL/min during the few seconds it takes for the iodinated contrast to pass through the arteries. A tagged RBC study does not have this limitation, given the ability to image the patient continuously for 1–2-h intervals over up to 24 h if needed. Continuous imaging increases the likelihood of detecting an intermittent active bleed and allows for localization of the site of bleeding (small bowel, ascending colon, transverse colon, descending colon, or rectum).

Meckel's Scan

A Meckel's scan is aimed at identifying the presence of ectopic gastric mucosa in a Meckel's diverticulum in the small intestine, which is present at birth and is a vestigial remnant of the omphalomesenteric duct. It contains heterotopic rests of gastric mucosa, which may lead to peptic ulceration and bleeding. The typical patient is a young child who presents with GI bleeding. The radiopharmaceutical is ^{99m}Tc-pertechnetate, which is avidly taken up by the chief cells of the gastric mucosa. The study takes about 1.5 h and shows uptake in the right lower abdominal quadrant that appears simultaneously with normal gastric uptake and increases in activity over time (Fig. 37.3). Note that some Meckel's diverticula contain a different tissue type than gastric mucosa (i.e., pancreatic tissue). Diverticula that do not contain gastric mucosa cannot be identified by this scan, as the chief cells of the gastric mucosa are required for radiotracer extraction and subsequent visualization.

S: Ultrasound examination of the abdomen is usually performed first in a patient with fever, right upper quadrant pain, elevated WBC, and a positive Murphy's sign, as it provides no ionizing radiation and can be performed rapidly. If these findings are inconclusive or equivocal, the addition of other modalities that do involve ionizing radiation may be required.

A: Abdominal ultrasound is the most appropriate first examination to perform in the patient described above (ACR AC 9). Unfortunately, ultrasound findings can often be equivocal, especially when patients have received pain medication in the emergency department that renders the Murphy's sign unreliable. In these situations, cholescintigraphy (ACR AC 6) is an appropriate next step as it provides valuable physiologic information at a lower cost than MRI (ACR AC 6), does not

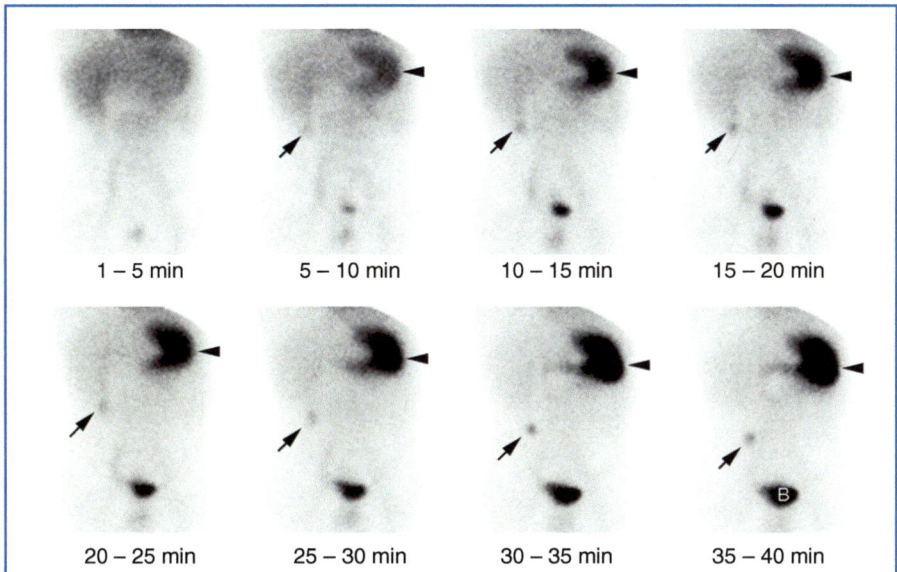

FIGURE 37.3 - MECKEL'S SCAN
Meckel's scan on a 3-year-old child with an episode of bright red blood per rectum 24 h ago. Radiotracer uptake is seen in the stomach (*arrowhead*) and in an extra-gastric focus (*arrow*) in the right mid-abdomen. Over time, both areas show progressively increasing activity that occurs simultaneously, consistent with a gastric mucosa containing Meckel's diverticulum. The extra-gastric focus moves during the acquisition, typical of a Meckel's diverticulum as it is rather mobile on a relatively long mesentery. There is normal physiologic excretion of tracer seen in the urinary bladder (*B*)

involve contrast of any type, and provides less radiation exposure than CT of the abdomen (ACR AC 6).

F: Absence of gallbladder filling with radiolabeled bile at the conclusion of 60 min of dynamic imaging is concerning of cystic duct obstruction and thus acute calculous cholecystitis in the appropriate clinical setting. To confirm this diagnosis and limit false-positive examinations, morphine can be administered (0.04 mg/kg) to contract the sphincter of Oddi and force bile back up into the cystic duct. If the gallbladder is not visualized at 30 min, the diagnosis can be made. In the presence of a morphine allergy, imaging of the patient should be performed in 4 h to confirm absence of gallbladder filling.

E: Findings consistent with acute calculous cholecystitis must be immediately relayed to primary clinical service via direct verbal communication to expedite surgical consultation and cholecystectomy. A definitive diagnosis by cholescintigraphy may help defer unnecessary radiation exposure looking for another cause of the patient's pain.

38 ONCOLOGIC NUCLEAR MEDICINE

Objectives:
1. Explain the principle of positron emission tomography (PET).
2. Describe the patient preparation for F-18 FDG PET/CT.
3. List the most common indications for F-18 FDG PET/CT.
4. State the most common PET pitfalls.
5. List common indications for lymphoscintigraphy.
6. Explain the concept of sentinel lymph node.
7. State the principle of radioactive iodine (RAI) whole-body scan and treatment for thyroid cancer.

Positron Emission Tomography (PET)

Positron emission tomography (PET) is an imaging method that depicts the distribution of positron-emitting radiopharmaceuticals within the body. Oncological imaging is currently the main clinical application of PET, but numerous other applications, such as cardiac imaging and others, are under continued development.

A positron is the positively charged counterpart of an electron (the antimatter equivalent). It is emitted from the nucleus during a decay process and undergoes an annihilation reaction with a free-floating electron, transforming their combined mass into energy. This energy is emitted as two 511 keV gamma photons traveling in directions directly opposite (i.e., 180°) from each other. These photons strike opposite sides of the PET scanner's ring of detectors simultaneously, and computational algorithms reconstruct the image by localizing the annihilation events from the collected data (Fig. 38.1).

The most commonly used positron-emitting isotope and radiopharmaceutical in medicine today are fluorine-18 (^{18}F) and ^{18}F-fluorodeoxyglucose (^{18}FDG). ^{18}FDG is

© Springer Nature Switzerland AG 2020
J. Kissane et al. (eds.), *Radiology Fundamentals: Introduction to Imaging & Technology*, https://doi.org/10.1007/978-3-030-22173-7_38

administered IV, and most facilities today use hybrid PET/CT cameras to image it (Fig. 38.2). [18]FDG is a glucose analogue whose cellular uptake is directly proportional to the metabolic demands of the cell. Unlike glucose, as hexokinase phosphorylates [18]FDG during the glycolytic process, it becomes trapped in the cell and can neither progress further along the glycolytic pathway nor escape the cell, allowing for its localization and measurement. An overwhelming majority of tumors have high metabolic demands that result in increased glycolysis and hexokinase activity to provide the energy required for rapid growth. This process is elegantly portrayed on the [18]FDG PET/CT images (Fig. 38.3).

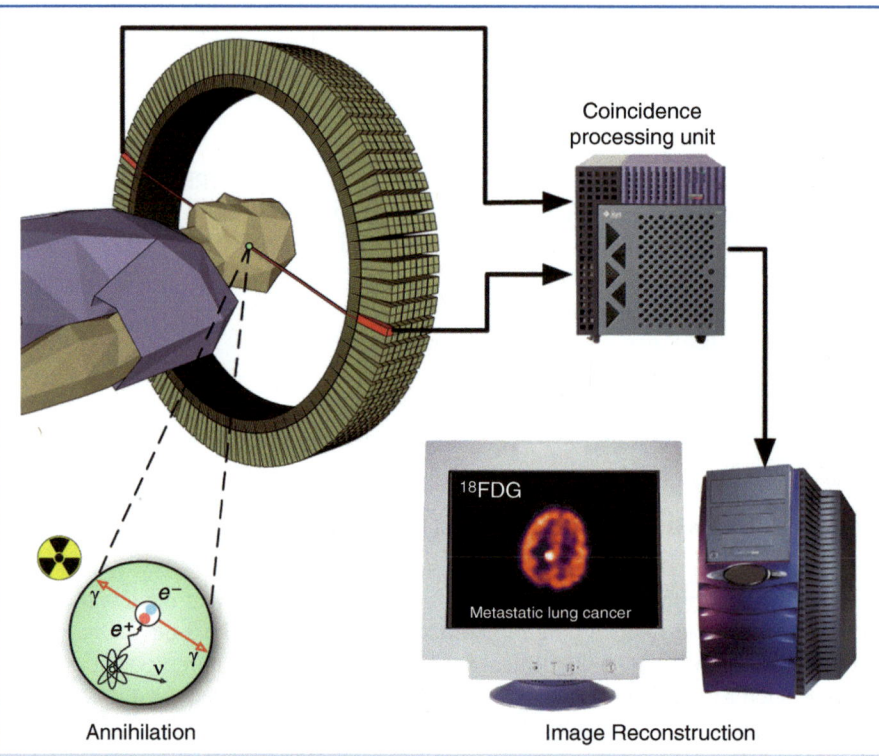

FIGURE 38.1 - PET PRINCIPLES
This diagram illustrates the processing principles of positron emission tomography (*PET*). A positron (e⁺) is emitted from the nucleus of the isotope and collides with an electron (e⁻), resulting in an annihilation event that transforms their mass into two gamma photons emitted in diametrically opposite directions. These photons are registered by the scanner's detector (the large ring surrounding the patient). After this event is registered, the data is forwarded to a processing unit which determines if the two events are coincident events (occurring at the same time) or not. All coincidences are forwarded to the image processing unit where the final image is produced via mathematical image reconstruction processes. (This figure is modified from the image released into the public domain by the author, Jens Langner)

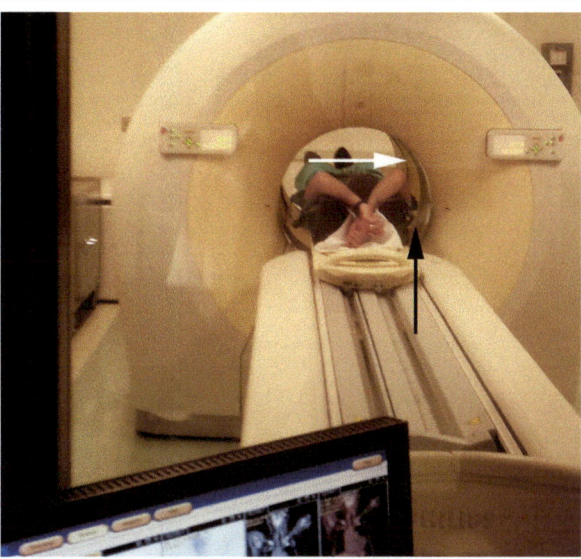

FIGURE 38.2 - PET/CT SCANNER
Photograph of a PET/CT scanner taken from the control room, which is separated from the scanner by leaded glass and a lead-lined wall to shield staff from CT-generated X-rays and patient-emitted gamma rays. The camera contains two imaging rings: the CT gantry (*black arrow*) and the PET detector (*white arrow*). Images are reconstructed by a dedicated imaging computer and checked by the technologist before submitting the study for evaluation to the interpreting physician

Careful patient preparation prior to the study is important for two main reasons: (1) to decrease ^{18}FDG uptake in a normal myocardium, which improves sensitivity for tumor detection in a myocardium or pericardium, and (2) to create a favorable environment for ^{18}FDG uptake in a tumor. Myocardium favors glycolysis for its energy needs but can also use fatty acids during carbohydrate deprivation. As such, patients are instructed to maintain a low-carbohydrate diet for a few days prior to the scan. They are also asked to fast for at least 6 h prior to ^{18}FDG injection. Fasting prevents the physiological movement of glucose and ^{18}FDG into skeletal muscles, which would limit the available ^{18}FDG for tumor uptake. Special care is needed in preparing patients with diabetes mellitus for their scan, as high glucose levels (usually above 200 mg/dL) can competitively inhibit ^{18}FDG uptake by tumors. Furthermore, administration of insulin to decrease glucose levels within a few hours of the test causes similar ^{18}FDG movement into the skeletal muscle and must be avoided. Similarly, increased glucose utilization in brown adipose tissue can be stimulated by exposure to cold and is reflected by intense ^{18}FDG uptake. This can obscure findings and degrade test accuracy. Therefore, patients are encouraged to

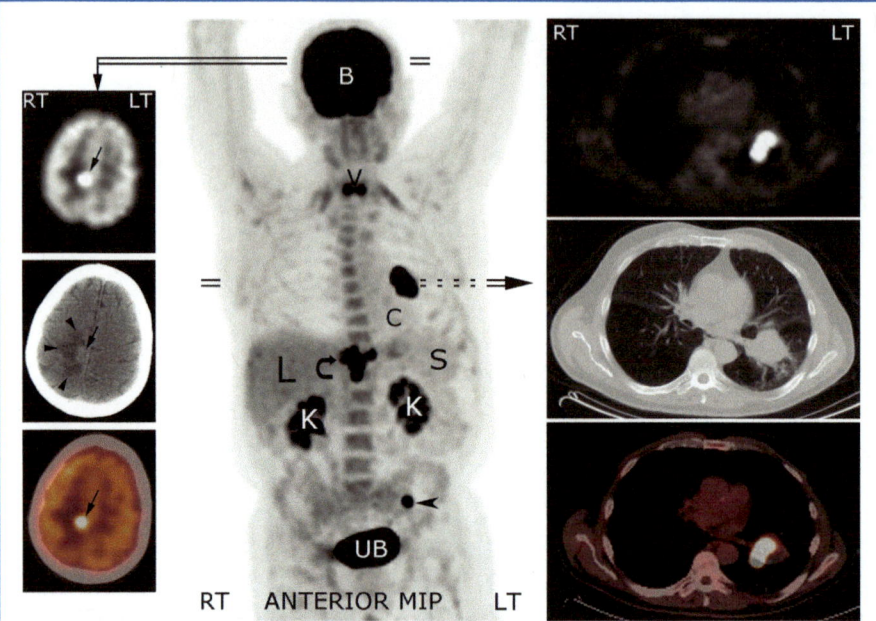

FIGURE 38.3 - PET/CT SCAN

Staging [18]FDG PET/CT of a 72-year-old male with new diagnosis of non-small cell lung cancer. Maximum intensity projection (MIP) image (center) shows normal biodistribution of [18]FDG: intense activity in the brain (*B*) and vocal cords (*V*), excretion of tracer by the kidneys (*K*) into the urinary bladder (*UB*), moderate activity in the liver (*L*), and subtle tracer in the spleen (*S*). There is expected lack of cardiac (*C*) activity due to carbohydrate deprivation diet and 8 h of fasting. On intensity-adjusted images of the brain (*double line arrow* leading left), there is a metastatic lesion at the corticomedullary junction (*arrow*), a typical metastatic location. Corresponding CT slice shows the lesion (*arrow*) and surrounding edema (*arrowheads*). Fusion image (color-coded PET on CT) allows for anatomic localization. Representative images of the lung (*dashed double line arrow* leading right) show intense [18]FDG activity within the primary lung tumor associated with a larger consolidation seen on CT. Fusion image confirms lack of activity within adjacent collapsed lung tissue. There are also skeletal metastases in the lower thoracic spine (*curved arrow*) and the left iliac bone (*concave base arrowhead*)

wear warm, comfortable clothing and use warm blankets while in the imaging facility.

The first [18]FDG PET/CT indication approved for payment by Medicare was to evaluate solitary pulmonary nodules for the likelihood of malignancy. [18]FDG PET/CT is currently indicated to stage, restage, assess response to treatment, and conduct surveillance in a wide variety of malignancies. Prostate and renal cell cancers have variable [18]FDG uptake and, therefore, are not among the approved indications for this test. Because [18]FDG uptake is not specific for a malignant tumor, its uptake should not be used for the definitive diagnosis of malignancy. One of the most common benign causes of [18]FDG uptake is active inflammation. In fact, [18]FDG PET/CT has been used in many countries for the work-up of fever of unknown origin. Unfortunately, it is not currently approved for this indication by Medicare. Other benign causes of [18]FDG uptake include benign tumors, trauma, bone fracture, healing surgical sites, and hematomas. False-negative studies do occur with greater frequency in tumors that commonly display poor [18]FDG uptake, such as adenocarcinoma in situ and minimally invasive adenocarcinoma of the lung, marginal zone lymphoma, and mucinous colonic neoplasms.

Lymphoscintigraphy

Lymphoscintigraphy is a test that depicts lymphatic flow and nodal distribution. This is a useful test in identifying the first node that receives lymph from a tumor-affected region, also known as the "sentinel lymph node." The most commonly used radiopharmaceutical is ^{99m}Tc-labeled sulfur colloid injected intradermally in cases of skin cancer and in the subareolar region in breast cancer. If tumor spreads along the lymphatics, the sentinel node should be the first node to receive it, and lymphoscintigraphy has proven utility in the regional lymph node staging of breast cancer and skin cancer (e.g., melanoma). Because there is expected drainage to the axilla in breast cancer, 2D planar images are sufficient to provide guidance to surgeons who are well familiar with axillary anatomy (Fig. 38.4). Since melanoma can involve various skin regions with less predictable lymphatic drainage, SPECT/CT is used to localize the sentinel node anatomically, which helps to locate it at surgery. The test takes about 1–1.5 h and is usually done within 24 h of planned surgery.

Previously, radical lymphadenectomy was done in these cancers to determine the presence of tumor (staging) and to remove regional tumor spread; however, this caused significant morbidity (e.g., lymphedema). Identifying and removing only the sentinel lymph node markedly decreases the extent of the surgery and minimizes potential morbidity, particularly when no tumor is found in the sentinel node.

Whole-Body Radioactive Iodine (WB RAI) Scan

The whole-body radioactive iodine (WB RAI) scan is a test that uses iodine isotopes to define RAI avidity in differentiated thyroid cancer (DTC). Iodine uptake makes DTC amenable to RAI imaging, treatment, and surveillance (Fig. 38.5). The most commonly used gamma-emitting isotopes for imaging are ^{131}I and ^{123}I, which are given orally in the form of sodium iodide. Some DTC is incidentally found and subcentimeter in size, which may only require a thyroidectomy. A larger DTC requires additional RAI therapy after the surgery. Because surgery cannot remove all of the thyroid tissue safely, the first RAI treatment completes the thyroidectomy by mainly targeting the benign remnant thyroid tissue, which is called RAI *ablation*. Ablation

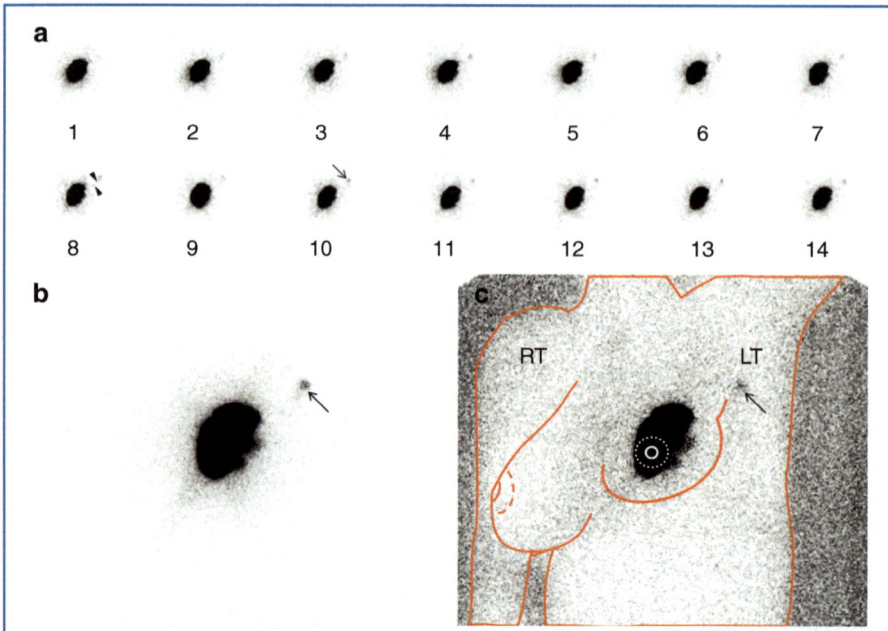

FIGURE 38.4 - LYMPHOSCINTIGRAPHY SCAN
(a) Following left breast subareolar injection (the intense focal activity on frame 1), dynamic images of the chest in the 35° left anterior oblique (*LAO*) projection are obtained for 1 minute per frame. The images show migration of the radiotracer into the left axillary lymph node (*arrow*) at the end of a channel seen on frames 3–8 (*arrowheads*). (b) A static image in the same LAO view obtained at 30 min after injection shows a clear focus of activity consistent with a sentinel node. (c) To better appreciate its location, a transmission view is obtained in the same LAO projection. The transmission image is similar to a radiograph, but in place of the X-ray tube is a flat and uniform source of radioactivity that is placed behind the patient's back. The drawn-in outline of the patient's body (*orange line*) helps to appreciate that the left (*LT*) breast is pulled up and displaced medially, fixed in place by adhesive tape, so it does not block or obscure localization within the axilla. The right (*RT*) breast is naturally laying over the right axilla

allows a subsequent effective use of thyroglobulin (Tg) for DTC surveillance. Since Tg is produced by both normal and cancerous thyroid cells, ablation is necessary for the detection of residual or recurrent DTC (i.e., we then know that any rise in Tg is due to a growing tumor).

One of the critical prerequisites to using RAI for either diagnosis or treatment is depleting the body of iodine prior to the scan or treatment. This markedly improves RAI uptake by the tumor. Thus, the patient is placed on a low-iodine diet for 2 weeks (a challenging diet to follow). The other critical prerequisite for iodine uptake is to have thyroid tissue stimulated with either intrinsic thyroid-stimulating hormone (by stopping hormone replacement, which causes iatrogenic hypothyroidism) or a human recombinant TSH analogue administered by IM injection.

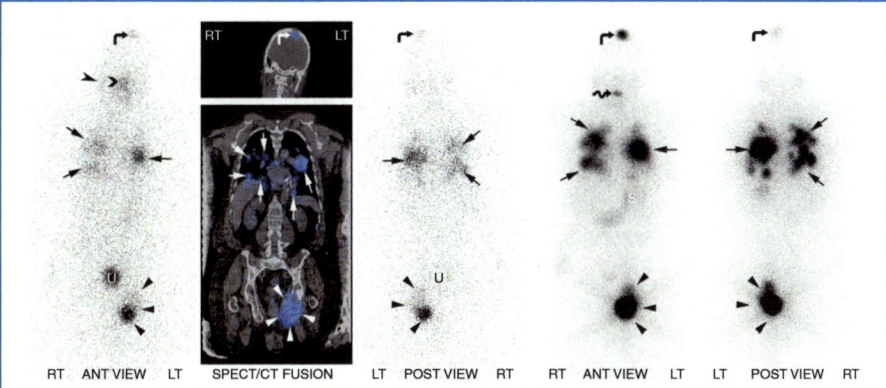

RT   ANT VIEW   LT   SPECT/CT FUSION   LT   POST VIEW   RT   RT   ANT VIEW   LT   LT   POST VIEW   RT

FIGURE 38.5 - I-131 SCAN
Diagnostic images obtained in whole-body planar mode and SPECT/CT at 48 h after a 5 mCi I-131 dose are shown to the left of the vertical divider line. There is abnormal activity in the lungs (*arrows*), left pelvis (*arrowheads*), and cranial vertex (*curved arrow*), confirmed on SPECT/CT fusion image (*color-coded blue*). There is physiologic activity in the nasopharynx (*open arrowhead*), salivary glands (*concave arrowhead*), and urinary bladder (*U*). Images to the right of the vertical divider line show a repeated whole-body scan 7 days post administration of a treatment dose of 100 mCi I-131, demonstrating the same sites of uptake and additional sites of pulmonary metastatic disease. There is physiologic activity in the stomach (*S*). Most of the salivary activity has cleared with some remaining in the mouth (*squiggly arrow*). Urinary activity is not well seen due to near-complete excretion of the remaining blood pool activity

S: The administration of radioactive iodine (RAI) for the treatment of differentiated thyroid cancer requires that the patient follows a series of stringent radiation precautions after the treatment is swallowed. Radioactive iodine is eliminated from the body mainly through the saliva and urine. Thus, it is imperative that the patient wash their hands frequently, always use separate utensils (e.g., plates and glasses), and use a separate bathroom, flushing twice after toilet use.

A: Thyroid cancer must first be treated surgically, requiring a total thyroidectomy and a bilateral cervical lymph node dissection. In the presence of well-differentiated thyroid cancer (and thus iodine avid thyroid cancer), the patient should then be evaluated with a whole-body scan with radioactive iodine. Whether or not to then treat with radioactive iodine, with what dose, and under what preparation (synthetic TSH stimulation vs hormone withdrawal) is of some debate at present; however, RAI has been shown to be an effective and safe agent for residual thyroid ablation and for the treatment for metastatic thyroid cancer.

F: The normal biodistribution of radioactive iodine includes the salivary glands, stomach, liver, bowel, and urinary system. Uptake within the thyroid bed on first postoperative examinations is also an expected finding, as it is extremely difficult to remove all of the thyroid tissue at surgery. Foci of uptake within the lateral neck usually signify lymph node involvement, as well as uptake within the adjacent major nodal basins. SPECT/CT scanning is useful in localizing abnormal uptake, particularly when present within the bones, lungs, or abdomen.

E: Foci of uptake that are concerning for metastatic disease usually necessitate treatment with radioactive iodine. While thyroid cancer is usually a slowly growing cancer, patient preparation for whole-body scanning that may require treatment (either through synthetic TSH administration or hormone withdrawal) is such that there is a window in which administration is optimal. Every effort should be made to ensure that the patient is treated within a timely fashion.

39 PULMONARY NUCLEAR MEDICINE

Objectives:
1. Define ventilation-perfusion lung scintigraphy.
2. Define the radiopharmaceuticals used in lung perfusion and ventilation scans and the physiologic rationale for this examination.
3. Describe the differences in probability-based and trinary systems of interpretation of ventilation-perfusion lung scans.
4. Describe the principles of quantitative (differential) lung scintigraphy.
5. List the main indications of quantitative (differential) lung scintigraphy.

The *ventilation-perfusion (or ventilation/quotient [V/Q]) scan* is an imaging technique aimed at interrogating the physiology and, to a lesser degree, the anatomy of these respective functions. It is mostly indicated for *pulmonary embolism* (PE) or *thromboembolism*.

Assessment of ventilation is performed following inhalation of either a radioactive gas (e.g., xenon-133) or aerosol (e.g., ^{99m}Tc-DTPA aerosol dispensed by a nebulizer) through a tightly fitted face mask. This allows for regional assessment of pulmonary airflow. The ventilation part of the V/Q scan is usually done first, as the radiotracer used during ventilation is either eliminated through expiration or given in a small enough activity that the radiotracer used during perfusion overrides the residual activity from the ventilation portion of the study. The perfusion imaging is done following intravenous injection of *^{99m}Tc-macroaggregated albumin* (MAA), which consists of small particles (average size of 15–30 μm). These particles are larger than the pulmonary capillary vasculature (about 7 μm); thus, nearly all radiolabeled particles are filtered out by the lungs during its first pass in proportion with the regional pulmonary artery blood flow. The test can be performed using planar (the most common method in contemporary practice) or SPECT imaging [1].

© Springer Nature Switzerland AG 2020
J. Kissane et al. (eds.), *Radiology Fundamentals: Introduction to Imaging & Technology*, https://doi.org/10.1007/978-3-030-22173-7_39

Perfusion is imaged after an I.V. injection of about 300,000–500,000 ^{99m}Tc-MAA particles. There are 300–500 million alveoli in the lungs that are surrounded by a capillary network. A conservative estimate is that less than 1 in 1000 capillaries would be occluded, which is generally very safe. An exception to this is a patient with severe pulmonary arterial hypertension that is associated with marked reduction in alveoli and capillaries. Blocking additional capillaries with ^{99m}Tc-MAA can precipitate right heart failure in these patients; therefore, the amount of particles administered is generally reduced in severe pulmonary hypertension, and caution is advised in cases of signs of right heart strain. A contraindication for this study is hypersensitivity to human albumin products (note that this is very rare).

The essential V/Q scan principle for detecting pulmonary embolism (PE) is based on detecting perfusion defects with normal ventilation, termed a *V/Q mismatch*. The larger the perfusion defect and the greater their number, the higher is the probability of PE. At least two large segmental mismatches are needed to be reasonably convinced that the patient has a PE (called a *positive study for PE*). If a perfusion defect is matched by a ventilation abnormality, then the likelihood of PE is low. Such findings often reflect airspace-based disease that causes regional hypoxia-mediated vasoconstriction, which in turn can result in a *matched V/Q defect*. Different patterns on a V/Q scan are comprised of variations in size, number, distribution, and corresponding chest X-ray (CXR) findings. Those patterns can be grouped into three categories: *negative study for PE*, *positive study for PE*, and *inconclusive or indeterminate*. This system of interpreting is called a *trinary approach*.

Pregnancy is a specific concern in V/Q scans, as the whole body receives radiation exposure (albeit small) particularly from ^{99m}Tc-DTPA which is cleared from the alveoli into the bloodstream and eventually into the urinary bladder (which is in close proximity to the uterus). Therefore, the ventilation portion of the examination should be initially omitted in pregnant patients and the perfusion done with lowest possible activity. If perfusion images show suspicious defects, ventilation can be done later (Fig. 39.1).

Spiral CT pulmonary angiography (CTPA) supplanted V/Q scanning as the initial diagnostic imaging for PE. However, concern has been raised recently that it may be too sensitive, resulting in overdiagnosis and overtreatment. Its major strengths include (a) ready availability around the clock in most hospitals, (b) quick performance time, and (c) simple interpretation with results that are positive, negative, or indeterminate (which is usually for technical reasons).

The indeterminate or inconclusive V/Q result is least helpful in clinical management and is most likely in the presence of CXR opacities; in this case, a CTPA would be favored. V/Q scanning may take several hours to obtain, or even longer if ordered after regular work hours, as a technologist often needs to be called in from home and radiopharmaceuticals must be freshly prepared. Contraindications to CTPA include contrast allergy and renal insufficiency (at which point V/Q scan becomes the preferred modality). Pulmonary hypertension from chronic PE is another circumstance where V/Q may be more sensitive than CTPA [2]. Pulmonary angiography still remains the gold standard for the diagnosis of PE and may be

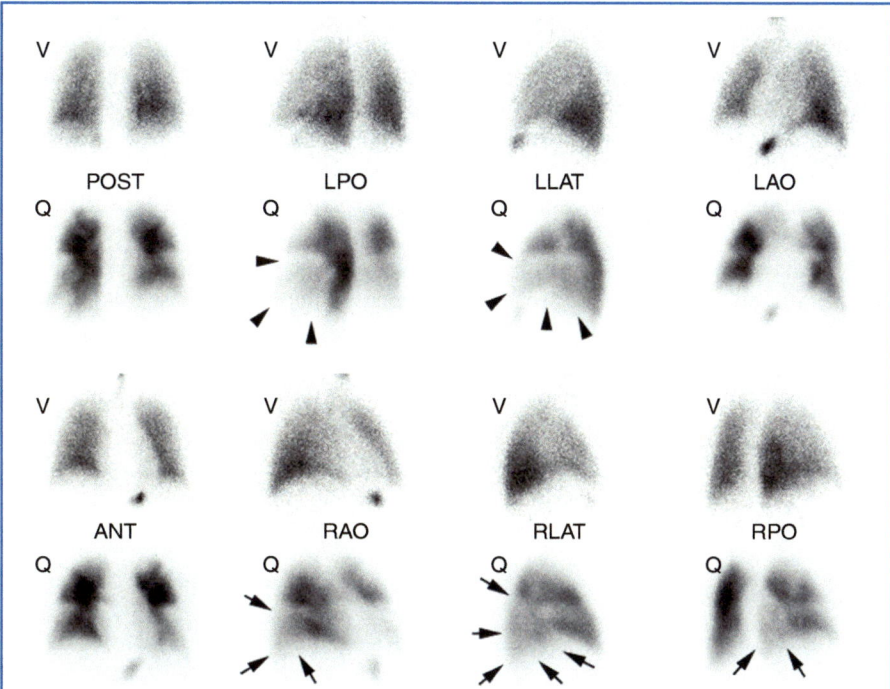

FIGURE 39.1 - HIGH PROBABILITY V/Q SCAN

The ventilation (*V*) obtained with ^{99m}Tc-DTPA aerosol is on the top and perfusion (*Q*) obtained with ^{99m}Tc-MAA IV is on the bottom, paired according to the eight standard views: posterior (*POST*), left posterior oblique (*LPO*), left lateral (*LLAT*), left anterior oblique (*LAO*), anterior (*ANT*), right anterior oblique (*RAO*), right lateral (*RLAT*), and right posterior oblique (*RPO*). The ventilation (V) images show normal physiological distribution of activity. The perfusion (Q) images show a large segmental perfusion defect (photopenia) in the left lower lobe (*arrowheads*) and a second large segmental defect in the right lower lobe (***arrows***). As both of these areas have normal ventilation, this is a "mismatch" and renders the study positive for pulmonary embolism. Of note, the chest X-ray was normal

necessary if the diagnosis remains in doubt after V/Q or CTPA scans are performed.

Quantitative lung scintigraphy or *differential pulmonary function scan* is performed to (1) predict pulmonary function after lung surgery (pneumonectomy or lobectomy) and (2) to quantify asymmetry in patients with compromised pulmonary artery flow, usually as part of a congenital heart syndrome. The common principle for both indications is based on the fact that perfusion images performed with ^{99m}Tc-MAA are the best correlates for both lung blood flow and lung respiratory gas exchange function. It has been shown that performing a ventilation study does not add significant information over perfusion alone in quantifying gas exchange function, likely because the blood flow and gas exchange functions are coupled.

The critical question in patients with lung cancer and abnormal baseline lung function (i.e., severe bullous emphysema) is whether the remaining lung function after surgery would be sufficient for patient survival, particularly during the perioperative period when the patient is first weaned off ventilator support. The essential lung function parameters in this context that would predict complications are preoperative and predicted postoperative forced expiratory volume in one second (FEV1). The example in Fig. 39.2 demonstrates how predicted postsurgical FEV1 is calculated.

Pulmonary artery stenosis is often part of congenital heart disease and is typically unilateral. These patients have procedures, such as balloon angioplasty and stenting, which can correct or improve it. The asymmetry in pulmonary blood flow can be detected, quantified, and followed for the surveillance of restenosis using the same left versus right whole-lung quantification on the ^{99m}Tc-MAA images.

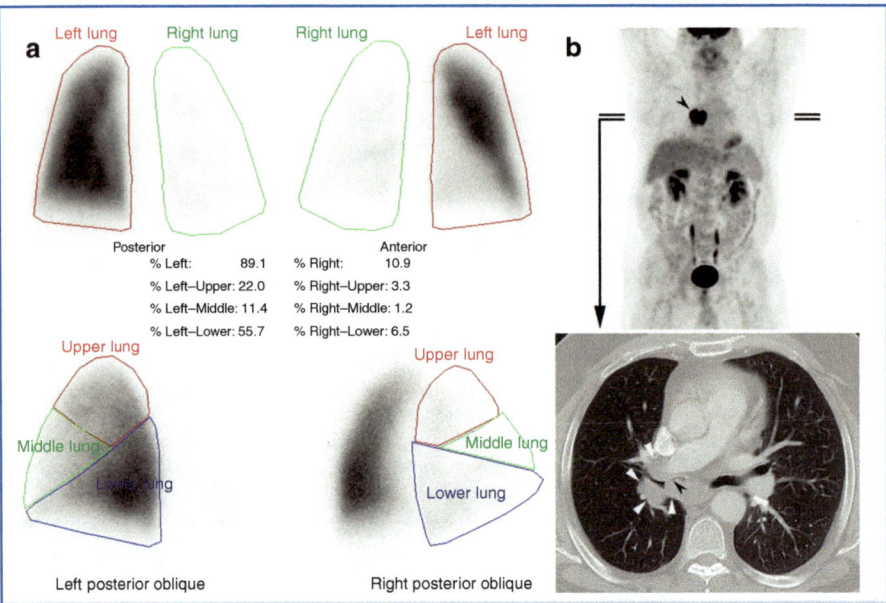

FIGURE 39.2 - QUANTITATIVE LUNG FUNCTION SCAN
This patient with right lung cancer had FEV1 of 1.92 L/min, which would be concerning for pneumonectomy clearance and requires further evaluation. (**a**) Perfusion images in anterior and posterior projections allow for count-based calculations of each lung contribution to lung function. Proportional calculations predict a post-right pneumonectomy FEV1 of 1.71 L/min, which is adequate to maintain gas exchange after surgery. The lower panel shows posterior oblique images that allow calculation of individual lobe contributions to the overall pulmonary function and can be used for prediction of post-lobectomy function. (**b**) The patient's non-small cell lung cancer was at the right hilum as seen on the top PET/CT MIP image (*arrowhead*) without metastases. The tumor (outlined by *white arrowheads* on CT) compressed the right mainstem bronchus (*black arrowhead*) and main branch pulmonary arteries, responsible for the severely decreased ventilation and perfusion to the right lung

S: Reducing radiation exposure is especially important in the pregnant patient. While the patient and fetus will be exposed to radiation by both CTPA and V/Q scanning, V/Q imparts less radiation, especially when performed as a low-dose perfusion-only scan (without the Tc99m-DTPA ventilation portion, which is eliminated by the kidneys and into the bladder).

A: Chest radiography (CXR) is the most appropriate first test to perform in the setting of suspected pulmonary embolus (ACR AC 9), as the patient usually presents with shortness of breath and chest pain. This is an inexpensive modality that can be obtained quickly and provide initial diagnostic information to assist in informed decision-making. If pulmonary embolus is still suspected, especially in the setting of a normal CXR, CTPA or V/Q scanning should then be obtained, as appropriate.

F: V/Q scans consist of two separate administrations of radiotracer which evaluate the ventilation (a map of the areas of lung that receive air effectively) and perfusion (a map of the areas of the lung that receive blood effectively). The diagnosis of a pulmonary embolus is suspected when a "mismatch" is encountered, in which an area of the lung is ventilated but not perfused. In the appropriate clinical setting, this is concerning for a pulmonary embolism as the cause of the mismatch.

E: The diagnosis of suspected pulmonary embolism requires emergent verbal notification of the primary clinical service to ensure prompt initiation of appropriate anticoagulation therapy to limit morbidity and mortality or possibly the placement of an IVC filter by Interventional Radiology.

References

1. Reinartz P, Wildberger JE, Schaefer W, Nowak B, Mahnken AH, Buell U. Tomographic imaging in the diagnosis of pulmonary embolism: a comparison between V/Q lung scintigraphy in SPECT technique and multislice spiral CT. J Nuc Med. 2004;45(9):1501–8. Official publication, Society of Nuclear Medicine.
2. Tunariu N, Gibbs SJ, Win Z, et al. Ventilation-perfusion scintigraphy is more sensitive than multidetector CTPA in detecting chronic thromboembolic pulmonary disease as a treatable cause of pulmonary hypertension. J Nuc Med. 2007;48(5):680–4. Official publication, Society of Nuclear Medicine.

40

SKELETAL NUCLEAR MEDICINE

Objectives:
1. Describe the physiological rationale for tracer uptake on a bone scan.
2. Describe the sensitivity and specificity of the bone scan.
3. List the common causes of locally increased radiotracer uptake.
4. Describe the advantages of SPECT/CT over SPECT and planar bone scans.

Bone scan or bone scintigraphy (*BS*) is among the earliest diagnostic applications in nuclear medicine imaging that remains useful today. Current bone-seeking radiotracers can be divided into those emitting gamma rays (imaged with gamma cameras) and those emitting positrons (imaged with PET/CT). The former group is collectively called ^{99m}Tc-polyphosphonates (^{99m}Tc-PPs), which include ^{99m}Tc-methylene diphosphonate (^{99m}Tc-MDP) and ^{99m}Tc-hydroxymethylene diphosphonate. The latter group includes ^{18}F-labeled sodium fluoride (Na^{18}F). They are all administered intravenously and taken up by the skeleton through a process called *chemabsorption*, whereby the tracer is incorporated into the calcium hydroxyapatite crystal (CHAC) matrix of the bone which is laid down by osteoblasts. Through this process, bone-seeking radiotracers reflect skeletal osteoblastic activity [1]. Sometimes the radiotracers can localize to pathological or dystrophic calcium depositions in soft tissues such as calcified metastatic liver lesions from colorectal cancer, calcium deposits in the lungs, or stomach in hyperparathyroidism.

^{111}In-labeled white blood cells (WBCs) can be used with ^{99m}Tc-PPs as an adjunct radiotracer to increase specificity to identify osteomyelitis (Fig. 40.1). Because of significant differences in emissions of the two isotopes, the images of both can be obtained simultaneously in their respective energy windows.

© Springer Nature Switzerland AG 2020
J. Kissane et al. (eds.), *Radiology Fundamentals: Introduction to Imaging & Technology*, https://doi.org/10.1007/978-3-030-22173-7_40

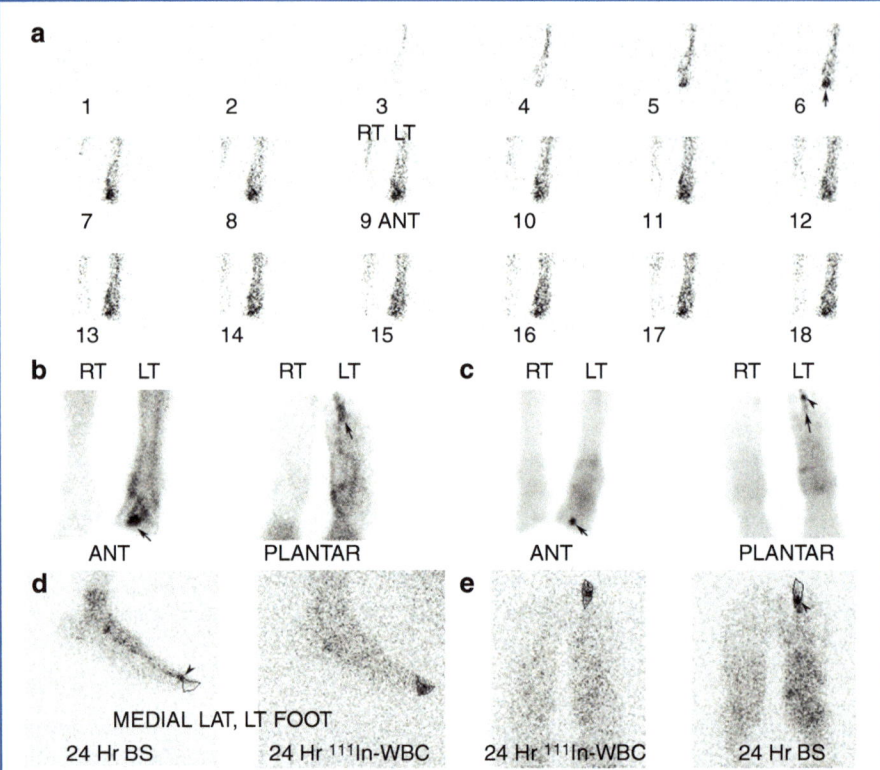

FIGURE 40.1 - THREE-PHASE BONE SCAN

Three-phase limited ^{99m}Tc-PPs bone scan (*BS*) in a patient with suspected osteomyelitis of the left second toe. The arterial or blood flow phase (first phase) is 3 seconds per frame dynamic imaging (**a**) obtained in the anterior view (*ANT*). The tracer appears in the left foot on frame 3 with intense focal activity (frame 6, *arrow*) corresponding to the affected toe. On frame 7, there is normal activity arriving to the unaffected side. The most intense focal activity is seen during the arterial phase (frames 4–9), and the intensity decreases during the venous phase (frame 10 onward). Frame 9 is annotated to show the left (*LT*) and right (*RT*) feet. The blood pool (second) phase (**b**) shows similar findings in the ANT view (*arrow*). The plantar view is obtained with feet placed flat on the camera detector which best isolates the affected toe. The hyperemia is moderate over the entire left foot and intense focally at the toe (*arrow*). Delayed phase (3 h) spot images (**c**) show focal intense activity in the toe (*arrow*) on the ANT view. The plantar view reveals the intense focus (*arrowhead*) in the distal third of the toe, with milder activity proximally (*arrow*). There is less activity distally, correlating with bone destruction on the radiograph and increased activity on the ^{111}In-labeled white blood cell (*WBC*) scan (**d, e**). It is the increased pressure of inflammation at that focus (*irregular black outline* on the ^{111}In- WBC scan) which decreases osteoblastic activity. The lateral (*LAT*, d) and plantar (**e**) views are orthogonal projections that best represent the distribution of the findings

Alternatively, ^{99m}Tc-WBCs can be used, but must be performed on a different day from the bone scan due to use of the same isotope label (^{99m}Tc), precluding differentiation of one from the other on simultaneous imaging. The advantage of the former approach is that the BS and ^{111}In-WBC scan may be acquired concurrently and inherently co-registered to each other. Accordingly, drawing a region of interest on the ^{111}In-WBC focus makes it possible to place it on the identical location of the BS image. In osteomyelitis, it would overlie the bone (Fig. 40.1d, e), whereas in cellulitis, it would fall on the soft tissues away from the bone.

^{99m}Tc-PPs are the most commonly used radiotracers for bone scintigraphy and the term "bone scan" is thus often synonymous with gamma-camera scanning. Although maximum uptake of ^{99m}Tc-PPs in bone is reached within the first 20–30 min after injection, the high background noise created by interfering activity from the blood pool and soft tissues would preclude good skeletal visualization at this time frame. As the radiotracer is cleared by the kidneys, skeletal visualization improves and reaches optimal quality by 2–3 h. Drinking fluids during this time improves tracer clearance and the sharpness, or contrast, of skeletal visualization.

The uptake of radiotracers depends on two variables: (1) blood flow and (2) the amount of amorphous (newly formed) CHAC. Skeletal regions with increased blood flow (hyperemia) receive greater delivery of the radiotracer, resulting in greater uptake. Osteoblasts lay down amorphous CHAC in actively growing, metabolizing, or repairing bone, which offers greater surface area for chemabsorption, leading to greater uptake of the bone-seeking radiotracer.

Common indications for bone scanning include primary skeletal tumors, benign neoplasms, metastatic skeletal disease (e.g., prostate cancer, non-small cell lung cancer, breast cancer, osteosarcoma, etc.), osteomyelitis, active facet arthropathy in patients with back pain, stress fractures, occult fractures, and metabolic bone diseases (e.g., Paget's disease, fibrous dysplasia, etc.). An abnormality on the scan is not specific in and of itself. The combination of the pattern (location, distribution, intensity, etc.), correlation with other imaging modalities, and the patient's clinical presentation allow the interpreter to offer a list of likely specific diagnoses (a differential). A differential can be narrowed by applying other correlative imaging findings and/or by obtaining more detailed history and physical findings.

Gamma imaging is most often performed using planar scintigraphy. But depending on clinical indication and a specific clinical dilemma, the imaging procedure (protocol) can vary. Three-phase imaging includes (1) dynamic arterial blood flow sequence obtained immediately after injection (Fig. 40.1a), (2) static imaging of the blood pool that is obtained during the first 5–15 min after injection (Fig. 40.1b), and (3) static delays that are obtained 2–3 h later (Fig. 40.1c). This method is most useful in evaluating traumatic injuries (fractures, stress fractures, etc.) and osteomyelitis (Fig. 40.1). Because those indications typically involve small parts of the skeleton, the spot images should be sufficient. This type of scan is often referred to as "limited," referring to the area of concern. For the detection of skeletal metastatic disease, only the static delay images are required and are usually obtained using the whole-body imaging mode (Fig. 40.2). See Introduction to NM for additional details.

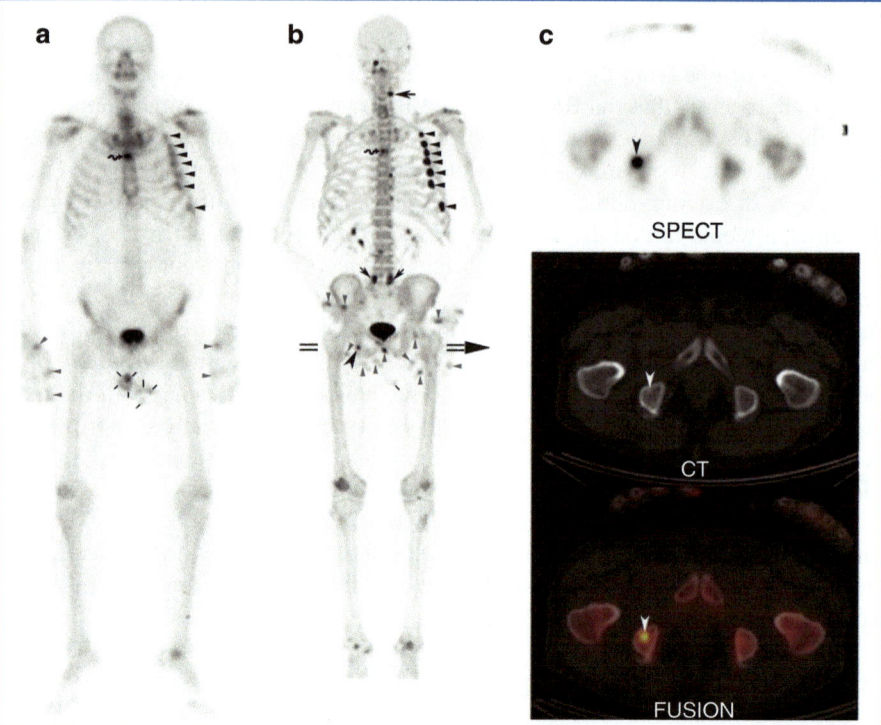

FIGURE 40.2 - METASTATIC DISEASE ON BONE SCAN

A 65-year-old male with a history of treated prostate cancer was found to have newly elevated prostate-specific antigen on laboratory surveillance. Anterior projection of the ^{99m}Tc-PPs whole-body bone scan (**a**) showed multiple mild foci of uptake in the left chest (*black arrowheads*), distributed in a pattern typical for rib fractures (corroborated by local pain and history of fall). Joint-centered areas of uptake in the cervical and lumbar spine (*concave-base arrows*), hands (*gray arrowheads*), sternomanubrial joint (*squiggly arrow*), knees, left ankle, and elbow are typical of osteoarthritis. Amorphous activity in the groin is due to urinary contamination (*gray lines*). Anterior maximum intensity projection image of the Na^{18}F scan a few days later (**b**) show uptake in the right inferior ramus of the pelvis (*concave-base arrowhead*). Multiple small spots scattered over the pelvis (*gray arrowheads*) correlate with arthritic foci in the hands placed over the pelvis. Axial CT through the pelvic lesion (*double line arrow* to the right) (**c**) shows the intense lesion on PET images in the inferior ischial ramus correlates with a small blastic lesion on CT, corroborated by fusion imaging (Images courtesy of Dr. Andrei H Iagaru)

Hybrid SPECT/CT is particularly useful in the work-up of back pain. It allows precise anatomical localization of active bone metabolism in facet arthropathy (Fig. 40.3) and/or spondylolysis on the CT portion, which is obtained with a significantly lower radiation dose as compared to the diagnostic CT. Before the advent of hybrid imaging, differentiating between those two pathologies on SPECT alone presented a significant challenge with precise anatomical positioning of a focal

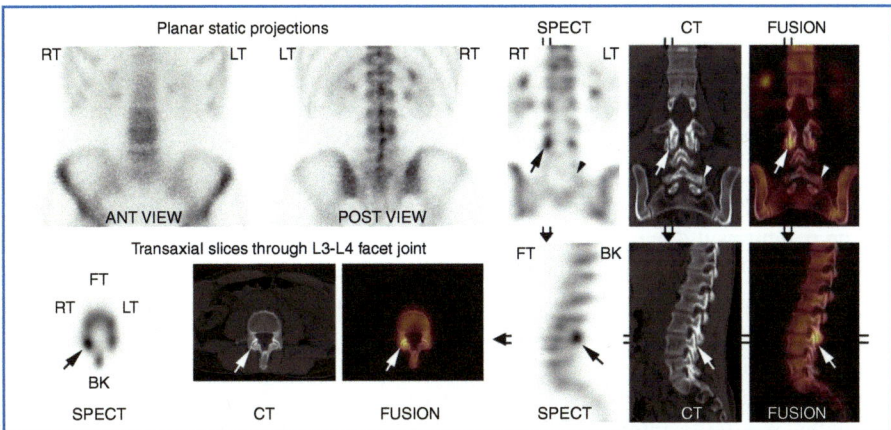

FIGURE 40.3 - DEGENERATIVE SPINE DISEASE ON BONE SCAN
Three-phase limited planar bone scan and SPECT/CT of a 56-year-old male with back pain. Blood flow and pool images were normal (not shown). Spot images in anterior (*ANT*) and posterior (*POST*) views show no obvious abnormality. Coronal slices through the lumbar spine (top right) demonstrate intense focal uptake (*arrow*) in the right L3/L4 facet joint. There is mild uptake in the left L3/L4 facet joint, which is less significant. For comparison, notice normal activity (*arrowheads*) at the L5/S1 facets. Sagittal section (bottom right) and axial section (bottom left) through the intense focus confirm the finding at the right L3/L4 facet

abnormality. It was necessary to correlate with a CT obtained at a separate visit. SPECT and SPECT/CT are more sensitive than planar bone scans for scintigraphic lesion detection because of better contrast resolution. Both facet arthropathy and spondylolysis can present either asymptomatically, such as in chronic and stable states when these are discovered incidentally, or symptomatically. While normal or minimal radiotracer uptake is usually seen in the former clinical circumstance, the latter is typically associated with increased accumulation of $Na^{18}F$ (Fig. 40.2) and ^{99m}Tc-PPs (Fig. 40.3).

Despite its nonspecific nature, the bone scan is very useful because of its high sensitivity. Bone turnover and osteoblastic activity increases well before there is either bone loss (lytic lesion) or formation of pathologically increased density (blastic lesion). Therefore, metastatic disease can be seen on a bone scan in advance of its appearance on plain radiographs and, at times, before any CT abnormality becomes obvious. The other advantage of the bone scan is its ability to image the whole body with a single radiotracer injection, leading to relatively low radiation exposure. In comparison, CT is more specific for skeletal conditions but typically exposes patients to a greater radiation burden, which increases with coverage of additional body areas (note that this is not applicable to a bone scan that has radiation exposure determined by injected radiotracer and independent of the number of obtained images).

S: ^{99m}Tc is produced via a ^{99}Mo "generator" in which a column of ^{99}Mo decays to its metastable product of ^{99m}Tc and detaches from its aluminum surface. It can then be extracted from the system by flushing saline across the column. ^{99m}Tc can be used on its own or attached to additional compounds as part of other radiopharmaceuticals. It is imperative that the solution first be checked to verify that no (or extremely little) ^{99}Mo has also been extracted with the ^{99m}Tc. This is important because ^{99}Mo would impart a very large (and unnecessary) radiation exposure to the patient as it decays via beta decay (ejects a high energy electron in the range of 700 keV) versus the much lower isomeric transition of ^{99m}Tc (releasing a gamma photon at 140 keV). Every extracted sample from the generator (colloquially known as "milking") must be checked for high energy decay radiation to ensure patient safety.

A: Bone scans are generally performed using a radiopharmaceutical known as methylene diphosphonate (MDP) attached to ^{99m}Tc. It is among the most appropriate tests that should be performed in the evaluation of metastatic bone disease (ACR AC 9), particularly for stage 2 metastatic breast cancers and for prostate cancer in patients with a PSA <20 mg/ml.

F: A small amount ^{99m}Tc-MDP adsorbs to the hydroxyapatite matrix of all bone, which allows visualization of the entire normal skeleton when scanned. Areas of increased uptake above this background activity are abnormal and indicate that the radiopharmaceutical is being incorporated into new bone formation (and/or delivered to bone in a higher proportion by hyperemia) in reaction to an abnormal process. The differential for abnormal uptake is broad, including everything from a healing fracture to metastatic disease, and consideration of the abnormal pattern within the current clinical context is imperative for correct interpretation.

E: In the evaluation of metastatic disease to bone, particularly in the cases of breast and prostate carcinoma, it is imperative to determine if the patient has recently started a new therapy. An overall pattern of increased uptake in previously identified areas of metastatic disease could be due to a flare (i.e., inflammatory) response to a new therapy and misdiagnosed as metastatic disease. Calling the ordering provider directly in cases of suspected flare response is often an invaluable step toward arriving at the correct diagnosis.

Reference

1. Wong KK, Piert M. Dynamic bone imaging with 99mTc-labeled diphosphonates and 18F-NaF: mechanisms and applications. J Nucl Med. 2013;54(4):590–9.

PART VI
INTERVENTIONAL RADIOLOGY

41 DIAGNOSTIC ARTERIOGRAPHY

Objectives:
1. Describe in detail the technique for arterial groin and arm punctures.
2. Discuss how catheter design helps in the performance of arteriography.
3. Discuss the complications of arteriography and their relative frequency.

Arteriography involves the placement of a catheter into the arterial system with injection of contrast while obtaining X-ray images. Various catheters and wires are used in combination to cannulate the desired arteries (Fig. 41.1).

Femoral, Radial, and Brachial Artery Access

Access to the femoral, radial, or brachial artery is performed at the level of the femoral head, the distal radius, or in line with the humerus above the elbow, respectively. Access is achieved at these points for two reasons. First, the artery in these locations is easy to palpate and therefore easier to locate and puncture. Second, the artery is adjacent to a bony structure; when the catheter is removed, hemostasis can be achieved by compressing the artery against the bone directly behind it (Fig. 41.2). Special care must be taken to ensure an intact palmar arch (with collateral supply to the arch from the ulnar artery) prior to radial artery access.

Once access to the artery is obtained with a needle, a floppy-tipped guidewire is advanced through the needle under fluoroscopy until a sufficient length of the stiffer portion of the guidewire is intraluminal. This allows for stable exchange of the needle for either a catheter or a vascular sheath. This is called the Seldinger technique. A vascular sheath is a device which has a hemostatic valve on the portion of

© Springer Nature Switzerland AG 2020   289
J. Kissane et al. (eds.), *Radiology Fundamentals: Introduction to Imaging & Technology*, https://doi.org/10.1007/978-3-030-22173-7_41

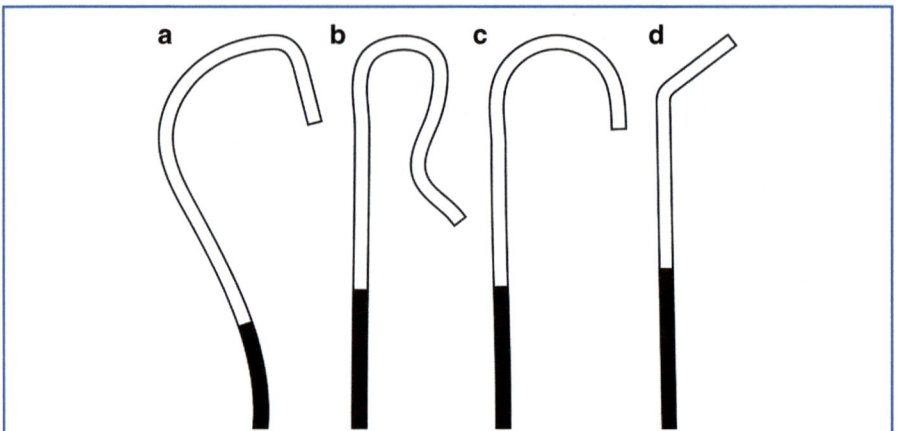

FIGURE 41.1 - CATHETERS AND WIRES
Various catheters and wires are used in combination to cannulate the desired arteries: (**a**) Cobra, (**b**) Simmons, (**c**) RC-1, (**d**) Berenstein

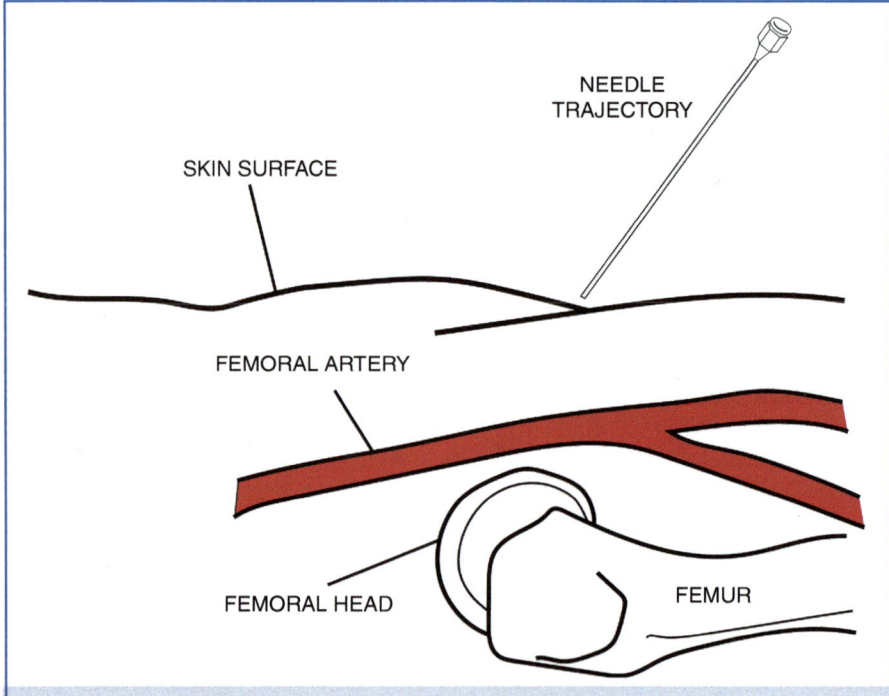

FIGURE 41.2 - COMMON FEMORAL ARTERY ACCESS
In the lateral view, the femoral artery lies just on top of the femoral head. At this point, it is easy to palpate and easy to compress after the catheter is removed

the sheath that remains outside of the patient. The sheath remains in the artery at the access point, and through the sheath, catheter exchanges can be accomplished with minimal blood loss. A disadvantage of using a sheath is its larger outer diameter and the larger hole it makes in the artery compared to a catheter alone.

If "flush" arteriographic studies are to be performed, particularly of large vessels, a catheter with multiple side holes is used to evenly distribute the contrast in the blood pool. A typical example of this would be aortography using a "pigtail" or "tennis racket" catheter. If selective arteriography is needed, then an appropriately shaped catheter, usually with a single end hole, is used with a guidewire to select the desired arteries and then inject contrast (Fig. 41.1).

Once the catheter is in appropriate position, contrast is injected either by hand or with a power injector using a known rate and pressure. Images are obtained with digital subtraction angiography (DSA) imaging (see Chap. 9). Diagnostic images are reviewed. Either the study is concluded at that time or, if appropriate, an intervention is undertaken.

At the completion of the procedure, the sheath and/or catheter is removed, and hemostasis is obtained at the puncture site by compressing the artery against the underlying bony structure. Compression is usually held for 15–20 min. Once hemostasis is obtained, the patient must lie flat for 6 h after femoral access, maintain the elbow extended for 6 h after brachial access, or wear a compression band at the wrist for 1–3 h after radial access. Access sites and associated extremities must be checked frequently to make sure no bleeding or neurovascular compromise has occurred. Using an arterial closure device at a femoral artery access site can shorten the bedrest period to 3 h.

Arteriography Complications

Complications of arteriography include:

1. *Groin or arm hematoma*
   In the groin, a hematoma is not uncommon, occurring up to 5–13% of the time, however requires minimal additional treatment. In the upper arm, it can be much more dangerous because of possible compression of the neurovascular bundle within the medial brachial fascial compartment requiring urgent attention.
2. *Infection*
   Infection is almost unheard of in arteriography. Because of the small access points and the sterile draping and technique, it occurs in less than 1% of all cases.
3. *Contrast reaction*
   Injection of contrast media in anyone may result in a contrast reaction. The most common reaction clinically is the onset of itching and hives. Treatment is nearly always successful using known drug algorithms. If a patient has a known contrast allergy, he or she must be pretreated with oral or intravenous steroids (e.g., oral

prednisone 50 mg) at 13, 7, and 1 h before the procedure. The patient should also be given Benadryl 50 mg IV or PO 1 h prior to the procedure. The most important steroid dose is the dose given 13 h before the procedure. The mechanism of protection is thought to be the stabilization of mast cell membranes, thereby preventing the degranulation and release of histamine. Shortened regimens can be used in emergent conditions. Under certain circumstances, carbon dioxide (CO_2) may be used in lieu of iodinated contrast in those known to have contrast allergy. The body naturally produces CO_2 as a by-product of cellular respiration; thus, when CO_2 is introduced into the body during interventional procedures, it is transported to the lungs where it is removed from the body in exchange for oxygen. Of note, CO_2 should only be used in arteries below the diaphragm to avoid gas embolism to the brain given the potential neurotoxicity of CO_2.

4. *Contrast-induced nephrotoxicity (CIN)*
   Current literature suggests the main risk factors for CIN include pre-existing renal insufficiency, diabetes mellitus, and, in some cases, severe congestive heart failure. When ordering an arteriogram (or any study with contrast), the increased risk for CIN should be considered.

5. *Vessel dissection or pseudoaneurysm formation*
   Any time a blood vessel is entered traumatically (as with a puncture for arteriography), there is a definite but small risk of vessel injury, pseudoaneurysm, or arteriovenous fistula formation.

S: The risks of an invasive procedure such as arteriography should be weighed against the information that cannot be obtained by noninvasive means. Increasingly, arteriography is both diagnostic and therapeutic, and so the risks of an invasive procedure are significantly outweighed by the benefits. Absolute contraindication to arteriography includes evaluation that will not change management or can be obtained by noninvasive imaging. Relative contraindications include iodinated contrast allergy, severe hypertension, hypotension, uncorrectable coagulopathy, renal insufficiency, congestive heart failure, and certain connective tissue disorders.

A: Successful arteriography evaluation involves gaining access to the artery, choosing the appropriate catheter, obtaining a complete set of images (i.e., including angiographic orthogonal obliquities), and accurate timely interpretation of the findings.

F: An example of complete diagnostic arteriography of the kidney involves imaging from the abdominal aorta to the renal parenchyma with dedicated vascular angiographic orthogonal obliquities.

E: Diagnostic arteriography remains the gold standard in instances in which noninvasive imaging is not possible, inconclusive or before therapy. Examples include evaluation and ability to isolate small caliber vascular anomalies as well as the capability to render endovascular therapies such as coiling, stenting, thromboembolectomy, and chemoembolization. Adjunctive noninvasive imaging may be performed post-intervention for follow-up as clinically indicated.

42

PULMONARY ARTERIOGRAPHY AND IVC FILTER PLACEMENT

Objectives:
1. List the indications for pulmonary arteriography.
2. Describe the technique for pulmonary arteriography including the contraindications.
3. Describe the technique for inferior vena cava filter placement including what is appropriate for an inferior cava larger than 28 mm.

Although still considered the gold standard for the diagnosis of pulmonary embolism, pulmonary arteriography has largely been supplanted by CT pulmonary angiography (CTPA). Nevertheless, pulmonary arteriography may still be indicated in patients with a high clinical suspicion for pulmonary embolism and:

1. A low probability or indeterminate V/Q scan or CTPA
2. An indeterminate V/Q or CTPA and contraindication to anticoagulation
3. Prior to catheter-based pulmonary embolectomy or lysis

Conventional pulmonary arteriography is accomplished from the right common femoral vein or the right internal jugular vein. Access is obtained in a fashion similar to that described in the arteriography section. Once access has been obtained, a pulmonary artery catheter is advanced to the level of the right atrium. The catheter is gently advanced across the tricuspid valve and, while pushing forward, is rotated (Fig. 42.1). As it crosses through the right ventricle to the pulmonary outflow tract, it is gently pushed farther, usually into the left pulmonary artery. The catheter position in each pulmonary artery is confirmed with a minimal amount of contrast, and *pulmonary artery pressures are recorded*. The contrast injection is tailored, based on the pulmonary artery pressures. If the pressures are normal or only mildly elevated, a standard pulmonary arteriogram is performed. If the pressures are elevated, the contrast injection volume is decreased or a subselective angiogram is performed.

© Springer Nature Switzerland AG 2020
J. Kissane et al. (eds.), *Radiology Fundamentals: Introduction to Imaging & Technology*, https://doi.org/10.1007/978-3-030-22173-7_42

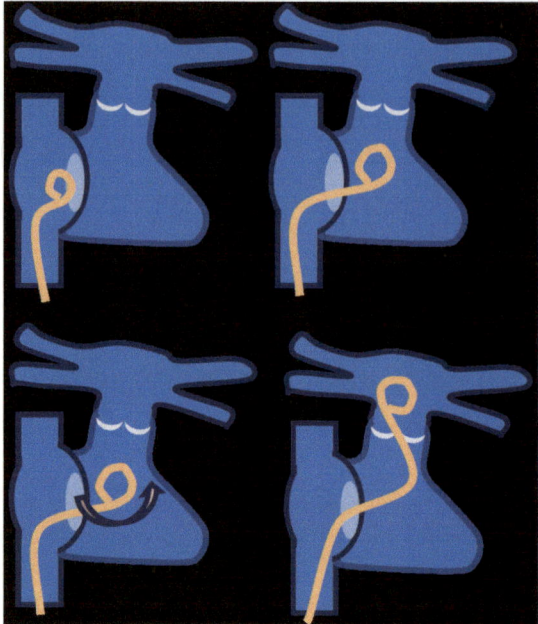

FIGURE 42.1 - TECHNIQUE FOR PULMONARY ARTERY CATHETERIZATION
Diagram depicts technique required to pass the pulmonary artery catheter across the right heart valves and into the main pulmonary artery

Once images have been obtained on the left, the catheter is then manipulated to the right side.

Images are obtained in the AP and opposite oblique (i.e., for a left pulmonary arteriogram, an AP and right anterior oblique study are performed). If there remains a question, selective magnification views of the area of concern can be performed. Angiographic findings of acute pulmonary embolism include "wormlike" filling defects (clots that are casts of the lower leg veins) that are often draped over vessel bifurcation points, tram-tracking of contrast around clots that are nearly occlusive in the vessel, and complete vessel occlusions characterized by cutoffs with a meniscus.

IVC Filter Placement

Although often thought of as separate entities, deep vein thrombosis (DVT) and pulmonary embolism (PE) are the beginning and ultimate final end result of a single disease process known as venous thromboembolic disease (VTED). The primary treatment of choice of VTED is anticoagulation therapy. Anticoagulation therapy prevents new clot formation and allows the body's *own mechanisms* to dissolve the blood clot. (Note—anticoagulation therapy does not dissolve clot itself.) It is a generally safe, effective, and affordable means of preventing a DVT from progressing to a PE.

Inferior vena cava (IVC) filters are metal devices placed in the inferior vena cava that prevent a large embolus from traveling from the lower extremities or pelvis to the pulmonary arteries via a mechanical barrier. Although IVC filters are effective in preventing PE, they remain as second-line therapy for several reasons:

1. IVC filters do nothing to help resolve existing clot and, in some cases, may worsen underlying DVT.
2. IVC filters are associated with complications that become more likely the longer the device stays in place. These include:

   (a) Filter fracture
   (b) Perforation of filter elements through the cava and into adjacent structures
   (c) Filter migration/embolization
   (d) Caval thrombosis

3. Some studies suggest that over time, IVC filters lose their protective value [1]. After 2 years, when compared with patients who receive anticoagulation, patients with IVC filters have the same rate of recurrent PE with twice the rate of recurrent DVT.

Indications for the placement of an IVC filter in patients with VTED include:

1. Contraindication to anticoagulation
2. PE despite adequate anticoagulation (failed anticoagulation therapy)
3. Significant risk of complication from anticoagulation therapy (e.g., fall risk, planned elective surgery)
4. Trauma with injury patterns known to place the patient at high risk for VTED, such as long bone fracture and spinal cord injuries

Many different filter designs are available in the North American and European markets, but in general, they all fall into one of two categories: permanent and retrievable (Fig. 42.2). A permanent filter, as the name implies, is intended to stay in place permanently. A retrievable filter (also sometimes referred to as an "optional" filter) can be used as a permanent device but has design features that allow it to be removed using percutaneous techniques. These devices are sometimes referred to as "optional" filters because they are permanent devices with the option to be removed.

The rationale for having such a device is simple. Because IVC filters are good at preventing PE in the short term but lose their effectiveness while increasing their complication rate over time, it makes sense to have a device that can be placed to protect a patient during a period of high risk that can then be removed once the risk returns to normal.

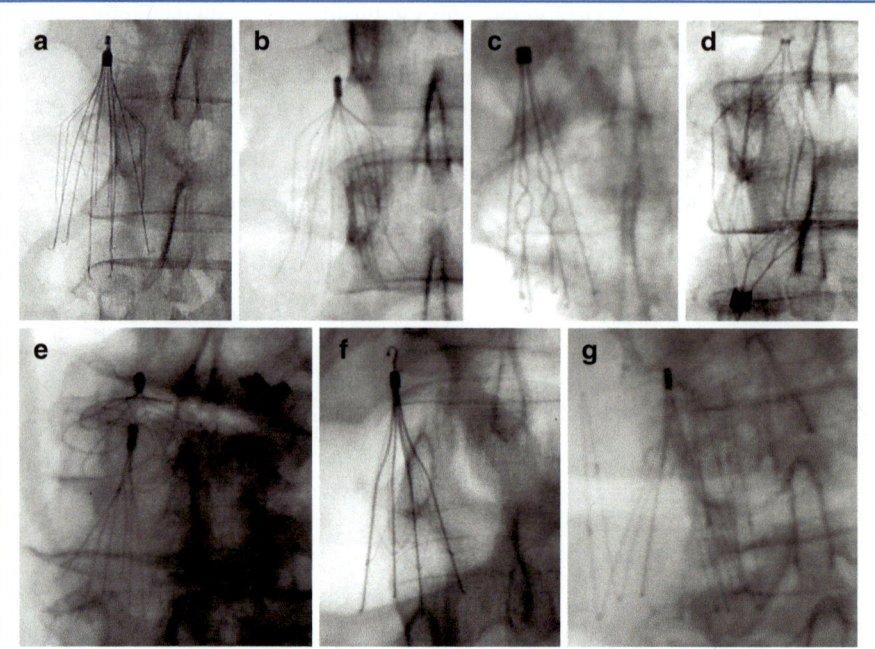

FIGURE 42.2 - EXAMPLES OF SEVERAL IVC FILTERS AVAILABLE TODAY
Clockwise starting from the *upper left*: (**a**) Denali (removable), (**b**) G2 (removable), (**c**) Greenfield (permanent), (**d**) Optease (removable), (**e**) Simon Nitinol (permanent), (**f**) Tulip (removable), (**g**) Vena Tech LP (permanent)

IVC filters are placed via internal jugular or common femoral vein access. A marker catheter (a catheter with radiopaque markers at an exact distance, usually 20 mm) is placed via a common femoral or right internal jugular vein approach and positioned in the left common iliac vein. A power-injection inferior vena cava study is performed, paying close attention to the iliac vein confluence and the inflow from the renal veins. Most IVC filters are designed to be stable in vena cavas 28 mm or less in diameter. The marks on the catheter serve as a reference distance and allow for accurate measurement of the caval diameter accounting for magnification. The appropriate filter is chosen (based on caval size and configuration) and delivered into position inside of a long deployment sheath. Rather than being pushed out the end of the sheath, the filter is deployed by withdrawing the outer sheath, allowing the filter to expand in place, usually just below the renal veins (Fig. 42.3). A follow-up study is performed to confirm the filter's position.

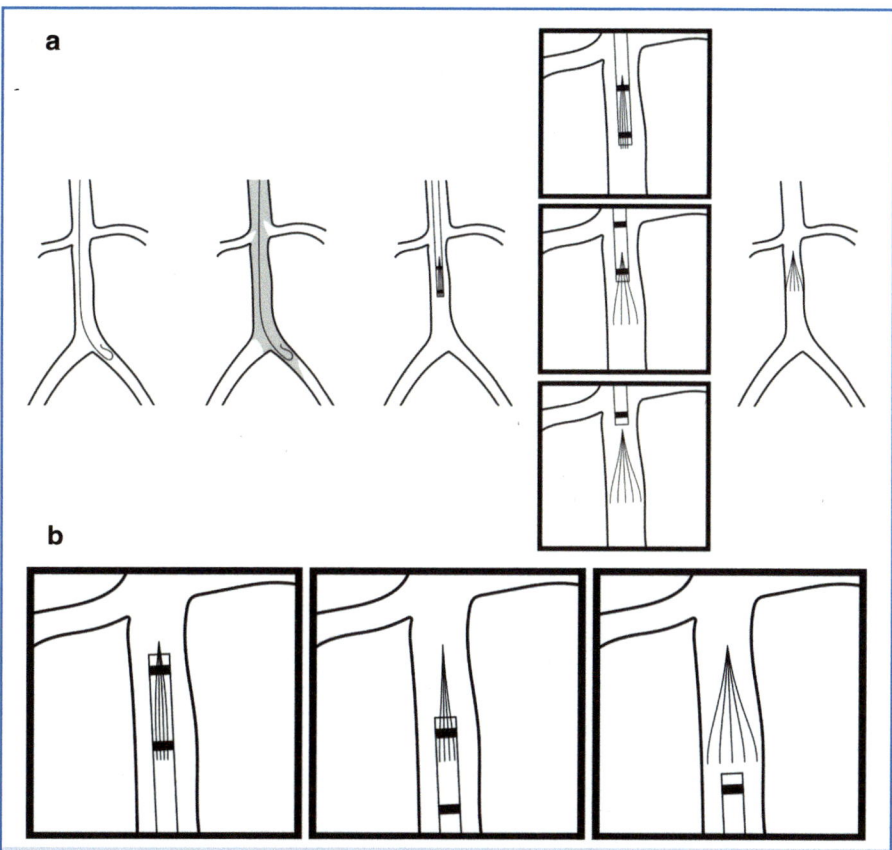

FIGURE 42.3 - DEPLOYMENT OF A VENA CAVA FILTER
(a) On the *left*, a venogram of the inferior vena cava is obtained prior to filter deployment to identify where the renal veins, accessory renal veins, and iliac vein confluence are, to ensure optimal deployment. Next, a deployment sheath with the introducing cannula is advanced over a wire. The cannula is then removed, and inside the sheath, the filter is advanced to the tip of the sheath. The sheath is then pulled back (subset of images within black boxes) and the filter self-deploys. Figure (**b**) depicts sheath advancement and filter deployment from a femoral approach

S: In patients who require an IVC filter, the appropriate indication is critical. During the procedure, it is important to identify variant anatomy that may impact placement of the filter.

A: In patients with recurrent DVTs who are fall risks where anticoagulation significantly increases the risk of intracranial hemorrhage, IVC filters can reduce the risk of PE from DVT.

F: Cross-sectional imaging and angiography can be used to confirm post procedural positioning as well as filter and IVC integrity.

E: In those at significant risk of pulmonary embolism who are not able to be treated with anticoagulation, timely identification and placement of the IVC filter are important. When the utility of the IVC filter is outweighed by the risk of remaining in place (fracturing, embolization, DVT), then removal should be performed.

Reference

1. Decousus H, Leizorovicz A, Parent F, et al. A clinical trial of vena caval filters in the prevention of pulmonary embolism in patients with proximal deep vein thrombosis. N Engl J Med. 1998;338(7):409–15.

43

GENITOURINARY INTERVENTIONS

Objectives:
1. Describe indications for common genitourinary interventions
2. Identify relevant renal and pelvic anatomy related to genitourinary interventions
3. Understand types of renal collecting system catheters and the indications for each

Percutaneous Nephrostomy Placement

Percutaneous renal collecting system access is most commonly performed for the relief of urinary obstruction due to calculi, urothelial malignancy, or extrinsic compression. Additional indications for percutaneous nephrostomy or ureteral stenting include access for diagnostic or therapeutic interventions and urinary diversion in the setting of collecting system trauma or inflammatory pelvic fistulous disease.

Renal vascular anatomy plays a large role in the technique and location of percutaneous nephrostomy placement. The main renal artery is located at the renal hilum with subsequent branches decreasing in caliber; because of this, primary collecting system access into the renal pelvis or an infundibulum is discouraged due to increased risk of bleeding complications. The junction of the anterior and posterior segmental renal arteries along the posterolateral aspect of the kidney is a relatively avascular plane, known as the plane of Brödel (Fig. 43.1), which is theoretically safe to obtain access. Additionally, the interventional radiologist must be aware of adjacent structures that could complicate nephrostomy placement, particularly the relationship of the kidneys with the neighboring pleura, colon, liver, and spleen.

© Springer Nature Switzerland AG 2020
J. Kissane et al. (eds.), *Radiology Fundamentals: Introduction to Imaging & Technology*, https://doi.org/10.1007/978-3-030-22173-7_43

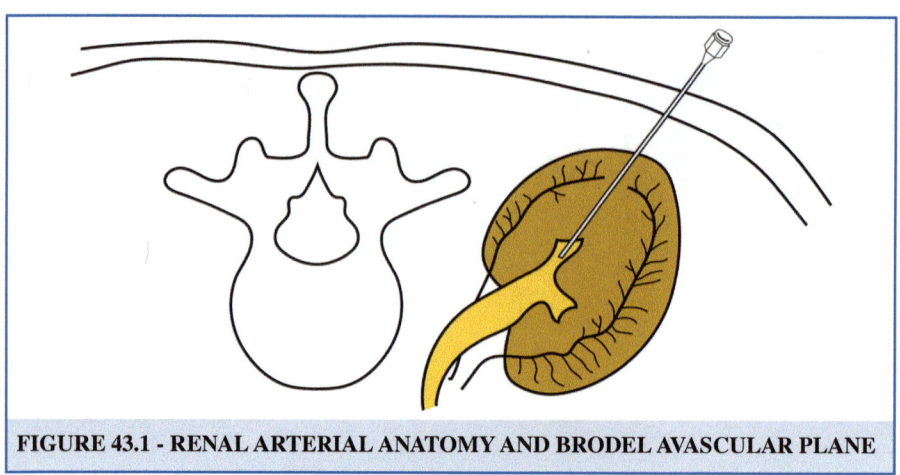

FIGURE 43.1 - RENAL ARTERIAL ANATOMY AND BRODEL AVASCULAR PLANE

Percutaneous nephrostomy placement is typically performed with the patient in a prone position under ultrasound or fluoroscopic guidance. Ultrasound guidance offers direct visualization of the collecting system and helps direct access, particularly in the setting of hydronephrosis, when dilated calyces are readily visualized. Ultrasound is also the modality of choice when there is a desire to reduce ionizing radiation, i.e., in children or a pregnant patient.

Access to the renal collecting system can be described as either initial or definitive. *Initial access* is usually obtained using a small caliber needle with the goal to delineate collecting system anatomy in the patient with a non-dilated system. In this situation, initial access is directed toward the renal pelvis, a radiopaque renal calculus, or excreted contrast if given intravenously to aid in target demarcation. Once access is confirmed, air is slowly injected into the renal pelvis utilizing the principle that air will collect in the nondependent posterior calyces. The air-filled posterior calyces can then be targeted under fluoroscopic guidance to obtain *definitive access* via a second needle. Using the Seldinger technique (as discussed in prior chapters) through the posterior calyx access, a wire is advanced into the ureter, and the skin tract is serially dilated before placing a catheter into the renal pelvis. Percutaneous nephrostomy catheters are equipped with a locking pigtail mechanism to help ensure appropriate positioning throughout patient motion and breathing (Fig. 43.2).

Percutaneous nephrostomy tubes are placed initially in the setting of obstruction or infection with the goal to decompress the collecting system, allow patient recovery from acute illness, and ensure adequate position and function prior to replacement or conversion to alternate urologic access. If ureteral access is desired for management of distal collecting system stricture or obstruction, a nephroureteral drain or an internal double-J ureteral stent can be placed through the percutaneous nephrostomy site. Nephroureteral drains allow continued external access to the collecting system with the differentiating factor between a nephrostomy tube being

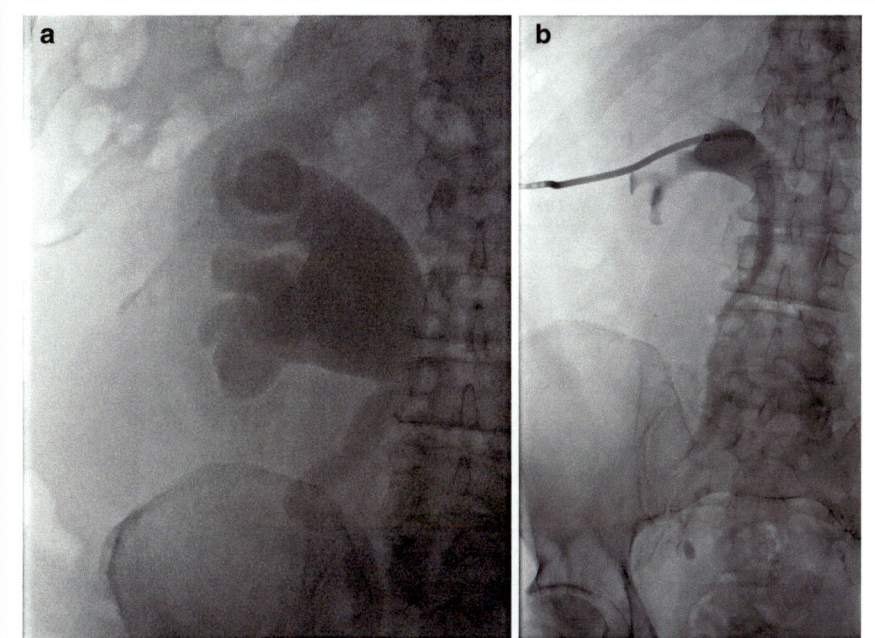

FIGURE 43.2 - HYDRONEPHROSIS SECONDARY TO URETEROLITHIASIS
Scout fluoroscopic abdominal image demonstrates a dilated renal collecting system visualized secondary to excreted intravenous contrast from prior CT (**a**). Post-percutaneous nephrostomy placement shows decompression of the collecting system with loop in the renal pelvis (**b**). Note the radiopaque distal ureteral calculus

ureteral extension from the renal pelvis to the distal ureter or bladder. A double-J ureteral stent provides drainage from the proximal renal collecting system to the bladder similar to the nephroureteral drain; however, external access is abandoned. Finally, if the patient has undergone surgical urinary diversion and requires access due to obstruction from anastomotic stricture or recurrent malignancy, a retrograde nephroureteral drain can be placed through a urinary ostomy with the pigtail loop positioned in the renal pelvis (Fig. 43.3).

Gonadal Vein Embolization

Gonadal vein embolization can be used in either the male or female population for different indications. In males, gonadal vein embolization is a treatment option for the management of varicoceles. Typical symptoms of varicoceles include infertility

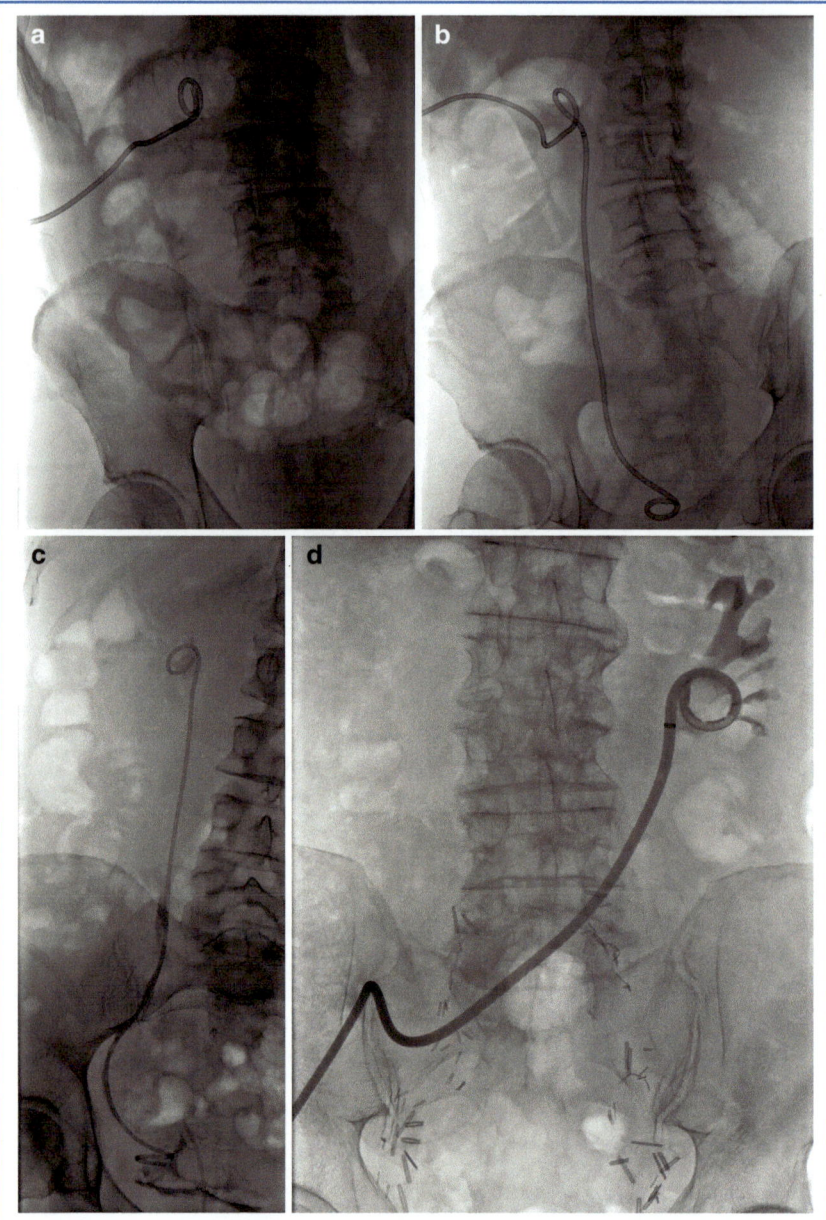

FIGURE 43.3 - EXAMPLES OF DIFFERENT GENITOURINARY ACCESS AND DRAINAGE CATHETERS
A percutaneous nephrostomy tube (**a**), nephroureteral drain (**b**), internal double-J ureteral stent (**c**), and reverse nephroureteral drain through a right lower quadrant ostomy (**d**). Note multiple pelvic surgical clips following cystectomy and pelvic lymph node dissection for treatment of bladder carcinoma

and pain. The incidence of varicocele in adult males is up to 17%; however, in the male infertility population, varicocele can range to almost 27%.

In females, gonadal vein embolization can be used in the management of pelvic congestion syndrome. Pelvic congestion results from pelvic varices and can cause significant and chronic pelvic pain. Typical symptoms of pelvic congestion syndrome include dull pain that worsens with prolonged standing or walking, dyspareunia, dysfunctional uterine bleeding, and urinary or gastrointestinal symptoms (Fig. 43.4).

Gonadal vein anatomy plays a large role in the laterality of varicocele. The left gonadal vein drains into the left renal vein, while the right gonadal vein drains directly into the inferior vena cava. Because of the circuitous route and the potential for slower flow, left-sided varicocele occurs in approximately 90% of cases. Conversely, if a unilateral right-sided varicocele is encountered, additional imaging should be pursued to identify the cause such as situs inversus or an abdominal mass resulting in caval or gonadal vein compression.

Venous access is typically obtained via a common femoral or internal jugular approach. Using the Seldinger technique (as described in previous chapters), a catheter is advanced into the inferior vena cava and left renal vein. Contrast is then injected to document venous valve incompetence and reflux into the gonadal vein.

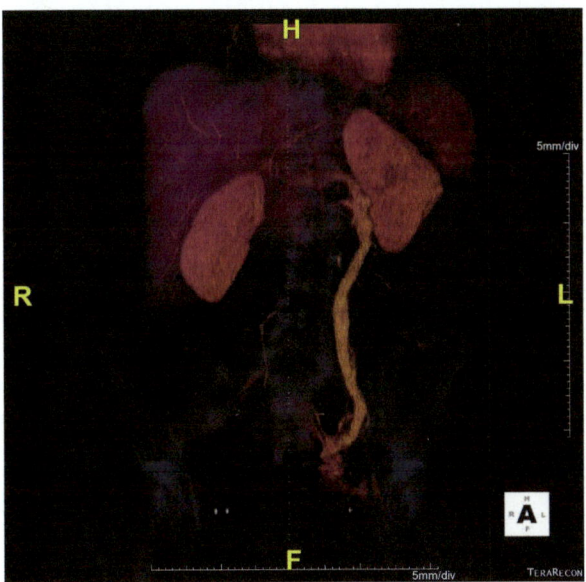

FIGURE 43.4 - PELVIC CONGESTION SYNDROME
Coronal 3D reconstructed CT images show a dilated left ovarian vessel draining into the left renal vein with multiple prominent pelvic collateral vessels in a patient with pelvic congestion syndrome

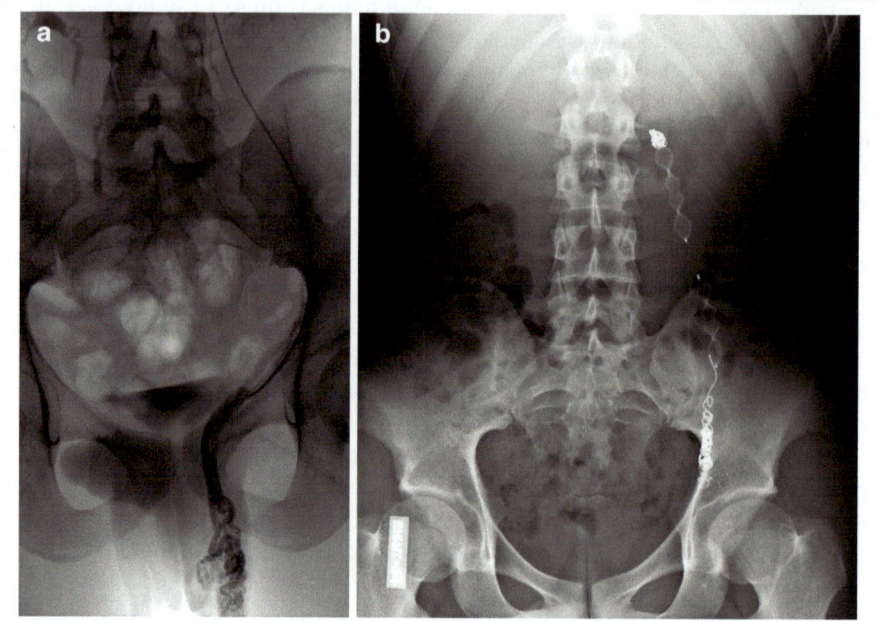

FIGURE 43.5 - LEFT GONADAL VEIN EMBOLIZATION IN A MALE
Intraprocedural left gonadal venogram shows dilated, tortuous vessels within the left scrotum
(**a**). KUB following gonadal vein embolization show embolization coils and Amplatzer plugs
within the left gonadal vein (**b**)

Once confirmed, the catheter is further advanced into the gonadal vein, and emboli-zation is performed of one, or both, gonadal veins. If right gonadal vein access is desired, catheter-based cannulation, venography, and embolization are performed from the inferior vena cava rather than the renal vein in cases of classic gonadal vein anatomy (Fig. 43.5).

Multiple studies have reported a significant improvement in pelvic pain in roughly 85% of female patients who underwent gonadal vein embolization for pelvic con-gestion syndrome. Alternatively, improvement in semen parameters was seen in approximately 25–75% of men following gonadal vein embolization for the treat-ment of infertility due to varicocele.

Uterine Fibroid Embolization

Uterine fibroid embolization (UFE) is a treatment option for patients who have symptomatic leiomyomas. Common symptoms of uterine fibroids include menor-rhagia, pelvic pain, urinary frequency, or obstruction. Careful selection of patients requires exclusion of a current pregnancy or further workup if there is suspected malignancy (i.e., vaginal bleeding in a postmenopausal patient or abnormal imaging suggesting malignant fibroid degeneration).

The uterine artery arises from the anterior division of the internal iliac artery in just over 50% of women. In approximately 40% of the remaining female population, the uterine artery arises from a trifurcation at the internal iliac artery.

Arterial access is obtained through either a femoral or radial approach. Typically, contralateral femoral arterial access is achieved, and a catheter is advanced over the aortic bifurcation to the opposite common iliac artery. The catheter can then be advanced over a wire into the internal iliac artery followed by selection of the uterine artery. Following confirmation of position by injection of contrast, embolization can be performed to complete, or near complete, stasis. Care should be taken to avoid embolization of proximal branches to decrease the likelihood of non-target embolization and associated treatment-related complications such as ovarian dysfunction or dyspareunia (Fig. 43.6).

Between 85% and 90% of patients reported improvement in clinical symptoms such as menorrhagia and pelvic pain at 1 and 3 years following UFE. Additional studies showed similar outcomes in health-related quality of life between patients having undergone uterine fibroid embolization compared to hysterectomy patients. While complication rates were similar between embolization and hysterectomy patients, UFE patients had a greater likelihood of reintervention.

Fallopian Tube Recanalization

The majority of female infertility is due to either ovulatory disorders or fallopian tube dysfunction. Pelvic inflammatory disease endometriosis, adhesions, debris, mucous plugging, and salpingitis isthmica nodosa are several different tubal pathologies that can result in infertility. Initial evaluation includes hysterosalpingography (HSG), which involves cannulation of the cervix and injection of contrast in the uterine cavity. In the setting of tubal patency, contrast extends through the fallopian tubes and spills into the peritoneal cavity. Fallopian tube recanalization is indicated in cases where HSG fails to demonstrate free intraperitoneal spillage of contrast due to fallopian tube obstruction. It is imperative to exclude pregnancy and active pelvic inflammatory disease prior to proceeding with fallopian tube recanalization.

Fallopian tube obstruction amenable to transcervical recanalization involves the proximal tube, also known as the interstitial portion. The distal, or fimbriated, fallopian tube segment is typically managed surgically or with in vitro fertilization.

The patient is placed in the lithotomy position, and a speculum is inserted to visualize and cannulate the cervix. Following this, an HSG is performed, and selective recanalization is directed toward the obstructed tube(s). An angled-tip catheter helps gain access to the interstitial portion of the fallopian tube. A hydrophilic guidewire and microcatheter can then be advanced through the fallopian tube to

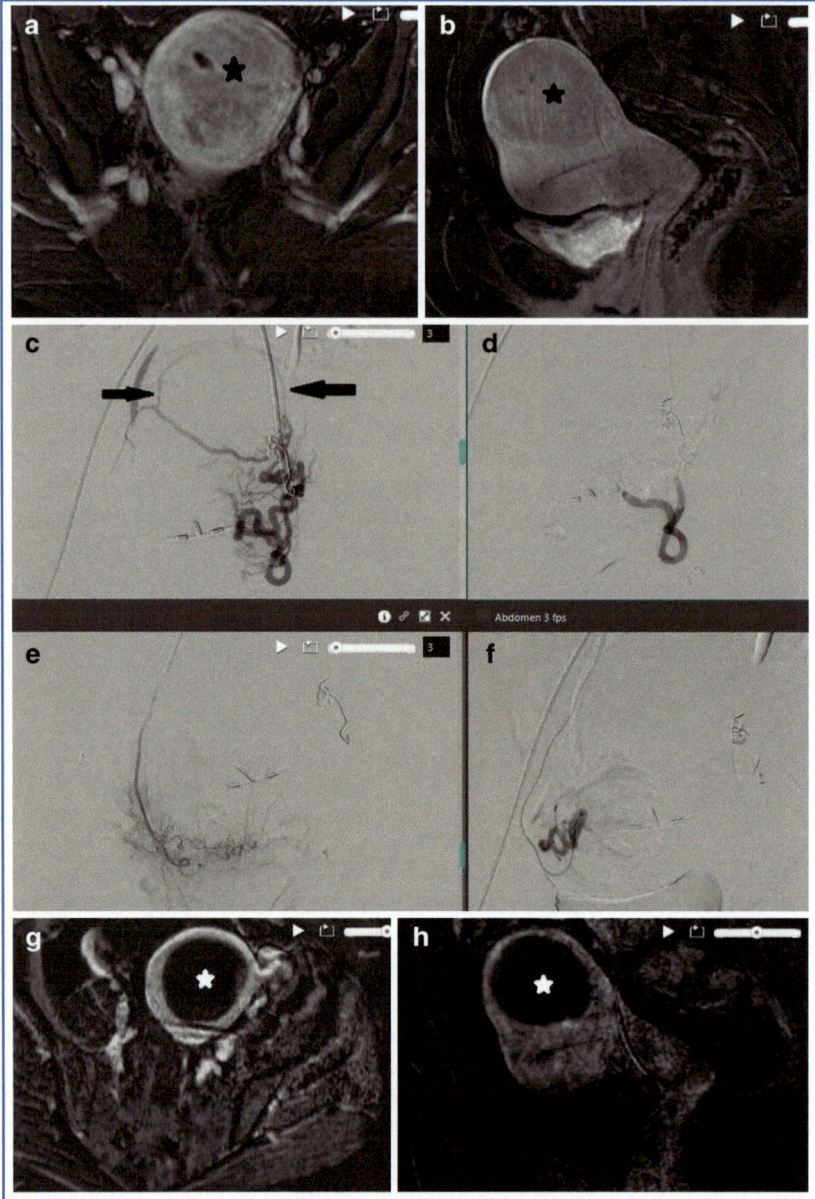

FIGURE 43.6 - UTERINE ARTERY EMBOLIZATION
Pre-embolization T1-weighted post contrast coronal (**a**) and sagittal (**b**) MRI shows a large enhancing fundal fibroid (*black stars*). Four images from intraprocedural arteriogram (top row: left uterine artery treatment (**c, d**), bottom row: right uterine artery treatment (**e, f**)) demonstrate blood flow to the large fibroid predominantly arising from the left uterine artery (*arrows*). Post-embolization T1-weighted post contrast coronal (**g**) and sagittal (**h**) MRI non-enhancement of the large fibroid (*white stars*)

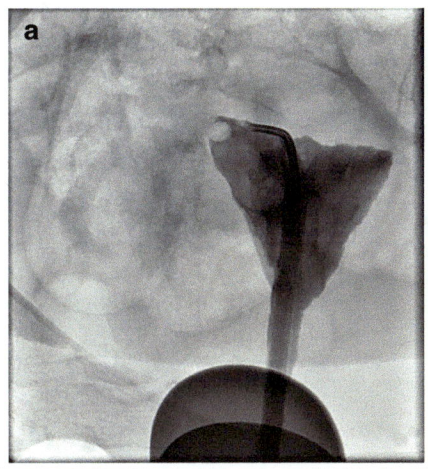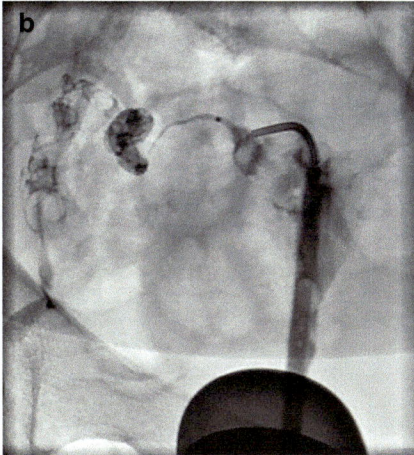

FIGURE 43.7 - FALLOPIAN TUBE RECANALIZATION
Hysterosalpingogram shows an angled-tip catheter within the uterine cavity and contrast opacification of the cavity without visualization of either fallopian tube (**a**). Intraprocedural fluoroscopic image demonstrates advancement of a microcatheter into the right fallopian tube. Contrast injection reveals opacification of the fallopian tube with free intraperitoneal spillage of contrast, indicating successful recanalization (**b**)

restore patency. Posttreatment HSG is repeated to document free intraperitoneal spillage of contrast (Fig. 43.7).

Technical success rates of fallopian tube recanalization are high, reported at 80–90%. Average unaided pregnancy rates following fallopian tube recanalization are approximately 30%; however, up to 60% of patients develop repeat tubal obstruction following intervention.

S: Invasive procedures anywhere in the genitourinary system need to be judged on the risk/benefit balance for those procedures. For instance, urinary sepsis is quite dangerous, and so despite the risks of placing a nephrostomy tube, the benefit can be life-saving. For a fallopian tube recanalization, the benefit is limited; however, the risk is limited as well, and so, the risk-benefit ratio is acceptable. Similar to all interventional procedures, the indications and patients' medical history must be carefully reviewed. Preprocedural workup should include review of any patient variant anatomy, coagulation abnormalities, and infection.

A: The judicious use of fluoroscopy for any of the GU procedures is very important. Since some of the procedures can take significant time, the interventional radiologist has to be cognizant of the amount of fluoroscopy time used.

F: For invasive procedures, documentation of the reason for the initial consult can help guide subsequent procedures. For example, demonstrating the obstructing stone in a patient who is septic can be beneficial.

E: When presented with genitourinary pathology, consultation with the interventional radiologist is the most appropriate next step. For some patient presentations, urgent consultation is needed in order to expedite the treatment (i.e., urosepsis).

Suggested Reading

Lee, Michael, et al. "Chapter 22: Percutaneous Genitourinary Intervention." *Vascular and Interventional Radiology: the Requisites*, Elsevier, 2014, pp. 485–510.

Kogut, Matthew, et al. "Chapter 23: Urologic and Genital Systems." *Vascular and Interventional Radiology*, Saunders Elsevier, 2006, pp. 684–717.

Stokes, LeAnn, et.al. "Chapter 146: Percutaneous Nephrostomy, Cystostomy, and Nephroureteral Stenting." *Image-Guided Interventions*. Saunders/Elsevier, 2014, pp. 1076-1089.

Griene, Bryan, et.al. "Chapter 79: Management of Male Varicocele." *Image-Guided Interventions*. Saunders/Elsevier, 2014, pp. 559-563.

Kies, Darren, et.al. "Chapter 80: Management of Female Venous Congestion Syndrome." *Image-Guided Interventions*. Saunders/Elsevier, 2014, pp. 563-569.

Grieme, Bryan, et.al. "Chapter 79: Management of Male Varicocele." *Image-Guided Interventions*. Saunders/Elsevier, 2014, pp. 559-563.

Neiderberger, Craig. "Chapter 24: Male Infertility." *Campbell-Walsh Urology*. Elsevier, 2016, pp. 556-579.

Spies, James, et.al. "Chapter 76: Uterine Fibroid Embolization." *Image-Guided Interventions*. Saunders/Elsevier, 2014, pp. 542-548.

Hall, Lee, et.al. "Chapter 150: Fallopian Tube Interventions." *Image-Guided Interventions*. Saunders/Elsevier, 2014, pp. 1117-1127.

44 TRANSJUGULAR INTRAHEPATIC PORTOSYSTEMIC SHUNT

Objectives:
1. List the indications and contraindications for TIPS.
2. Describe the relevant anatomy for TIPS.
3. Describe the steps needed to create a TIPS.
4. Described the follow-up and complications of TIPS.
5. Discuss how TIPS placement alters long-term survival.

TIPS Indications

1. Variceal hemorrhage which is refractory to medical management
2. Prophylaxis for recurrent variceal bleeding
3. Ascites or hepatic hydrothorax which is refractory to medical management
4. Budd-Chiari syndrome

TIPS Contraindications

1. Severe hepatic insufficiency
2. Severe uncontrolled encephalopathy
3. Severe heart failure
4. Polycystic liver disease
5. Hypervascular hepatic tumor

© Springer Nature Switzerland AG 2020
J. Kissane et al. (eds.), *Radiology Fundamentals: Introduction to Imaging & Technology*, https://doi.org/10.1007/978-3-030-22173-7_44

TIPS-Relative Contraindications

1. Active bleeding
2. Active infection
3. Portal vein occlusion

Once placement of the TIPS has been deemed appropriate, several questions must be answered.

Has cross-sectional imaging (CT/MRI) been performed to evaluate anatomy? Is there portal vein thrombus noted by ultrasound, CT, or MRI scan? This can affect whether or not a TIPS is placed and the procedural approach taken. Has endoscopy been performed to confirm site of varices or bleeding and attempts made to stop bleeding? Endoscopic variceal ligation is typically the first-line therapy among other endoscopic methods and should be attempted prior to TIPS, if deemed safe.

Are the varices actively bleeding? If the varices are actively bleeding, TIPS is relatively contraindicated because of the high mortality associated with placement of a TIPS in an actively bleeding patient. Sometimes, however, it is the patient's only option when endoscopic methods fail. In these cases, ensure the patient has received adequate resuscitation with IV fluids, blood products, and pressor support. In addition, ensure the patient has received appropriate treatment for coagulopathies, placement of gastric balloon tamponade devices (i.e., Blakemore), and airway protection as indicated.

It is important to calculate the MELD (Model for End Stage Liver Disease) score as this dramatically influences survival.

$$\text{MELD} = 3.78 \times \ln\left[\text{serum bilirubin}\left(\text{mg}/\text{dL}\right)\right] + 11.2 \times \ln\left[\text{INR}\right] + 9.57 \times \ln\left[\text{serum creatinine}\left(\text{mg}/\text{dL}\right)\right] + 6.43$$

As would be expected, the higher the MELD score, the lower the overall survival [1]. MELD scores over 18 are associated with a significantly higher risk of early mortality following TIPS. The formula to calculate a MELD score using serum bilirubin, INR, and serum creatinine is shown above. Multiple online and app-based calculators are available. Additionally, the Child-Pugh score can be used to determine the prognosis of a patient based on several predictive factors indicating the level of decompensation in chronic liver disease as shown in Fig. 44.1.

Relevant Anatomy

Normal hepatic vein and portal vein anatomy is shown below in Fig. 44.2. It is important to review this anatomy prior to TIPS as a shunt between a hepatic vein and portal vein will be created, and there may be variants of normal anatomy

Diagnostic criteria	1	2	3
Encephalopathy	None	Moderate	Severe
Ascites	None	Moderate	Severe
Bilirubin	<2	2–3	>3
Albumin	>3.5	2.8–3.4	<2.8
PT	<14	15–17	>18

FIGURE 44.1 - CHILD-PUGH SCORE
This classification scheme is used to assess the prognosis of chronic liver disease. To calculate a score, add the points from each category together. A is 5–6 points, B is 7–9 points, while C is greater than 10 points

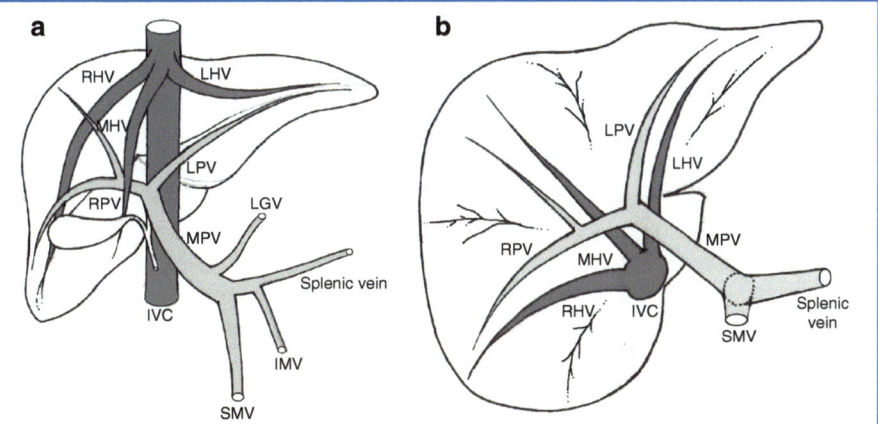

FIGURE 44.2 - HEPATIC VEIN AND PORTAL VEIN NORMAL ANATOMY
Left image (**a**) demonstrates the normal hepatic venous and portal venous anatomy in an AP-view, and the right image (**b**) demonstrates the anatomy in an axial (cross-sectional) view. The hepatic vein typically splits into a right, middle, and left. The portal vein typically splits into a right and left portal vein with the right bisecting the right and middle hepatic veins. RHV Right hepatic vein, MHV Middle hepatic vein, LHV Left hepatic vein, RPV Right portal vein, LPV Left portal vein, MPV Main portal vein, LGV Left gastric vein, SMV Superior mesenteric vein, IMV Inferior mesenteric vein, IVC Inferior vena cava

discovered. The shunt is typically from the right hepatic vein to the right portal vein, which lies anterior. Alternatively, a shunt from the middle hepatic vein to the right portal vein can be created if directing the shunt posteriorly from the middle hepatic vein. Additionally, imaging should be evaluated for portal vein patency and large volume ascites which should be drained prior to the TIPS.

TIPS Placement

For placement of the TIPS, the right internal jugular vein is used for access. Once access has been obtained, a large, long sheath (10 French) is placed with its tip in the right atrium. Using an angled catheter, access is obtained to the right hepatic vein (or sometimes the middle hepatic vein). Simultaneous pressures are obtained within the hepatic vein and the right atrium. Next the catheter is "wedged" as peripherally as possible in the hepatic vein. A wedged hepatic vein pressure to right atrial pressure gradient (similar to inflating the balloon of a Swan-Ganz catheter to obtain left atrial pressures) is determined. A hepatic venogram is then obtained. The angled catheter is exchanged for one of several transhepatic needle access systems.

A large, hollow, directional needle is used to gain access to the portal vein through the liver parenchyma, and via the needle, a wire is advanced into the portal vein. True simultaneous pressures are obtained across the liver in the hepatic vein and the portal vein. The tract is pre-dilated with an 8-mm balloon. A stent of appropriate length is deployed across the liver and dilated (Fig. 44.3). Simultaneous gradients are then obtained. If the gradient is too low, there can be a significant "steal" phenomenon from liver perfusion. If the gradient is too high, improvement in the varices or ascites/effusion may be inadequate. Pressure gradients greater than 12 mmHg are associated with an increased rate of variceal bleeding. If the pressure gradient remains elevated after TIPS placement, the stent may need to be dilated to a larger diameter to reduce the gradient to an acceptable level. Alternatively, if post-TIPS hepatic encephalopathy cannot be controlled, the TIPS may actually need to be occluded.

Follow-Up

An ultrasound is obtained prior to the patient's discharge and at subsequent regular intervals for follow-up after discharge to ensure patency of the TIPS.

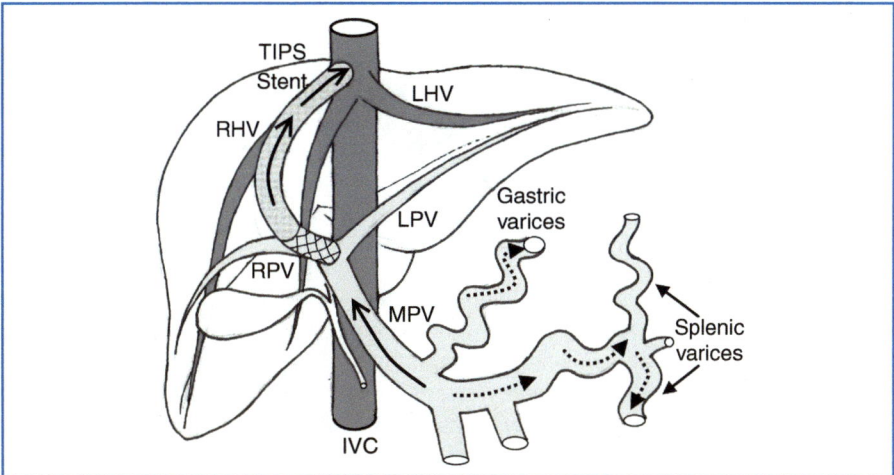

FIGURE 44.3 - DIAGRAM OF A TIPS
Portal hypertension causes portal venous flow to reverse and flow away from the liver (dashed arrows) leading to portovenous collateral development (varices) and splenomegaly. Through a percutaneous access from the internal jugular vein, the right hepatic vein is "connected" to the right portal vein branch via a transparenchymal tract. This tract is supported open utilizing a stent, frequently a Viatorr device. This allows the portal venous flow to decompress into the hepatic venous system and the associated varices to decompress (solid arrows). RHV Right hepatic vein, LHV Left hepatic vein, RPV Right portal vein, LPV Left portal vein, MPV Main portal vein, IVC Inferior vena cava

Complications

As with any interventional procedure, infection and bleeding are always a risk. In TIPS, the major risk of bleeding is from liver capsular rupture with intraperitoneal hemorrhage. Therefore, it is imperative to understand the cross-sectional and fluoroscopic anatomy to properly direct the portal vein access needle. Worsening hepatic encephalopathy is seen in 30–50% of patients with less than 10% being refractory to medical therapy [2]. Accelerated hepatic failure can be seen in 1–5% of patients, more commonly occurring in patients with a higher MELD score or hepatic arterial disease [3]. Normally, 75% of the blood supply and 50% of the oxygen demand come from the portal vein with the remaining supplied by the hepatic artery. Following TIPS the majority of blood flow is from the hepatic artery leading to hepatic ischemia if there is significant underlying hepatic arterial disease. Congestive heart failure from increased venous return from the shunting is uncommon with proper fluid and diuretic management. Stent thrombosis or occlusion is uncommon using modern covered stents with 1-year unassisted patency rates of 80–90% [4].

Long-Term Survival

TIPS placement is successful in 96% of cases. It is important to understand that TIPS placement does not alter the underlying liver disease. It only alters the manifestations of portal hypertension. Current transplant-free survival after a TIPS is 75.1% at 6 months, 63.1% at 12 months, 49% at 24 months, and 38.1% at 36 months [5]. As previously mentioned, it is important to calculate the MELD score as this dramatically influences survival.

S: Pre-procedural cross-sectional imaging such as CT or MRI can determine portal vein patency, hepatic artery patency, and volume of ascites and display relevant anatomy. Additionally, an echocardiogram can determine if the patient has significant heart failure or pulmonary artery hypertension. Pre-procedural imaging can affect the management and procedural approach, reduce procedural radiation dose, and reduce morbidity and mortality related to the procedure. It is important to recognize that many patients with cirrhosis will have renal impairment. Therefore, intravenous contrast should be used judiciously.

A: Post-procedure duplex ultrasound is indicated to determine patency and baseline characteristics of the TIPS. This should be performed 5–10 days post procedure as air within the stent graft inhibits adequate visualization of the TIPS on ultrasound immediately post placement. Prior to the use of stent grafts, imaging was performed 24 h post procedure as air was not present within bare-metal stents. Routine duplex ultrasound should be performed every 6–12 months thereafter. Using ultrasound for follow-up helps reduce the patients and physicians radiation exposure. A follow-up angiographic TIPS study should be performed if the ultrasound indicates TIPS dysfunction, but a revision should always be based on recurrence and management of symptoms.

F: For routine duplex ultrasound follow-up of TIPS, it is important to compare to a baseline study as TIPS measurements are highly variable and can be misleading. The most specific value for TIPS dysfunction is a main portal vein velocity lower than 30 cm/s. However, values should always be correlated with symptoms and TIPS revisions performed accordingly.

E: It is important to understand and identify the possible complications of a TIPS procedure such as liver capsular rupture, shunt stenosis, shunt thrombosis or occlusion, and pneumothorax on follow-up imaging. Complications should be communicated with the proceduralist in a timely fashion.

References

1. Ferral H, Gamboa P, et al. Survival after elective transjugular intrahepatic portosystemic shunt creation: prediction with model for end-stage liver disease score. Radiology. 2004;231:231–236.
2. Zuckerman DA, Darcy MD, Bocchini TP, Hildebolt CF. Encephalopathy after transjugular intrahepatic portosystemic shunting: analysis of incidence and potential risk factors. AJR Am J Roentgenol 1997; 169:1727–1731
3. Luca, A., Miraglia, R., Maruzzelli, L., D'Amico, M., & Tuzzolino, F. Early liver failure after transjugular intrahepatic portosystemic shunt in patients with cirrhosis with model for end-stage liver disease score of 12 or less: incidence, outcome, and prognostic factors. Radiology 2016; 280: 622–629.
4. Rossi P, Salvatori FM, Fanelli F, et al. Polytetrafluoroethylene-covered nitinol stent-graft for transjugular intrahepatic portosystemic shunt creation: 3-year experience. Radiology 2004; 231:820–830
5. Salerno F, Camma C, et al. Transjugular intrahepatic portosystemic shunt for refractory ascites: a meta-analysis of individual patient data. Gastroenterology. 2007;133:825–34.

45

CENTRAL VENOUS ACCESS

Objectives:
1. List the types of devices available and their indications for placement.
2. List the different methods of central venous access.

Maintenance of venous access is the cornerstone of many medical therapies. Durable venous access into the central venous systems is essential for most cancer regimens, extended antibiotic therapies, parenteral nutrition, and inotropic therapies. Durable central venous access for patients who require dialysis serves as a bridge until a dialysis fistula, dialysis graft, or peritoneal dialysis (PD) catheter is established or as a means of last resort when a graft, fistula, or PD catheter is no longer possible. Increasingly, the placement of a long-term central venous access device is performed using ultrasound and fluoroscopic image guidance and is most commonly performed by interventional radiology (Table 45.1).

There is a great deal of confusion concerning the different types of venous access devices. This situation is complicated by the common practice of referring to catheters by trade names, which are often ambiguous as to form and function. In general, catheters are classified by two attributes: non-tunneled versus tunneled and infusion versus exchange. An exception to this is subcutaneous devices (ports) which are almost always used for infusion therapy and can remain in place for extended periods of time (Fig. 45.1).

Non-tunneled catheters are generally intended for short-term use (days to weeks). These catheters have no subcutaneous tunnel, and their entry site goes directly through the skin and into the access vein. As the name implies, tunneled catheters have a subcutaneous tunnel between the skin entry site and the vein entry site. These devices include a cuff positioned along the tunnel that serves to provide a barrier to infection and eventually to assist in anchoring the catheter in place (Fig. 45.2). The tunnel and cuff system allows the device to stay in place for weeks to months.

© Springer Nature Switzerland AG 2020
J. Kissane et al. (eds.), *Radiology Fundamentals: Introduction to Imaging & Technology*, https://doi.org/10.1007/978-3-030-22173-7_45

Table 45.1 Central venous access. Indications and route of access for various central venous catheters

Catheter type	Duration	Route of access	Expected duration
Non-tunneled infusion catheter	Short term	IJ, subclavian, femoral	3–7 days
Non-tunneled dialysis catheter	Short term	IJ Femoral if inpatient Subclavian discouraged	2–4 weeks
PICC (peripherally inserted central catheter)	Short term	Upper extremity veins, usually basilic vein	2–6 weeks
Tunneled infusion catheter	Long term	IJ, subclavian	4–6 months
Tunneled dialysis catheter	Long term	IJ Subclavian discouraged	6–12 months
Chest port	Long term	IJ, Subclavian	12–18 months

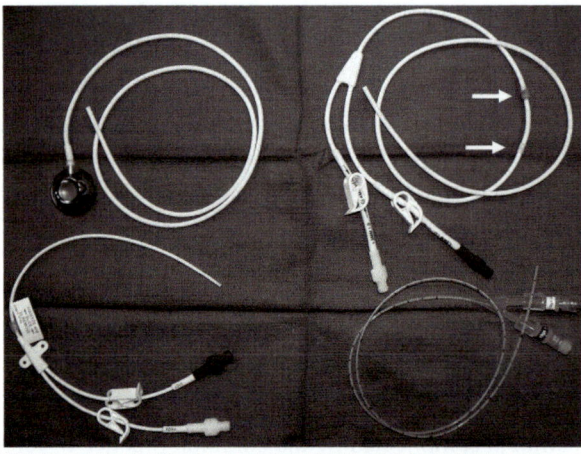

FIGURE 45.1 - EXAMPLES OF INFUSION CATHETERS
From *left* to *right* and *top* to *bottom*, they include a subcutaneous port, a tunneled infusion catheter, a non-tunneled infusion catheter (Hohn), and a peripherally inserted central catheter (*PICC*). Note the fabric cuffs on the midshaft of the tunneled catheter (*arrows*). (Image courtesy of F. Lynch MD, FSIR)

Subcutaneous ports (aka, mediports or port-a-caths) consist of an infusion catheter attached to a reservoir hub. The entire device is placed under the skin, and when accessed or used, a special needle is placed under sterile conditions through the skin into the reservoir. Once accessed, the port functions like any other infusion catheter. When not accessed, the port requires little care. These attributes make it ideal for

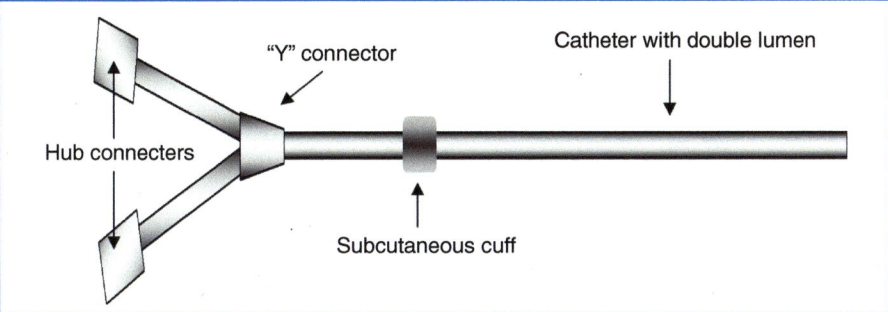

FIGURE 45.2 - TUNNELED CATHETER GENERAL DESIGN
In this dual lumen catheter, the main catheter has an extruded dual lumen. These are divided at the Y connector. The hub connectors are used for access, each equipped with a Luer-Lok device. The subcutaneous cuff seals the subcutaneous access tunnel when the surrounding tissues grow into the cuff, preventing movement of the catheter as well as advancement of skin flora up the tract into the central venous system

patients whose therapies are characterized by episodes requiring continuous venous access separated by periods where venous access is not required, e.g., chemotherapy.

Catheters intended for infusion therapy are generally small in diameter (5–10 Fr), may have one to three lumens, and have simple end-hole designs. Catheters intended for exchange therapy, such as hemodialysis or plasmapheresis, are much larger in diameter (11–16 Fr), have at least two lumens (one to withdraw and one to return blood), and have specially designed tips that prevent the blood that is returned from the catheter from being re-aspirated through the other lumen (Fig. 45.3). During exchange therapy, blood flows sometimes up to 600 ml per minute are required through these devices.

The subclavian vein is often used for short-term venous access because of the relative distance of the vein to the mouth reduces the likelihood of infection. Anatomically, the subclavian vein passes through a narrow space at the junction of the first rib and clavicle. This space is further compressed with movement at the shoulder. This compression, combined with the presence of the catheter, is associated with a high incidence of venous stenosis and even catheter fracture, also known as catheter pinch-off syndrome. Since subclavian vein stenosis may have long-term implications for future venous and hemodialysis access, the preferred site for long-term central venous access is the internal jugular vein.

The procedure for placement of central venous access is quite straightforward. A preliminary ultrasound of the vein to be accessed is performed to confirm its patency. The neck and the ipsilateral chest are then prepped appropriately. Access is obtained to the vein using vascular ultrasound guidance almost exclusively. Once venous access is established, an appropriate tunnel area is chosen. The tunnel is formed under the skin using a tunneling device, and the catheter is advanced through the

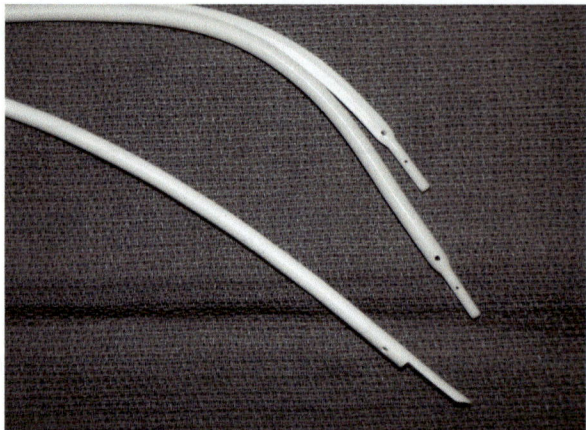

FIGURE 45.3 - EXCHANGE CATHETERS
Two examples of specially designed tips on exchange catheters that prevent recirculation of blood that has already been processed during dialysis or plasmapheresis

tunnel. Finally, the catheter is advanced into the vein. The ideal catheter tip position is at the cavoatrial junction, which is typically 3–4 cm below the carina (roughly equivalent to two vertebral bodies) on chest radiograph.

In unusual circumstances, when a patient may no longer have patent veins in the chest, central venous catheters can still be placed in other locations. Using similar techniques as described above, catheters can be placed in the common femoral veins or even directly into the inferior vena cava through the back. Trans-organ venous access can also be performed percutaneously through the kidneys or liver. Catheters placed in these sites carry high rates of complications and are therefore used as options of last resort for venous access.

S: In patients about to undergo tunneled central venous line placement, it is important for the INR to be under 1.5 in order to minimize bleeding risk.
A: Ultrasound evaluation of jugular and subclavian veins is a quick and inexpensive imaging modality to evaluate venous anatomy and patency without the use of ionizing radiation.
F: It is important to obtain a post procedural x-ray to evaluate line positioning.
E: It is imperative to quickly communicate any findings of line misplacement or migration and post procedural complications such as pneumothorax or hemorrhage with the clinical team for appropriate and timely management.

46 INTERVENTIONAL ONCOLOGY

Objectives:
1. Understand the basics of hepatic transarterial chemoembolization (TACE).
2. List the indications and contraindications of TACE.
3. Understand the basic hepatic arterial anatomy.
4. Describe the basic steps of performing a TACE.
5. Describe the follow-up, complications, and long-term outcomes of TACE.
6. Understand the similarities and differences of TACE and hepatic transarterial radioembolization (TARE).
7. Understand the basics of different ablative therapy options.

Hepatic Transarterial Chemoembolization (TACE)

Hepatic transarterial chemoembolization (TACE) is often used to treat unresectable hepatocellular carcinomas (HCC) and other hypervascular tumors. Normal liver parenchyma receives much of its blood supply from the portal vein with a smaller component derived from the hepatic artery. HCCs and other hypervascular tumors desire the highly oxygenated blood in the hepatic arteries and therefore are almost exclusively supplied by the hepatic artery. Because of this property, TACE can deliver the chemoembolization mixture directly to the hypervascular tumors. The chemoembolization cocktail is a mixture of one or more chemotherapy drugs, an embolic agent to slow blood flow to the tumor, and sometimes a special oil called Lipiodol to help visualize tumors on imaging.

© Springer Nature Switzerland AG 2020
J. Kissane et al. (eds.), *Radiology Fundamentals: Introduction to Imaging & Technology*, https://doi.org/10.1007/978-3-030-22173-7_46

Indications

The indications for TACE include:

1. Patients with unresectable tumors
2. To maintain a patient on the transplant list by controlling the tumor(s) size
3. To downsize a tumor(s) so that a patient can be placed on a transplant list

The Milan Criteria is used to determine if a patient is appropriate for transplant for HCC. Patients not meeting the Milan Criteria have a high rate of HCC recurrence following transplant, therefore are not eligible for transplant. These patients may still benefit from TACE or transarterial radioembolization (TARE) to slow progression of disease.

The Milan criteria for transplant eligibility are as follows:

1. Solitary tumor, diameter ≤5 cm
2. 3 tumors or less, each diameter ≤3 cm
3. No extrahepatic involvement
4. No major vessel involvement

Contraindications

Absolute contraindications:

1. Uncompensated end-stage liver disease (i.e., Child-Pugh score C).

   Please see Chap. 44, TIPS, for details on Child-Pugh score.

2. Poor performance status (ECOG score >2)

Relative contraindications:

1. Bilirubin greater than 4
2. Portal vein occlusion

Relevant Hepatic Arterial Anatomy

It is important to obtain cross-sectional imaging (CT or MRI) prior to TACE to determine the vascular supply of the tumors, determine if there is variant anatomy, and determine if the portal vein is patent. Normal hepatic arterial anatomy is shown in Fig. 46.1. Normal celiac artery terminates in a trifurcation giving rise to the splenic artery, left gastric artery, and common hepatic artery. Normal common

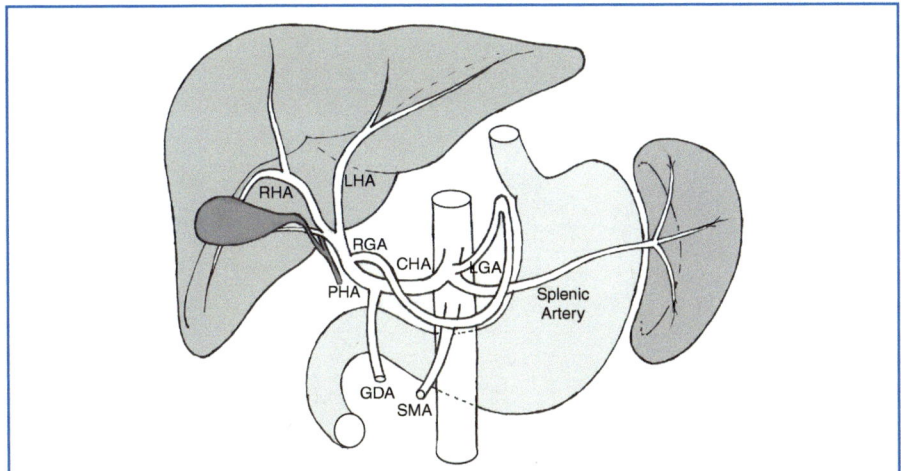

FIGURE 46.1 - RELEVANT HEPATIC ARTERIAL ANATOMY
Image demonstrates the normal hepatic arterial anatomy. RHA Right hepatic artery, LHA Left hepatic artery, PHA Proper hepatic artery, RGA Right gastric artery, GDA Gastroduodenal artery, CHA Common hepatic artery, SMA Superior mesenteric artery, LGA Left gastric artery

hepatic artery terminates in a bifurcation giving rise to the gastroduodenal artery and proper hepatic artery. The proper hepatic artery typically bifurcates into the left and right hepatic arteries following the portal triad of hepatic arteries, portal veins, and biliary ducts. However, there is a high percentage of variant hepatic arterial anatomy. The most common is the right hepatic artery arising from the superior mesenteric artery, termed "right hepatic artery replaced to the superior mesenteric artery," seen in approximately 15% of people. The second most common variant is the left hepatic artery replaced to the left gastric artery, with a prevalence of approximately 10%. The third most common is the common hepatic artery replaced to the SMA, seen in approximately 5% of people.

TACE Procedure

Vascular access is gained in one of the femoral arteries. A hepatic arteriogram is performed of the celiac artery to determine the hepatic arterial anatomy and arterial supply of the tumor(s). Then various wires and catheters are guided into a branch of a hepatic artery that supplies the tumor(s). Finally, the chemoembolization mixture is injected once the catheters are properly positioned (Fig. 46.2).

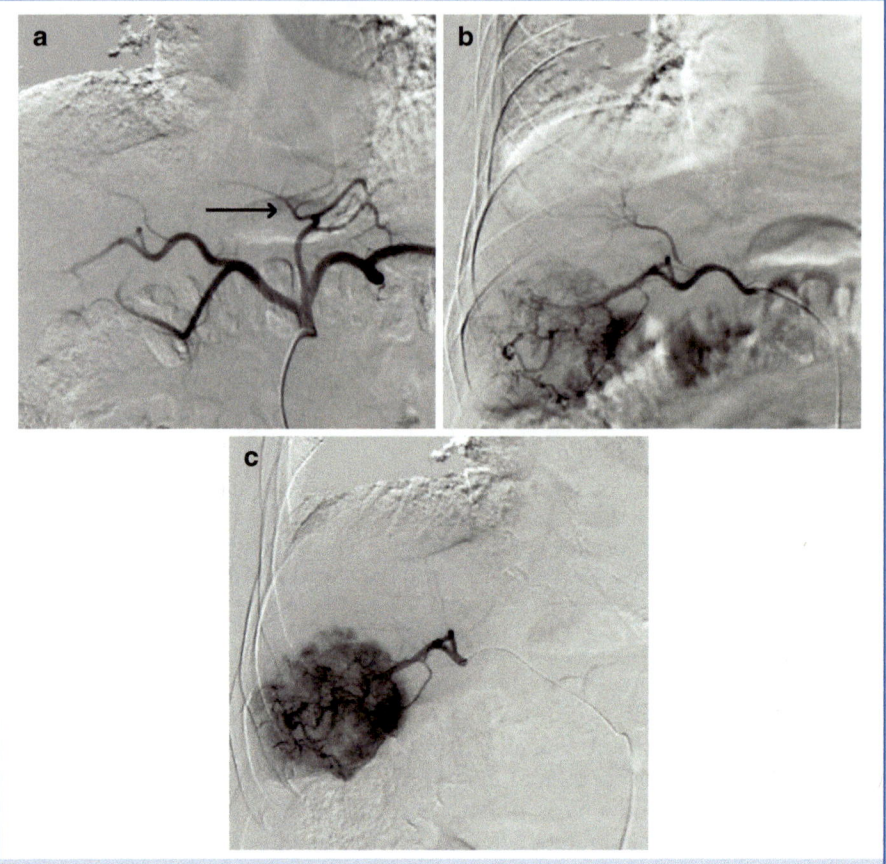

FIGURE 46.2 - TRANSARTERIAL HEPATIC CHEMOEMBOLIZATION
Celiac artery arteriogram (**a**) demonstrates a typical trifurcation and variant anatomy with a left hepatic artery replaced to the left gastric artery (arrow). Selective proper hepatic arteriogram (**b**) demonstrates a hypervascular right hepatic tumor. Post therapy angiogram (**c**) with a microcatheter positioned in the right hepatic artery shows accumulation of chemotherapy cocktail within the right lower lobe hypervascular tumor

Complications

With proper patient selection, the major risks are minimized. Major risks include progressive liver failure with encephalopathy, liver abscess, or nontarget embolization. Nontarget embolization is a phrase which refers to the delivery of chemoembolization mixture or radioembolization particles to unintended areas, particularly the stomach or bowel. This occurs due to reflux of the agent into other vessels, such as those that supply the stomach or bowel. Nontarget embolization to the stomach and bowel can cause severe bowel ulceration and/or perforation. Nontarget embolization can be avoided with judicious angiographic technique. As with any interventional procedure, infection and bleeding are always a risk, although minimal with careful technique.

Most patients experience some degree of post chemoembolization syndrome. This consists of a triad of abdominal pain, nausea, and fever and is secondary to the effect of embolization and not indicative of a true complication.

Follow-Up

Patients should have follow-up cross-sectional imaging in 4–6 weeks to determine response to therapy. Some patients may need several treatments to the same liver lobe or segment.

Long-Term Survival

Randomized controlled studies have shown a significant survival benefit increase at 2 years of approximately 50% (63% vs 27%) when compared to supportive care alone [1]. Despite prolonging survival it is important to understand that TACE and TARE do not cure HCC, and transplant is currently the only cure for HCC and cirrhosis in eligible patients.

Hepatic Transarterial Radioembolization (TARE)

Hepatic transarterial radioembolization (TARE) is a procedure similar to TACE. It is FDA approved to treat unresectable hepatocellular carcinoma or to treat HCCs as a bridge to transplant. It is also FDA approved for the treatment of hepatic metastases from colorectal carcinoma. The procedure is technically very similar to TACE. However, instead of a chemoembolization mixture, either glass or resin microspheres impregnated with a pure beta-emitting isotope called Yttrium-90 (Y-90) (half-life of 64 h, mean/max tissue penetration of 2.5 mm/10 mm) are injected into the tumor(s). Poor hepatic function with elevated bilirubin and poor ECOG performance status are again a contraindication.

The post chemoembolization syndrome seen frequently with TACE is uncommon with radioembolization. However, radioembolization is not free of complications. Nontarget embolization is a potential complication with either TACE or radioembolization, but it is associated with much greater morbidity with radioembolization due to the long half-life of Y-90. For this reason, radioembolization requires extensive pretreatment planning and meticulous attention to detail during treatment, factors that are beyond the scope of this discussion.

Ablative Therapy

Ablative technology is another rapidly growing and expanding modality for the treatment of locoregional lesions in malignant and benign diseases of the kidneys, liver, lung, breast, prostate, and bones. Historically, ablation therapy was limited to chemical ablation where either alcohol or acetic acid was injected into tumors in order to cause tissue necrosis. Currently, the most commonly used ablative therapies use extremes of temperature to cause tissue necrosis. The three most commonly used ablative therapies are radiofrequency ablation (RFA), microwave ablation, and cryoablation.

Radiofrequency ablation generates high temperatures by passing high-frequency electrical current through an electrode. Microwave ablation utilizes high-frequency electromagnetic waves to cause rapid vibration of molecules. The friction generated by the vibration causes extreme heat (temperatures greater than 50 °C). The heat generated by RFA and microwave ablation disrupts cellular activity and produces coagulative necrosis. Alternatively, cryoablation freezes tissues to less than −20 °C. Cellular injury and death results from direct injury from ice formation, shifting of cellular solutes and solvents resulting in dehydration and cell rupture, as well as microvascular thrombosis resulting in ischemia.

Each of these three techniques requires image-guided (CT, US, MRI, or fluoroscopy) placement of one or several probes, through which either electrical current, electromagnetic waves, or a cryogen is delivered to the probes in order to generate the desired temperature extreme for cellular destruction (Fig. 46.3).

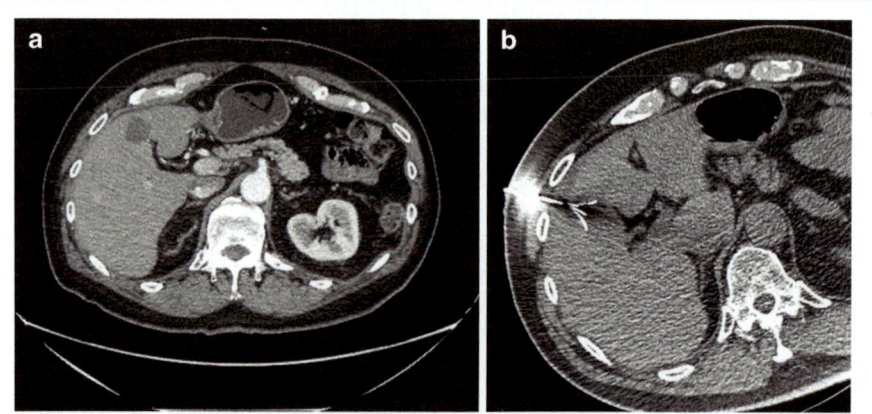

FIGURE 46.3 - RADIOFREQUENCY ABLATION
Image (**a**) demonstrates a round hypodensity in the liver. Image (**b**) shows a radiofrequency (*RF*) probe deployed into the lesion during ablation

S: Pre-procedural cross-sectional imaging such as CT or MRI can determine tumor location, tumor size, arterial blood supply, and portal vein patency and display other relevant anatomy. Pre-procedural imaging can affect the management and procedural approach, reduce procedural radiation dose, and reduce morbidity and mortality related to the procedure. It is important to recognize that many patients with cirrhosis will have renal impairment. Therefore, intravenous contrast should be used judiciously.

A: Post-procedure cross-sectional imaging is indicated to determine response to therapy. This should be performed 4–6 weeks after completion of treatment and every 3 months for 2 years or as needed. If no residual or recurrent disease is seen after 2 years of imaging, patients may return to routine HCC screening with annual CT or MRI. Contrast-enhanced US is an alternative in patients with contraindication to intravenous contrast although it is currently not recommended by the ACR due to lower sensitivity in detecting HCC.

F: For follow-up imaging, it is important to use the ACR LI-RADS criteria to describe lesions. Additionally, it is important to use the EASL or mRECIST criteria to describe response to therapy. These criteria simplify reporting based on clinical trial data and avoid unnecessary biopsies and procedures.

E: It is important to understand and identify the possible complications of a TACE procedure such as liver abscess, bowel ischemia, and arterial injuries such as dissection or pseudoaneurysm. Complications should be communicated with the proceduralist in a timely fashion.

Reference

1. Llovet, JM, Real MI, Montana X. (2002). Arterial embolization or chemoembolization versus symptomatic treatment in patients with unresectable hepatocellular carcinoma: a randomised controlled trial. *Lancet*, 2002; 359: 1734–1739.

PART VII
MUSCULOSKELETAL RADIOLOGY

47 FRACTURES 1

Objectives:
1. List five major categories of description when evaluating a fracture.
2. Identify internal and external rotation views of the shoulder.
3. Define normal and abnormal anatomy on the "Y" view of the shoulder.
4. Discuss the significance of a joint effusion in the elbow in the presence of acute trauma.
5. State the mechanism of injury in a Colles' fracture.
6. Discuss the concept of the "Scottie dog" in evaluating the lumbar spine.
7. Describe the "bony ring" principle and relate its importance to acute trauma involving the pelvis.

Fractures are ubiquitous in medical practice. Radiographs have been used to evaluate fractures from the earliest days of diagnostic radiology and remain a cornerstone of clinical care in the diagnosis and treatment of skeletal trauma.

The Simple Fracture

Figure 47.1 demonstrates an acute fracture of the fourth proximal phalanx in the left foot. Note the presence of a linear lucency, sharp edges without marginal sclerosis, and soft tissue swelling.

© Springer Nature Switzerland AG 2020
J. Kissane et al. (eds.), *Radiology Fundamentals: Introduction to Imaging & Technology*, https://doi.org/10.1007/978-3-030-22173-7_47

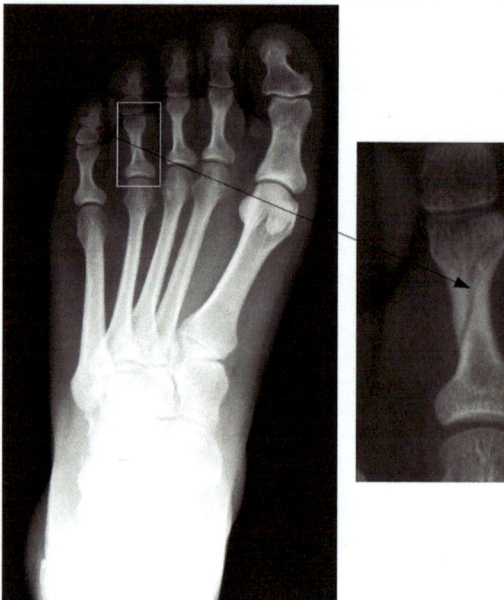

FIGURE 47.1 - SIMPLE FRACTURE
Oblique, nondisplaced fracture of the fourth proximal phalanx of the left foot

Fracture Nomenclature

It is important to verbally describe a fracture since you will often need to communicate the radiographic findings to other healthcare professionals. Features that must be mentioned include the following:

1. *Location:* The name and part of the bone involved. In long bones, the fracture can involve the epiphysis, metaphysis, diaphysis, and even the physis (growth plate). Other designations such as head, neck, body, waist, etc. (depending on the bone) may be employed (Fig. 47.2).
2. *Types of fracture:* Transverse, oblique, spiral, and butterfly are all appropriate descriptors. Comminuted is used when there are multiple fracture fragments. It is also important to note any intra-articular extension of the fracture (extension into the joint) and any associated incongruence at the articular surface (Fig. 47.3).
3. *Displacement (nonalignment of periosteal surfaces of the bone):* Displacement is described using the location of the distal fracture fragment with respect to the proximal fragment. Hence, if the distal fragment is medially displaced, the fracture is medially displaced. Open or compound fractures are fractures which penetrate the skin (Fig. 47.4).

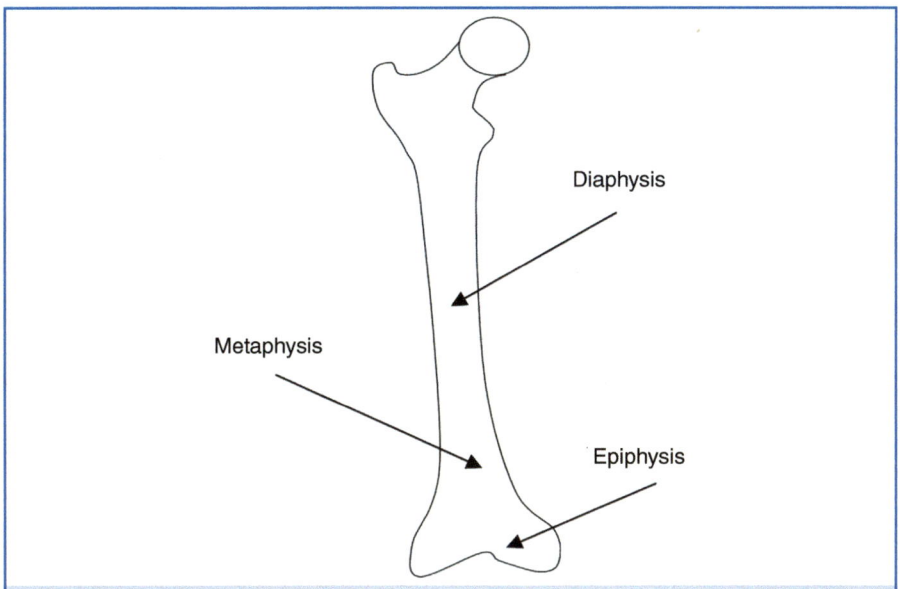

FIGURE 47.2 - BASIC LONG BONE ANATOMY
It is important to have familiarity with the long bone anatomy

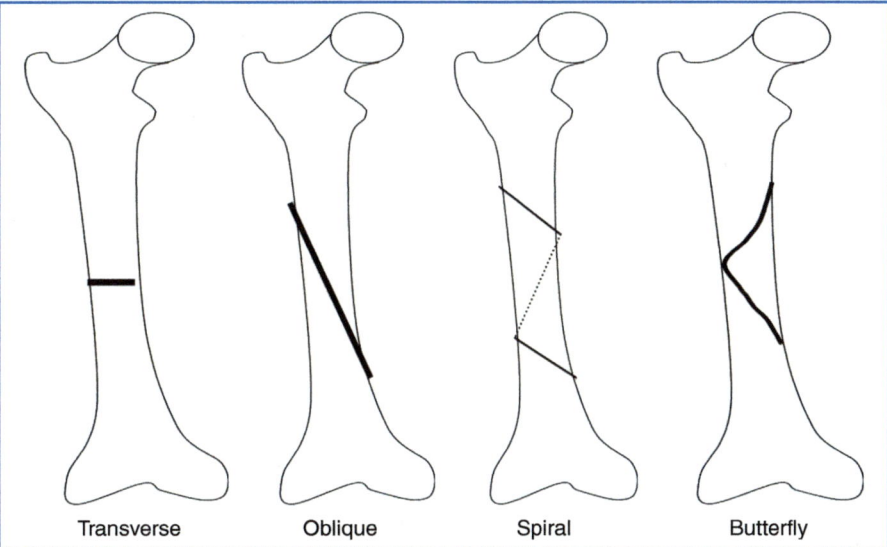

Transverse   Oblique   Spiral   Butterfly

FIGURE 47.3 - FRACTURE NOMENCLATURE
In describing fractures, the referring physician should be able to visualize the fracture without the x-rays. Knowing the nomenclature greatly facilitates this communication

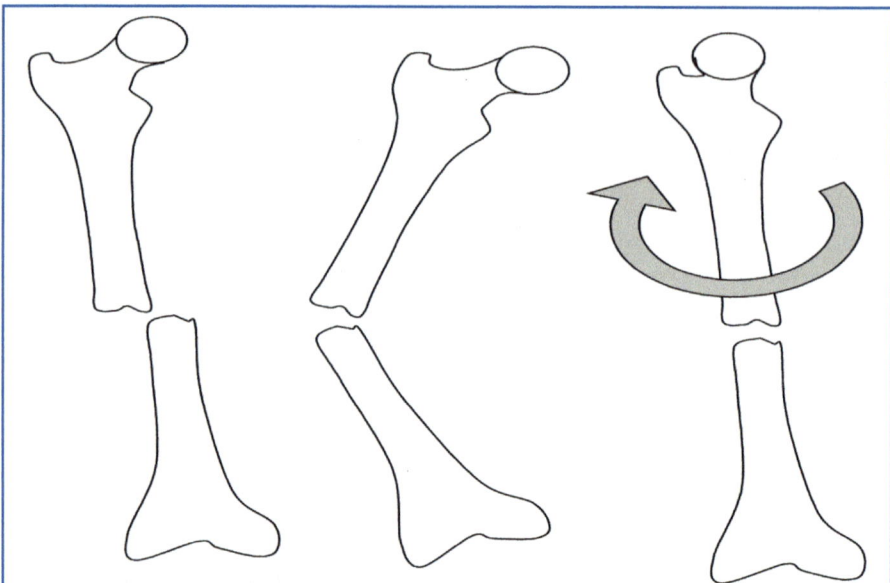

FIGURE 47.4 - FRACTURE FRAGMENT ORIENTATION
In the image on the *left*, there is one shaft width medial displacement of the distal fracture fragment. In the *middle* image, there is lateral angulation of the fracture apex. In the image on the *right*, there is rotation of the fracture fragments

4. *Angulation of the "apex" of the fracture:* The direction that the angle of the fracture points is used to describe the fracture position. A common phrase used would be "the apex of the fracture is directed laterally" (Fig. 47.4).
5. *Rotation of the distal fragment:* If the distal fragment is rotated relative to the proximal fragment, this should be included in the description (Fig. 47.4).

Note that at least two views are required to completely visualize and describe the position of a fracture. An example of a complete description of a fracture would be: "There is a comminuted fracture of the mid diaphysis of the left femur with medial displacement of the distal fragment, apex lateral angulation, and internal rotation of the distal fragment."

Shoulder Views

Figure 47.5 shows a normal two-view study of the shoulder as might be obtained in the emergency room.

Note the difference between the internal and external rotation views. On internal rotation views, the appearance of the humeral head is similar to the smooth round

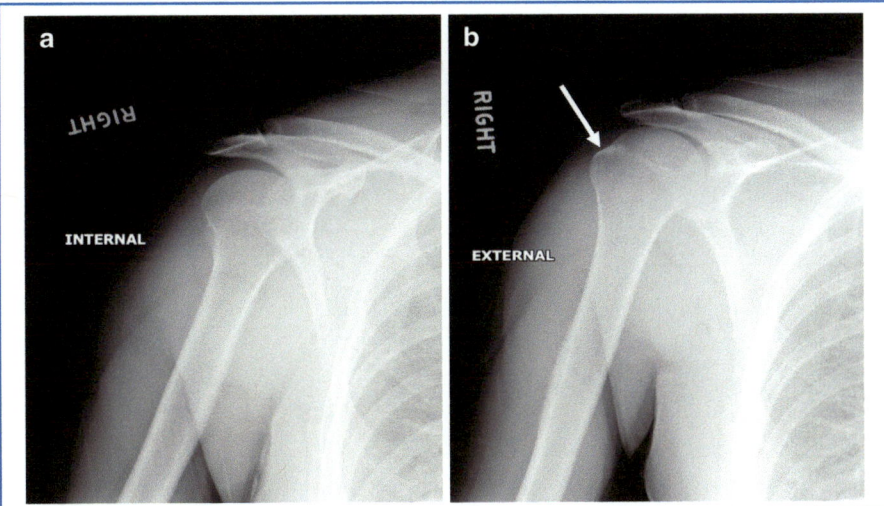

FIGURE 47.5 - INTERNAL (a) AND EXTERNAL (b) ROTATION VIEWS OF THE RIGHT SHOULDER
Arrow shows the greater tuberosity of the humeral head

top of an ice cream cone (Ice cream = Internal). On external rotation views, the greater tuberosity is seen clearly in profile. These two views will usually suffice to exclude a fracture. However, dislocation may be more difficult to exclude without views from another projection.

Figure 47.6 shows an axillary and scapular "Y" view of the shoulder. The axillary view is projected so that you are looking upward through the axilla toward the ceiling in a standing patient. You should be able to visualize the clavicle and acromion process anteriorly, the acromioclavicular joint, and the glenohumeral articulation. Because of the projection of the axillary view, anterior or posterior dislocations are usually well demonstrated. The problem with this view is that it is often very uncomfortable for a patient with an acutely injured shoulder.

A different way of imaging the shoulder in a plane perpendicular to the anterior-posterior projection is called a scapular Y view. In this case, the patient is obliqued slightly, and a "lateral view" of the shoulder is obtained. The stem of the Y is the scapular body, while the two upper arms of the Y are the acromion and coracoid processes. At the center of the Y is a circle corresponding to the glenoid fossa. The humeral head should project over the confluence of the three arms of the Y. If the humeral head is posterior to the intersection of the arms of the Y, a posterior dislocation may be diagnosed. Again, remember that a posterior dislocation may look normal in the AP view. Note that the scapular Y view is not as good as the axillary lateral view for assessing dislocations or subluxation.

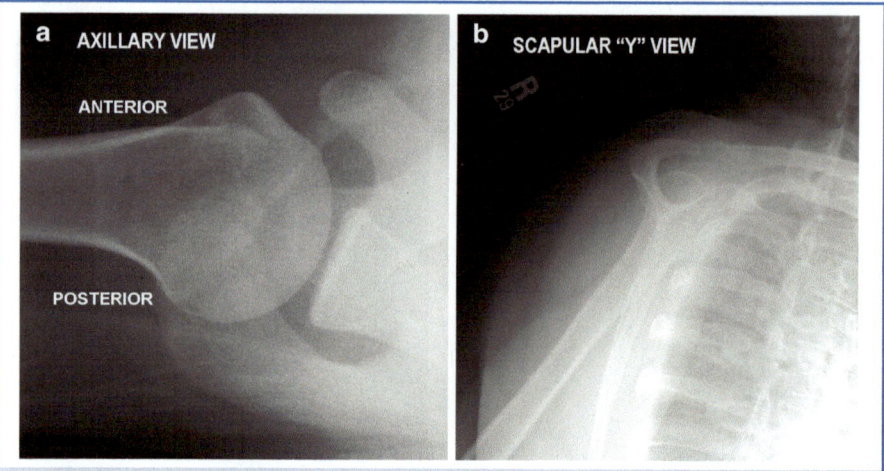

FIGURE 47.6 - (a) AXILLARY AND (b) SCAPULAR Y VIEWS OF THE RIGHT SHOULDER

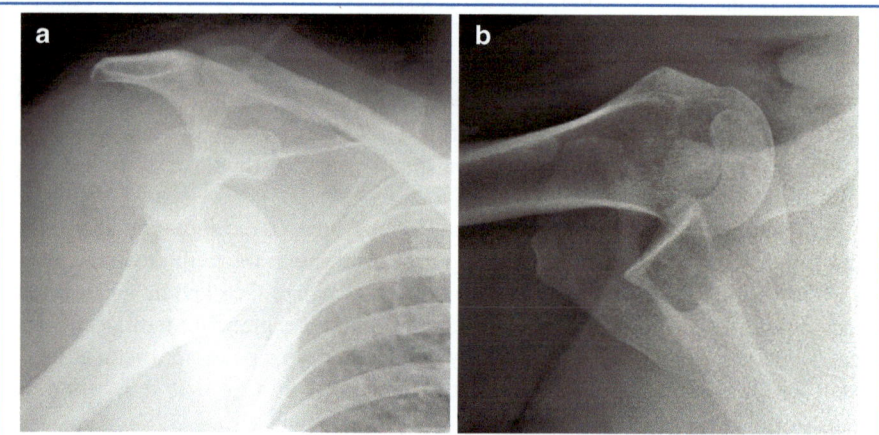

FIGURE 47.7 - ANTERIOR DISLOCATION OF THE SHOULDER
AP (**a**) and axillary (**b**) view of the shoulder demonstrating anterior dislocation

Shoulder Dislocation

Figure 47.7 shows a typical anterior (most common) dislocation of the humerus. In anterior dislocation, the humeral head moves inferiorly under the coracoid and slightly medially. This can usually be identified on the routine anterior views (a). The axillary view (b) demonstrates the humeral head anterior to the glenoid.

Figure 47.8 demonstrates a typical posterior dislocation of the humerus. The dislocation is hard to appreciate on the AP view (a), but in posterior dislocations the

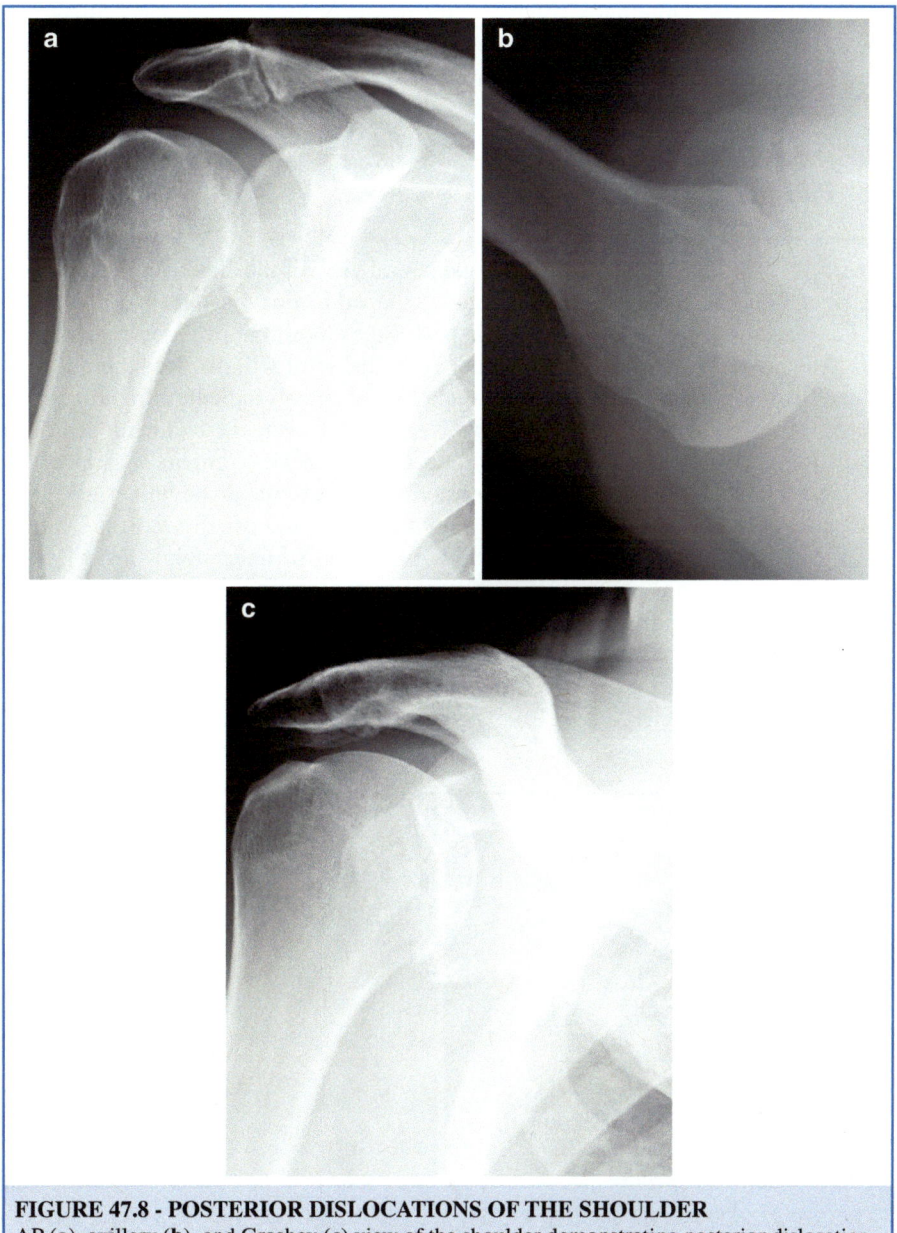

FIGURE 47.8 - POSTERIOR DISLOCATIONS OF THE SHOULDER
AP (**a**), axillary (**b**), and Grashey (**c**) view of the shoulder demonstrating posterior dislocation

humerus is always internally rotated (patient cannot externally rotate). Image (b) shows the axillary view with the humeral head posterior to the glenoid. The Grashey view (c) reveals overlap of the humeral head at the glenohumeral joint.

Fat Pad Sign

Figure 47.9 shows a normal and abnormal lateral view of the elbow. In the image on the right, note the presence of the triangular-shaped lucency just anterior to the distal humerus representing the anterior fat pad of the elbow. Fat pads serve as markers for elbow joint effusions. Fluid or blood within the joint will displace them. Elbow joint effusions in the setting of acute trauma almost always indicate a fracture. In the image on the right, no obvious fracture is seen. However, there is evidence of an elbow joint effusion since the anterior fat pad is displaced (compare to normal). In addition, a posterior fat pad along the posterior aspect of the distal humerus is seen. This always indicates the presence of a joint effusion and usually indicates a fracture, in the proper clinical situation. It is important to understand that while an anterior fat pad sign is more sensitive for joint pathology, a posterior fat pad sign is more specific for occult fracture.

The elbow is not the only joint in which fat pads can be useful. For instance, ankle injuries may reveal a fat pad anterior to the joint between the talus and tibia which may suggest fracture.

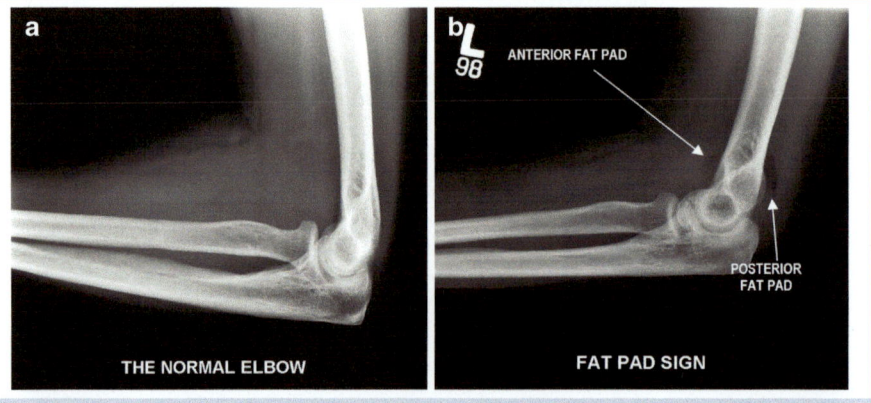

FIGURE 47.9 - NORMAL (a) AND ABNORMAL (b) VIEWS OF THE ELBOW AND FAT PAD SIGN
The image on the left is a normal lateral elbow. The triangular lucencies anterior and posterior to the humerus on the right image represent displaced fat (fat pad sign) when there is fluid in the elbow joint. Fluid in the joint can be seen in inflammatory conditions. In the setting of trauma, displaced fat pads have a high association with fracture even if the fracture is not immediately visualized

These fractures may be occult radiographically. Occasionally, a small fracture of the radial head can be demonstrated with a dedicated radial head view or follow-up views. Again, whenever an elbow joint effusion is seen in the setting of acute trauma (and in the absence of other preexisting reasons for an elbow joint effusion such as rheumatoid arthritis, hemophilia, etc.), the patient should be treated for a fracture.

Colles' Fracture

Figure 47.10 demonstrates one of the most common wrist injuries. The Colles' fracture is defined as a transverse fracture of the distal metaphysis of the radius with dorsal angulation of the distal fragment commonly caused by falling on an outstretched hand. Based on the previously described nomenclature, it would be appropriate to describe this fracture as apex volar (palmar) angulation. However, in the case of a fracture near an articular surface, the direction of the articular surface is used to describe angulation. Often a Colles' fracture will have an associated fracture of the ulnar styloid process.

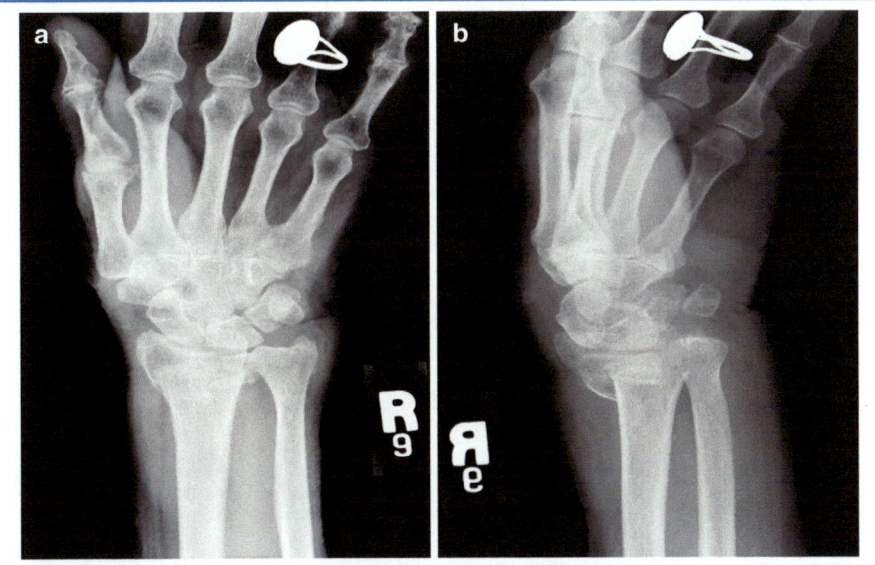

FIGURE 47.10 - COLLES' FRACTURE
AP (**a**) and oblique views (**b**) of the right wrist demonstrate a comminuted, impacted, and intra-articular fracture of the right distal radius, with approximately 20° of dorsal angulation of the distal fragment. Note that there is also deformity and marked soft tissue swelling at the site of injury

The Scottie Dog

Another term you should be familiar with is the Scottie dog. This refers to the outline of a dog that can be seen on an oblique view of the lumbar spine. As depicted in the figures below, the eye of the dog corresponds to the pedicle, the snout the transverse process, the neck the pars interarticularis, the ear the superior articular facet, and the front leg the inferior articular facet.

It is important to evaluate these structures, especially the pars interarticularis. A fracture or congenital defect in this region will manifest itself as a lucent (dark) line in the neck of the dog (it looks like a dog collar). This is termed spondylolysis. Spondylolysis can lead to spondylolisthesis which is a slippage of the superior vertebra on the inferior one, most often in the anterior direction. There is a grading system based upon what percentage of the vertebra has slipped forward, but for now, just understand the concept.

Roughly 5% of the population has L5 spondylolisthesis, and of those, roughly 5% are symptomatic. In general, spondylolysis with spondylolisthesis is more likely to be symptomatic (Fig. 47.11).

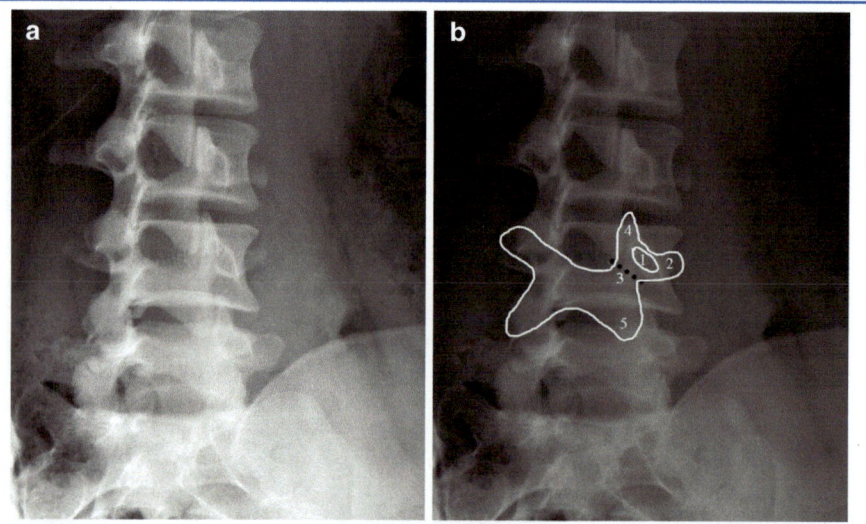

FIGURE 47.11 - THE SCOTTIE DOG CONCEPT
Oblique lumbar radiograph, without (**a**) and with annotation (**b**) demonstrating the Scottie dog concept: *1* pedicle, *2* transverse process, *3* pars interarticularis, *4* superior articular facet, and *5* inferior articular facet. The *dashed line* through the neck that looks like a collar represents what a pars fracture would look like

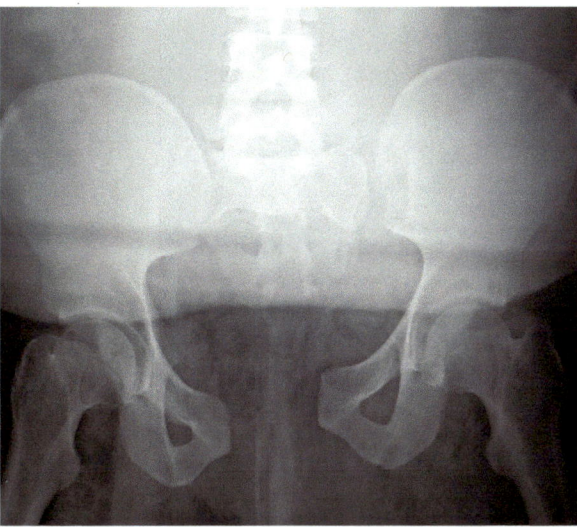

FIGURE 47.12 - PELVIC FRACTURE
There is marked widening of the left sacroiliac joint and the pubic symphysis. Also note that there is extensive soft tissue density in the pelvis consistent with hematoma

Pelvic Fractures

Evaluation of the pelvis is often a part of the radiographic evaluation of acute trauma patients. One helpful principle in looking for fractures of the pelvis is the "bony ring" concept. This concept states that a bony ring will always break in two places. A fracture or separation in a bony ring is usually associated with at least one other fracture in that ring. Figure 47.12 illustrates this principle. Remember that pelvic fractures also occur in the elderly with much less force of trauma secondary to osteoporosis.

S: The majority of fractures can be diagnosed with a two to three view radiographic series. Very little radiation is delivered to the patient and diagnosis can be made quickly for patient triage.

A: Radiographs are the most appropriate exam (ACR appropriateness criteria of 8–9) for suspicion of fracture. CT and MR are indicated for occult fractures or surgical planning.

F: At least two views should be obtained to completely describe fracture displacement, angulation, and rotation. When a fracture is diagnosed, surgery will routinely request images of the joint above and below the fracture.

E: Findings of an open fracture warrant verbal communication to expedite surgical management and antibiotic treatment to prevent infection.

48

FRACTURES 2

Objectives:
1. Describe the classification of femoral neck fractures.
2. Describe the radiographic features of a suprapatellar knee joint effusion.
3. Discuss the imaging of tibial plateau fractures and the significance of a fat fluid level within the knee joint space.
4. List the two main mechanisms of injury in ankle fractures.
5. Define Bohler's angle and its pathologic significance in regard to fractures of the calcaneus.
6. Define the phrase pathologic fracture.

Femoral Neck Fractures

The femoral neck is a very common site for acute skeletal trauma. Femoral neck fractures range from quite obvious both clinically and radiographically to very subtle abnormalities radiographically. Fractures are classified according to the site of the fracture within the proximal femur. The most common locations for femoral neck fractures are in the intertrochanteric area extending between the greater and lesser trochanters and in the subcapital region, that area of the femoral neck just distal to the femoral head. Mid-cervical or basi-cervical femoral neck fractures are less common. Internal rotation of the hip will improve evaluation of the femoral neck on AP radiographs (Fig. 48.1).

Fractures of the hip may be more extensive than is evident on plain radiograph alone, and further imaging, commonly with computed tomography, is often performed. Of course, as with all fractures, two plain film views are required to assess the fracture. A commonly used view with hips is called the cross-table lateral view. An example of this view is shown in Fig. 48.2.

© Springer Nature Switzerland AG 2020

J. Kissane et al. (eds.), *Radiology Fundamentals: Introduction to Imaging & Technology*, https://doi.org/10.1007/978-3-030-22173-7_48

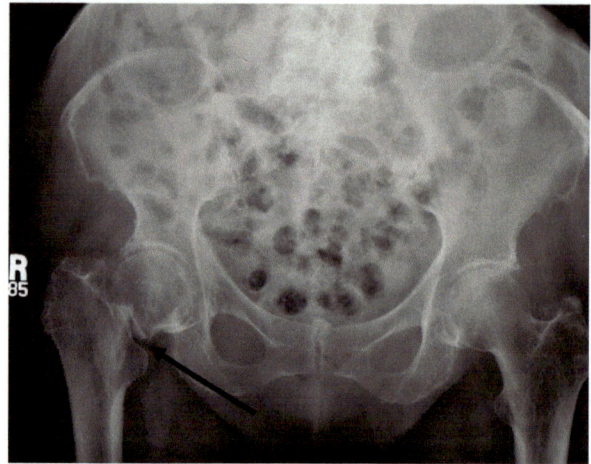

FIGURE 48.1 - FEMORAL NECK FRACTURE
Displaced subcapital fracture in an osteopenic elderly female. Femoral necks are best evaluated with the hips internally rotated

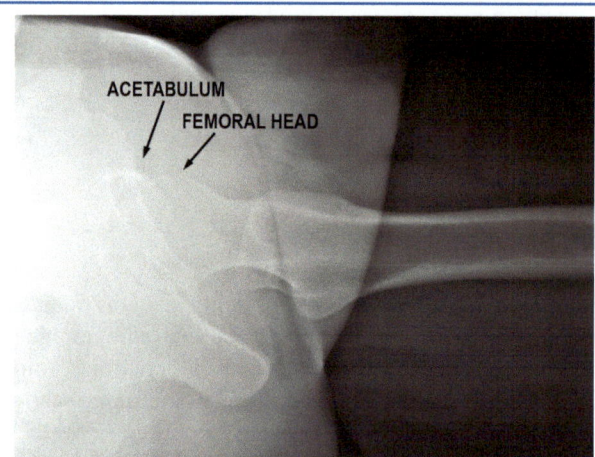

FIGURE 48.2 - CROSS-TABLE LATERAL VIEW OF THE HIP

Knee Joint Effusion

Many abnormalities of the knee are associated with a knee joint effusion. The relationship of effusion to fracture is not as strong as that discussed in a previous section in relation to the elbow. However, the presence of a knee joint effusion may be the

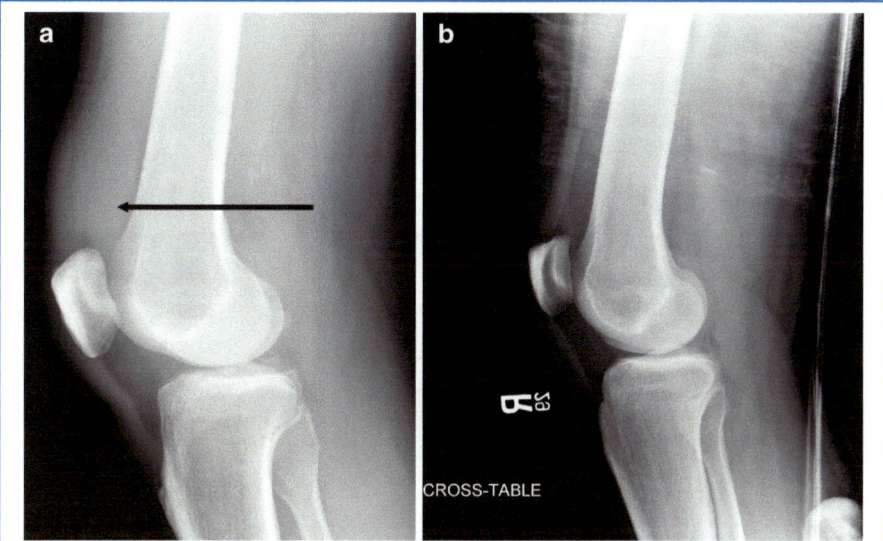

FIGURE 48.3 - KNEE JOINT EFFUSION
Large left knee joint effusion with associated soft tissue swelling (*arrow*) seen in (**a**) and a normal lateral knee radiograph (**b**) for comparison

only manifestation of a cartilaginous or ligamentous injury in the absence of fracture. On the lateral view, the suprapatellar fat pad is a dark triangle with its apex directed superiorly and its base situated along the superior aspect of the patella itself. The pre-femoral fat pad is a broad, anteriorly convex area of decreased density along the anterior aspect of the distal femur. The suprapatellar pouch of the knee joint is between these fat pads. When there is a knee joint effusion, these two fat pads are separated by more than 5 mm. It is important that on the lateral view, the knee be appropriately flexed at approximately 30° and that a true lateral view (non-rotated) be obtained when evaluating for a joint effusion (Fig. 48.3).

In some patients who have undergone significant trauma involving the knee, a cross-table lateral view may be performed with the knee straight. Sometimes a horizontally oriented transverse interface of differing densities may be seen within the joint effusion. This represents a fat-fluid level. Remember that fat is less dense (darker) radiographically than fluid. Also, fat is of lesser physical density than fluid and tends to rise to the top of the joint compartment, while the fluid sinks to the bottom. The fat represents marrow contents which have leaked into the joint space as the result of a fracture, usually of the proximal tibia, which involves the articular surface. In patients with a fat fluid level, an intra-articular fracture will invariably be present (Fig. 48.4).

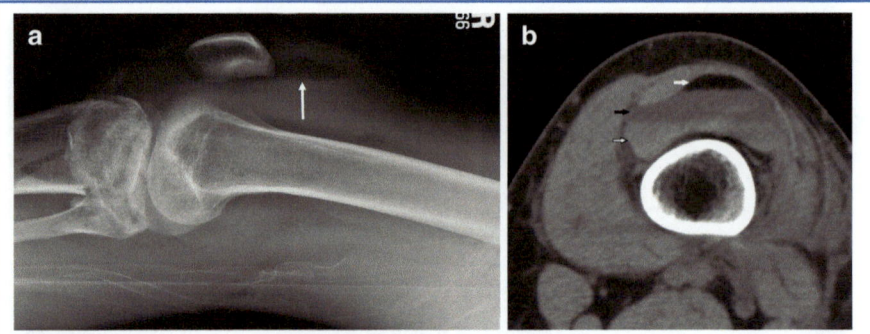

FIGURE 48.4 - LIPOHEMARTHROSIS
Image (**a**) shows a cross-table lateral view demonstrating a fat fluid level (*white arrow*). Image (**b**) shows the corresponding axial CT slice revealing lipohemarthrosis with fat (*top white arrow*), serum (*black arrow*), and hematocrit fluid levels (*bottom white arrow*)

Tibial Plateau Fractures

A common intra-articular fracture involving the proximal tibia is a so-called tibial plateau fracture. The lateral and medial tibial plateaus may be injured by impact from the femoral condyles. This results in a depression of the plateau with subsequent fracture of the underlying bone. The radiographic features of a tibial plateau fracture may be quite subtle with only a small cortical irregularity or plateau depression noted on plain radiographs. Further imaging with computerized tomography is commonly performed to delineate the true extent of the fracture which may be much more extensive than appreciated on the radiograph alone (Fig. 48.5).

Ankle Fractures

Figure 48.6 shows a trimalleolar fracture. There is an oblique fracture of the lateral malleolus (distal fibula), a transverse fracture of the medial malleolus, and, seen best on the lateral film, a fracture of the posterior malleolus. In some cases, there may only be a tear of the deltoid ligament (medial aspect of ankle). In these cases, only nonspecific soft tissue swelling may be seen on the radiograph.

During the injury process, different types of rotation stress can result in fractures of the mid or even high fibula. High fractures of the fibula are especially common in eversion (or pronation)-type injuries, are called Maisonneuve fractures, and can easily be missed if only ankle radiographs are taken. For this reason, understanding the mechanism of injury is important in deciding which radiographs should be performed.

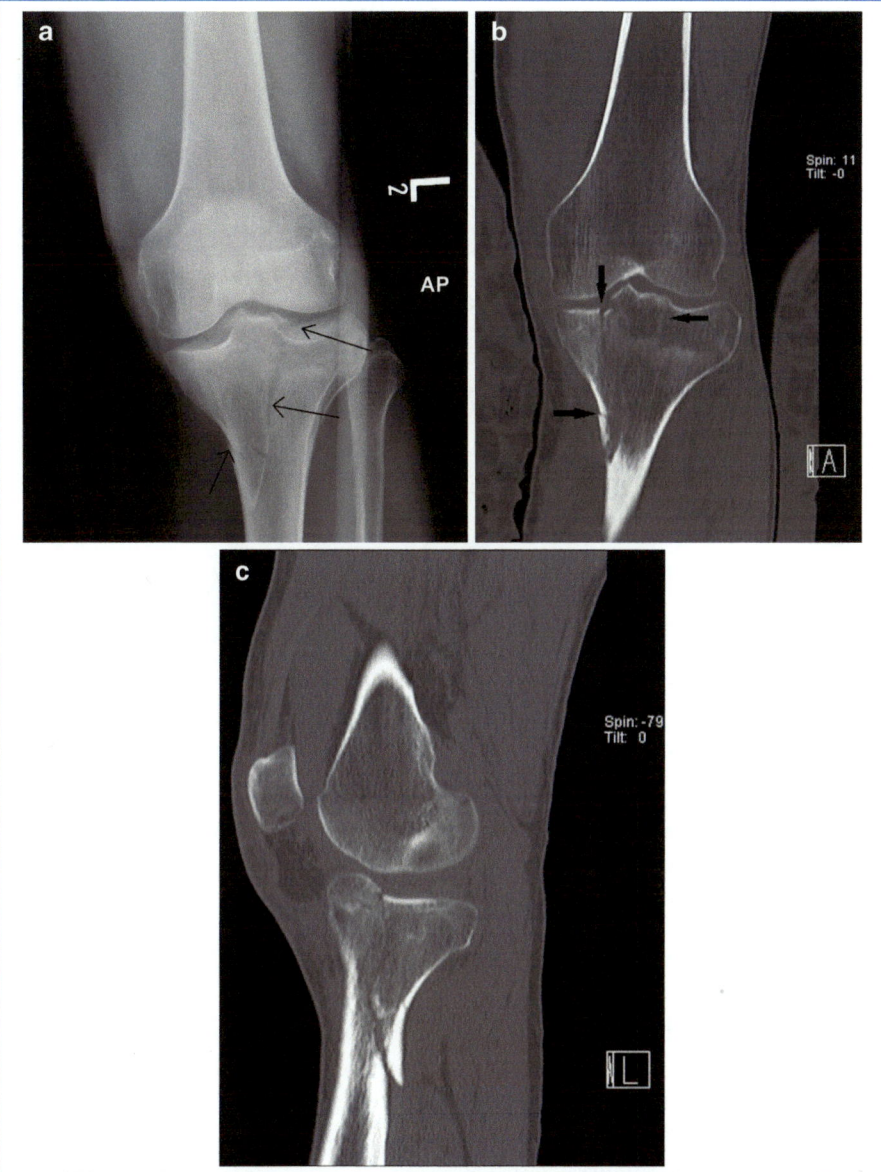

FIGURE 48.5 - TIBIAL PLATEAU FRACTURE
Comminuted intra-articular fracture of the medial and lateral tibial plateau with depression and posterior displacement of the fracture fragments as seen on AP radiograph (**a**), coronal CT (**b**), and sagittal CT (**c**)

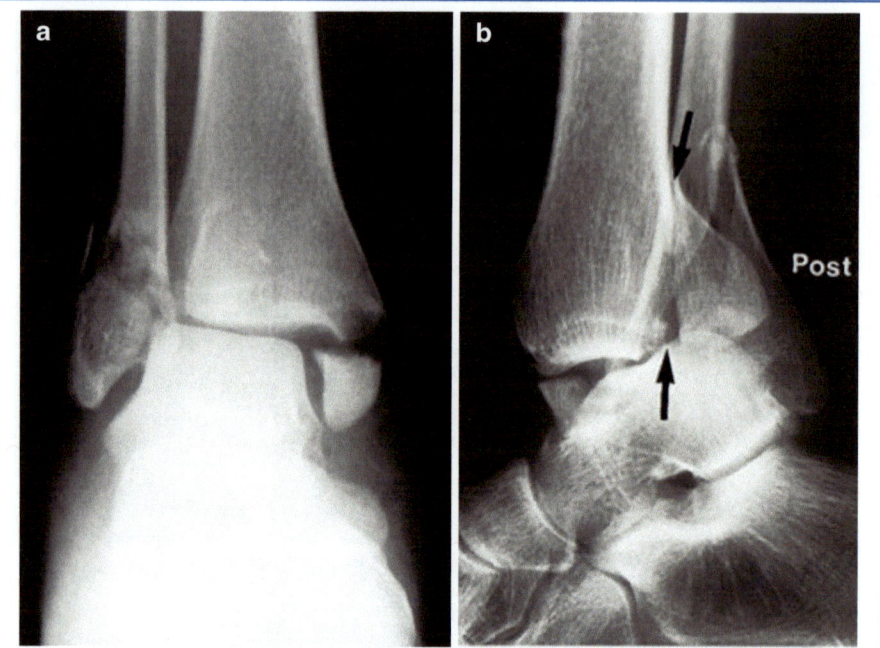

FIGURE 48.6 - AP (a) AND LATERAL (b) VIEWS OF A TRIMALLEOLAR ANKLE FRACTURE
Note that all three malleoli are fractured

Ankle injuries may be divided into inversion and eversion types. One can further subdivide these fractures into inversion (adduction) with or without rotation and eversion (abduction) with or without rotation. The most common type of "twisted ankle" is the inversion injury with rotation. From the location and appearance of the injuries, the mechanism of injury can be ascertained (Fig. 48.7).

There are four areas that are always important to check on a foot or ankle view because fractures can easily be missed in these areas.

They are:

1. Base of the fifth metatarsal
2. Lateral process of the talus
3. Superior part of the talus/talar neck
4. Anterior process of the calcaneus

Since ankle injuries are so common and often imaged, the Ottawa ankle rules were developed [1]. These are recommendations to determine when radiographs are necessary to evaluate an ankle injury based on physical exam findings. These recommendations have a sensitivity of nearly 100%. These rules do not apply to pregnant females, children under the age of 18, or patients that cannot follow the test commands (intoxication, dementia, cognitive deficit, etc.)

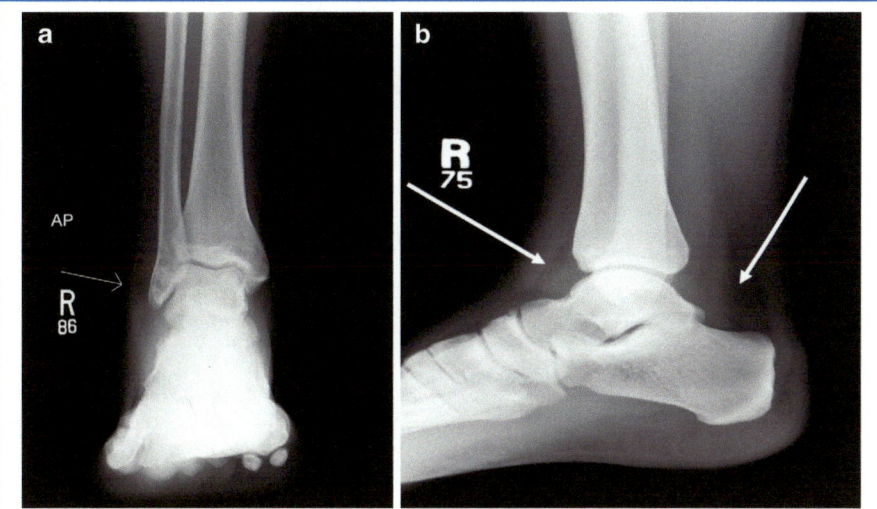

FIGURE 48.7 - ANKLE SPRAIN
This patient presented following an ankle sprain with significant soft tissue swelling about the lateral malleolus seen on AP view (**a**) and with significant soft tissue swelling over the anterior and posterior-lateral aspects of the ankle joint seen on lateral view (**b**)

Ankle radiographs are indicated if there is any pain in the malleolar zone and any one of the following:

1. Bone tenderness along the distal 6 cm of the posterior edge of the tibia or tip of the medial malleolus
2. Bone tenderness along the distal 6 cm of the posterior edge of the fibula or tip of the lateral malleolus
3. An inability to bear weight for four steps

The Ottawa foot rules are followed for assessing whether a foot X-ray series is indicated. Foot radiographs are indicated if there is any pain in the midfoot zone and any one of the following:

1. Bone tenderness at the base of the fifth metatarsal
2. Bone tenderness at the navicular bone
3. An inability to bear weight for four steps

A common foot injury occurs when a patient jumps from a high location, landing on his/her feet. Often the bone that bears the brunt of the initial impact is the calcaneus. The calcaneus may be evaluated on the lateral view by calculating Bohler's angle, with normal measuring between 20° and 40°. See Fig. 48.8 where the angle is reduced when a fracture is present. The fracture line(s) itself may not be evident on the radiograph.

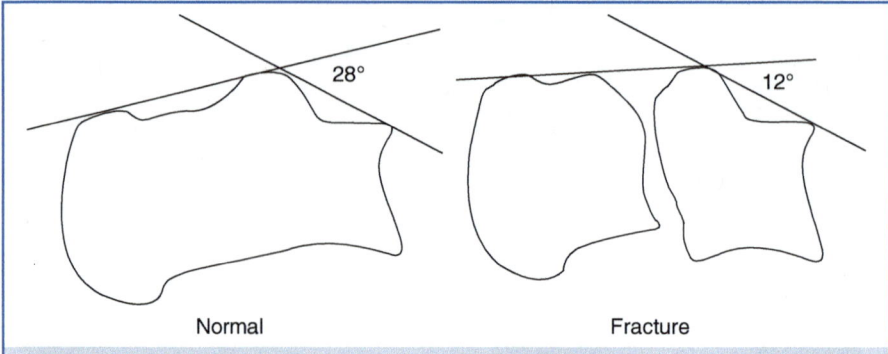

| Normal | Fracture |

FIGURE 48.8 - BOHLER'S ANGLE
On the *left*, the diagram demonstrates the normal angle of 28° formed by the intersection of the anterior and the posterior aspect of the calcaneus. With axial loading injuries (i.e., landing feet first), the calcaneus is fractured. The angle then is reduced and is noted to be less than 28°

Note that calcaneal injuries are often bilateral and can be associated with other axial loading injuries such as tibial plateau or thoracolumbar spine fractures.

Another term important to be familiar with is Lisfranc injury or fracture. The Lisfranc ligament connects the medial cuneiform to the bases of the first and second metatarsals. Lisfranc injuries tend to be quite difficult to evaluate with plain films. As with most radiographs, it is important to provide a good clinical history which can greatly help the radiologist when attempting to determine if an injury or fracture has occurred.

Pathologic Fracture

Figure 48.9 shows a patient with a lytic lesion in the bone as a result of metastatic lung cancer. Because this has thinned the cortex of the bone and weakened it structurally, a fracture has occurred. This is termed a pathologic fracture. A pathologic fracture is the result of normal stresses in an abnormal bone. The pathologic process can be benign or malignant.

A useful mnemonic for remembering which tumors spread to bone is PB KTL (Lead Kettle—remember lead's symbol is Pb).

P = Prostate
B = Breast
K = Kidney
T = Thyroid
L = Lung

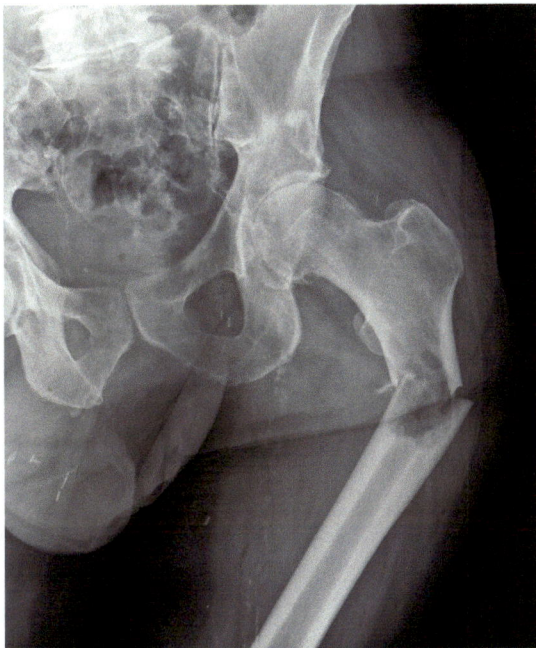

FIGURE 48.9 - PATHOLOGIC FRACTURE
Lytic lesion in the proximal left femoral metaphysis with a mildly comminuted pathologic fracture. Pathology at the time of fixation revealed metastatic squamous cell carcinoma of lung primary

Osteoporosis

Osteoporosis refers to decreased bone density which is most often associated with aging. Screening for osteoporosis is accomplished with a modality called dual-energy X-ray absorptiometry (DEXA). All women over age 65 are counseled to get a baseline DEXA exam. It is also recommended that men with a history of vertebral fracture or long-term corticosteroid use get a DEXA scan. A DEXA scan uses approximately 1/10th the radiation dose of a chest X-ray. Figure 48.10 shows an example of an osteoporotic vertebral column with a normal vertebral column for comparison. Note how lucent the vertebrae appear in Fig. 48.10a. Figure 48.11 shows an example of a DEXA scan printout.

The patient's bone mineral density (BMD) is compared to two norms. These are calculated as T-scores and Z-scores and reported as standard deviations. T-scores compare the patient's BMD to a healthy 35-year-old's BMD. Meanwhile, Z-scores

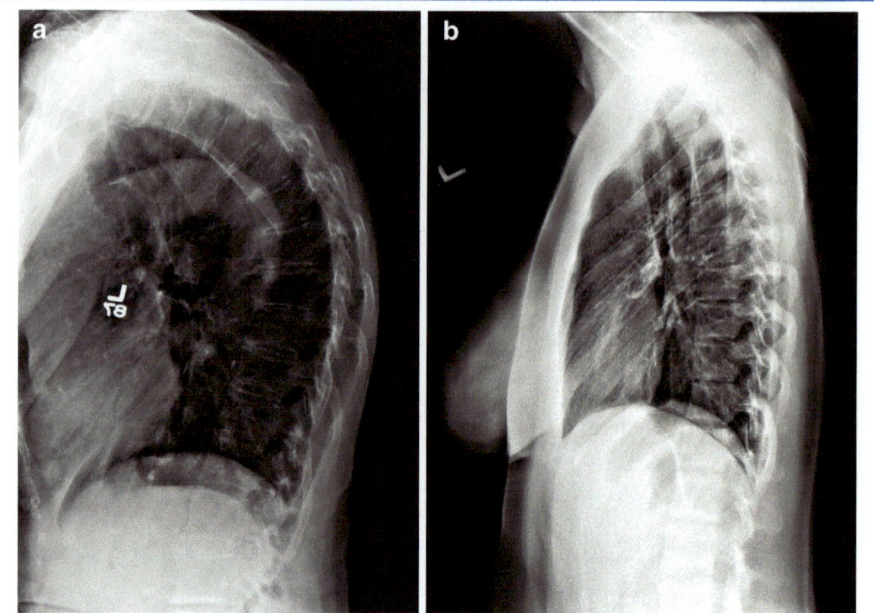

FIGURE 48.10 - OSTEOPOROSIS
Note the lucency of the vertebral column and resulting kyphotic deformity in (**a**) as compared with a normal thoracic spine (**b**)

compare a patient's BMD to an age-matched control. While a Z-score is often measured, the T-score is the number used to define osteopenia and osteoporosis. On the scale, anything above zero is normal. Negative 1 to negative 2.5 is considered osteopenia, which means low bone density. Anything more negative than negative 2.5 is defined as osteoporosis. A general rule of thumb is that for every standard deviation below normal, the risk of fracture doubles (T-score of negative 1 has double the risk, T-score of negative 2 has four times the risk).

Vertebral Fracture

Low back pain is an extremely common reason for physician visits and affects a majority of people over the course of their lifetime. A focused history and physical exam is critical to determine if imaging is warranted, and by what modality, as low back pain in most patients is a self-limiting condition. First-line treatment for uncomplicated acute and chronic low back pain or radiculopathy is an initial course

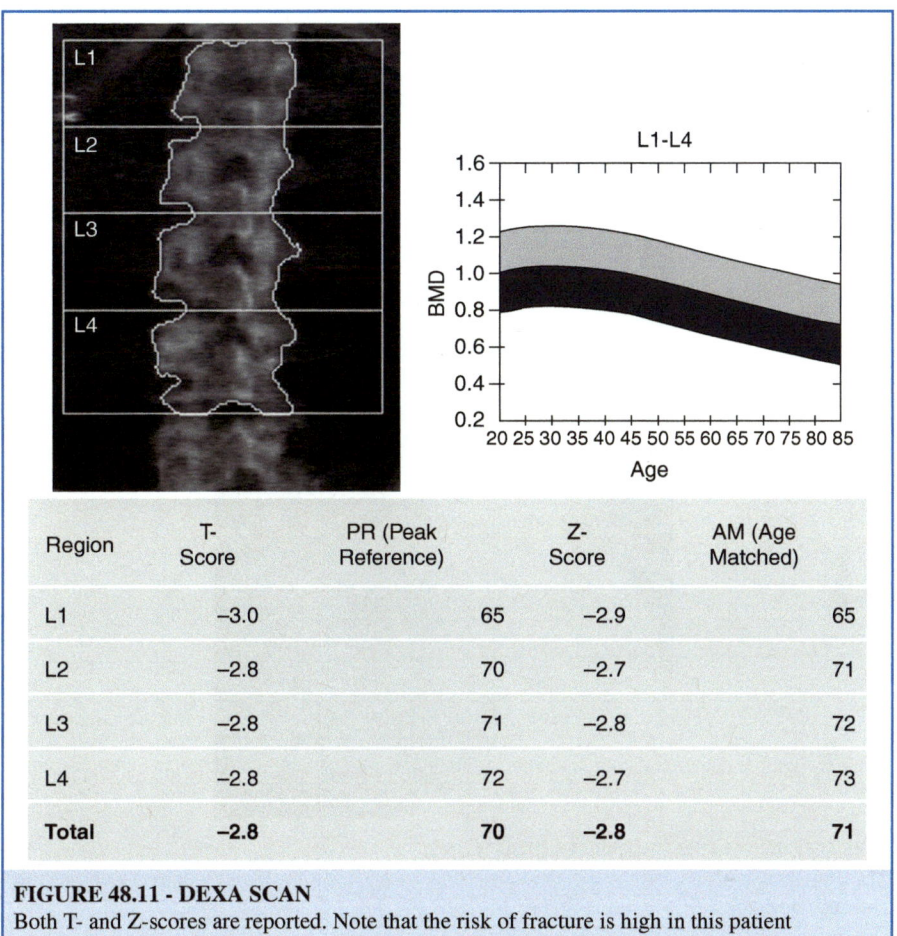

Region	T-Score	PR (Peak Reference)	Z-Score	AM (Age Matched)
L1	−3.0	65	−2.9	65
L2	−2.8	70	−2.7	71
L3	−2.8	71	−2.8	72
L4	−2.8	72	−2.7	73
Total	**−2.8**	**70**	**−2.8**	**71**

FIGURE 48.11 - DEXA SCAN
Both T- and Z-scores are reported. Note that the risk of fracture is high in this patient

of medical management and physical therapy. In elderly patients or patients with a history of low-velocity trauma, osteoporosis, or chronic steroid use, initial evaluation with radiographs is recommended (Fig. 48.12).

Imaging with MRI can be considered in patients who have persistent or progressive symptoms after 6 weeks of conservative management and are deemed candidates for surgery or perineural steroid injection. "Red flags" raising suspicion for serious underlying conditions, such as cauda equina syndrome, malignancy, or infection are another indication for MRI. Patients with recurrent back or spine pain and history of prior surgical intervention should be evaluated with contrast-enhanced MRI (Fig. 48.13). The patient should be screened for a history of allergic reaction to steroids or contrast prior to referral for perineural injection or contrast enhanced MRI.

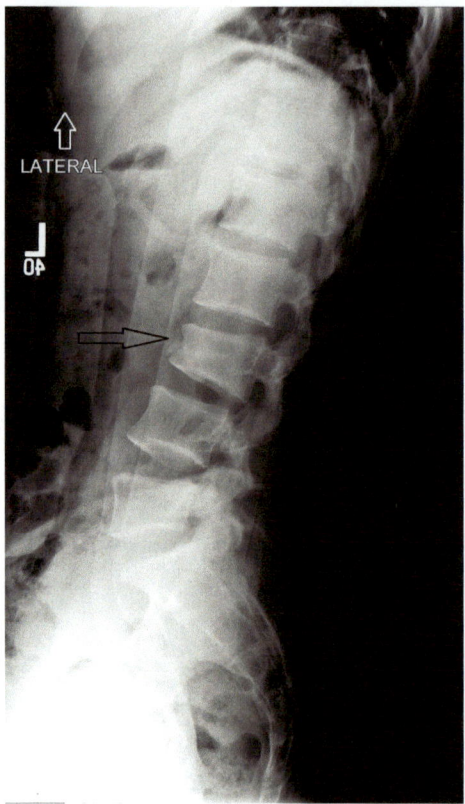

FIGURE 48.12 - COMPRESSION FRACTURE
Lateral lumbar spine radiograph demonstrating an L3 anterior wedge compression fracture (*black line arrow*)

Mineralization

There are four abnormal types of mineralization that you should be familiar with:

1. *Heterotopic ossification* is an abnormal deposition of true bone within soft tissues. It is formed by dormant osteoprogenitor cells in the soft tissue that are caused to differentiate into osteoblasts by a variety of bone morphogenetic proteins (BMPs) (Fig. 48.14a).

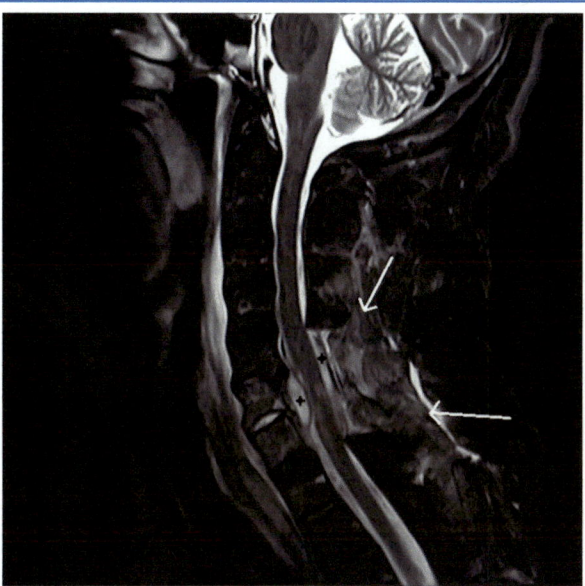

FIGURE 48.13 - EPIDURAL ABSCESS
Sagittal T2 sequence MRI of the cervical spine demonstrating an epidural abscess (*black stars*) spanning C5 through C7 with associated soft tissue inflammation (*white arrows*) post surgery

2. *Dystrophic calcification* refers to an accumulation of calcium salts in dying tissues (any area of necrosis, AVN, damaged heart valves). This calcification can become heterotopic. Serum calcium is normal (Fig. 48.14b).
3. *Metastatic calcification* refers to the deposition of calcium in tissues secondary to hypercalcemia. This may be due to increased parathyroid hormone, destruction of bone by tumors, chronic renal failure, and increased vitamin D (Fig. 48.14c).
4. *Calcific tendinosis/periarthritis* refers to the deposition of calcium hydroxyapatite in tendons or the soft tissues about a joint respectively. These deposits can incite an inflammatory response resulting in severe pain (Fig. 48.14d).

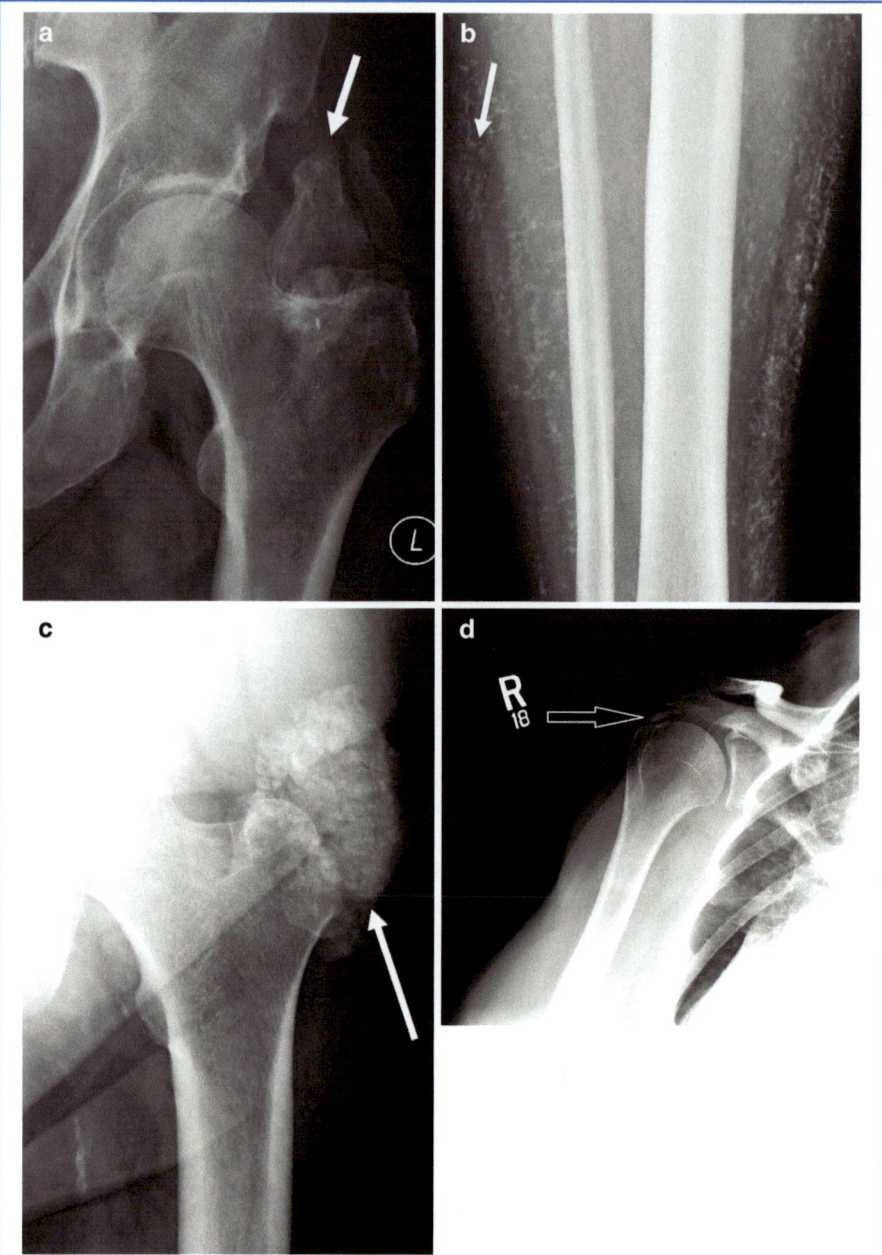

FIGURE 48.14 - SEVERAL TYPES OF CALCIFICATION
(**a**) Heterotopic ossification (*arrows*) (**b**) Dystrophic calcifications are noted in the skin of a patient with peripheral vascular disease (**c**) Metastatic calcification (tumoral calcinosis) is present above the greater trochanter in a patient with chronic renal failure on dialysis (*arrow*) (**d**) Calcific tendinosis of the rotator cuff (*white lined arrow*)

S: Deciding on the most appropriate method of initial imaging in the setting of possible fracture is critical to ensure both the appropriate coverage and the least amount of radiation exposure.

A: Imaging algorithms ensure the quickest and safest way to arrive at a diagnosis. Appropriateness is complex in extremity injuries and history, such as mechanism of injury, is essential. Algorithms such as the Ottawa Ankle Rule for ankle injuries and the American College of Radiology (ACR) Appropriateness Criteria for low back pain may suggest that imaging is not appropriate initially. The use of plain radiographs is essential to quickly evaluate areas of concern, and more detailed imaging, such as CT scanning that has a higher radiation dose, can be used for focused imaging.

F: A careful review of all the images, particularly in those who might be osteopenic, will allow for the correct diagnosis and direct advance imaging as needed.

E: Initial findings, particularly with displaced or complex fractures, must be reported to the ordering physicians as soon as possible, as there can be a limited window for operative repair.

Reference

1. Wofle M, Uhl T, Mccluskey L. Management of ankle sprains. Am Fam Physician. 2001;63(1):93–105.

49 BONE TUMOR CHARACTERISTICS

Objectives:
1. Name the two most important variables when creating a differential for bone tumors.
2. Name three lesional characteristics that further refine a differential of bone tumors.
3. Understand the difference between aggressive/nonaggressive and benign/malignant.

This chapter is not an exhaustive description detailing the characteristics of various types of bone tumors. It does however provide a list of characteristics to evaluate and classify types of bone tumors which allows for the creation of a useful differential diagnosis when a new bone tumor is encountered in clinical practice.

First, it is imperative to understand the concept that aggressive and nonaggressive are not synonymous with malignant and benign. Though an aggressive appearing lesion is more likely malignant, certain lesions can be aggressive and not malignant and vice versa. For example, osteomyelitis often appears aggressive but is not malignant, whereas a giant cell tumor may look nonaggressive but can be malignant.

The two most important aspects when evaluating a bone tumor lesion and creating a differential diagnosis are to note the age of the patient and the location of the lesion.

Skeletal maturity is the most important variable used to classify bone tumors. That is, certain tumors have a predilection for certain age ranges (less than 20 years old, between 20 and 40, and older than 40 years of age). For instance, primary bone

J. Kissane et al. (eds.), *Radiology Fundamentals: Introduction to Imaging & Technology*, https://doi.org/10.1007/978-3-030-22173-7_49

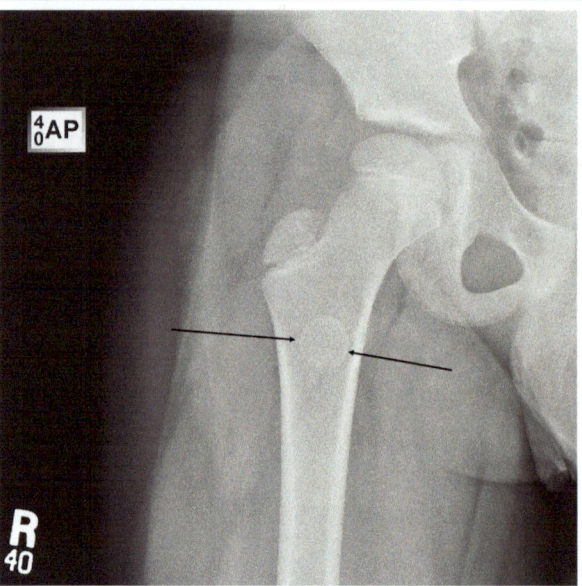

FIGURE 49.1 - NONAGGRESSIVE MARGINS
Thin white (sclerotic) rim margins indicate a nonaggressive lesion

malignancy is less common than metastatic disease or myeloma in a patient over 40. The second most important way to classify a bone tumor is based upon the tumor's location. Most tumors have a predilection for specific locations within the bone, i.e., diaphysis, metaphysis (site of rapid bone growth), and epiphysis. Axial skeleton versus appendicular skeleton or long versus flat bones are other important factors regarding location. As an example, a Ewing sarcoma follows the course of red marrow. Therefore, in children, it is often found in the diaphysis of long bones, and in young adults, it has a predilection for flat bones such as the pelvis reflecting the normal evolution of red marrow distribution.

Certain features of the lesion itself are quite important. Most notable is the margins of the lesion. The sharper the margins, especially if there is a sclerotic (white) rim, the less aggressive the lesion (Fig. 49.1). The more indistinct and ill-defined the margin, the more aggressive the lesion. The most aggressive lesions have a characteristic appearance called "moth eaten" or "permeative" (Fig. 49.2). These terms refer to small, patchy, ill-defined areas of destruction.

Furthermore, the presence of periosteal reaction and its appearance is an important characteristic in evaluating a bone lesion. A solid or unilamellar periosteal reaction signifies that a tumor is slow growing, allowing the bone to "wall off" the lesion (Fig. 49.3). A multi-lamellated appearance, also known as "onion skin appearance,"

360

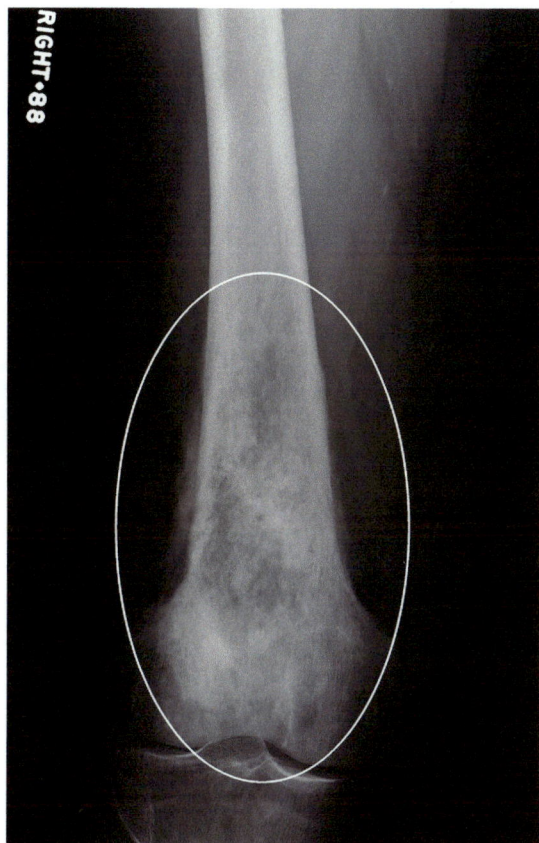

FIGURE 49.2 - AGGRESSIVE MARGINS
Example of permeative or "moth-eaten" appearance of an aggressive lesion

suggests an intermediate aggressiveness. Periosteal reaction that is spiculated in appearance, "hair on end," is the most aggressive type (Fig. 49.4). A Codman triangle refers to an elevation of the periosteum away from the cortex. This term is classically associated with an osteosarcoma but is not limited to this as any number of malignant or benign processes can cause this feature.

Some bone tumors produce mineralization. Evaluating the matrix mineralization of a bone tumor can help classify the lesion and further refine the differential diagnosis. A tumor producing new bone will have a fluffy or cloudlike amorphous matrix appearance (Fig. 49.5). Whereas a chondral (cartilaginous) tumor will have matrix

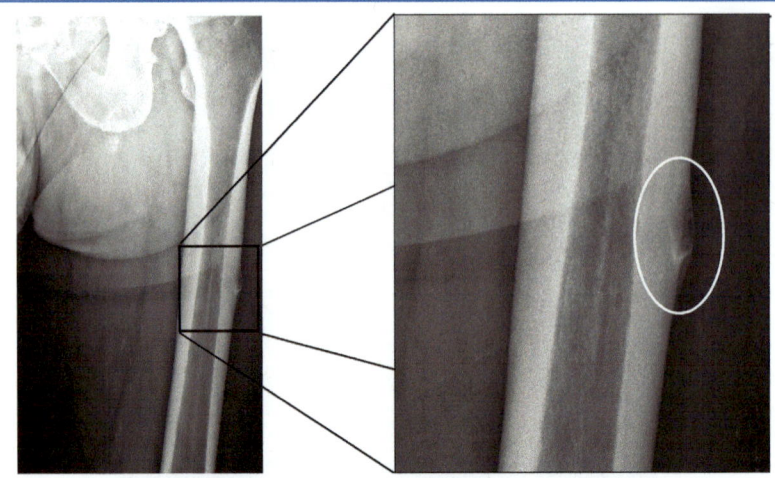

FIGURE 49.3 - NONAGGRESSIVE PERIOSTEAL REACTION
Unilamellated or solid periosteal reaction usually found with nonaggressive lesions

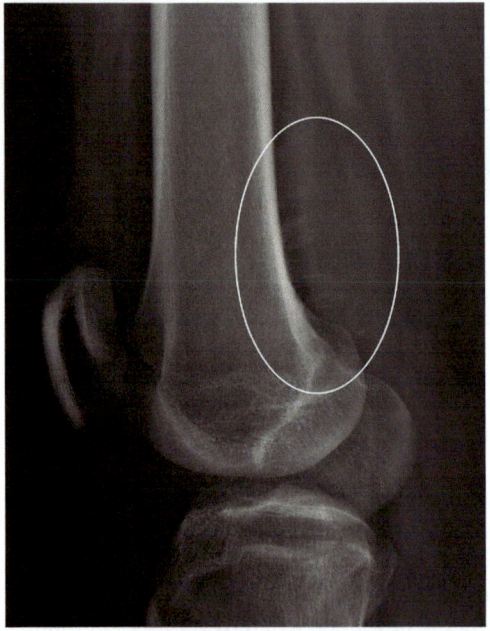

FIGURE 49.4 - AGGRESSIVE PERIOSTEAL REACTION
Radiographic appearance of the classic "hair-on-end" periosteal reaction characteristic of aggressive lesions

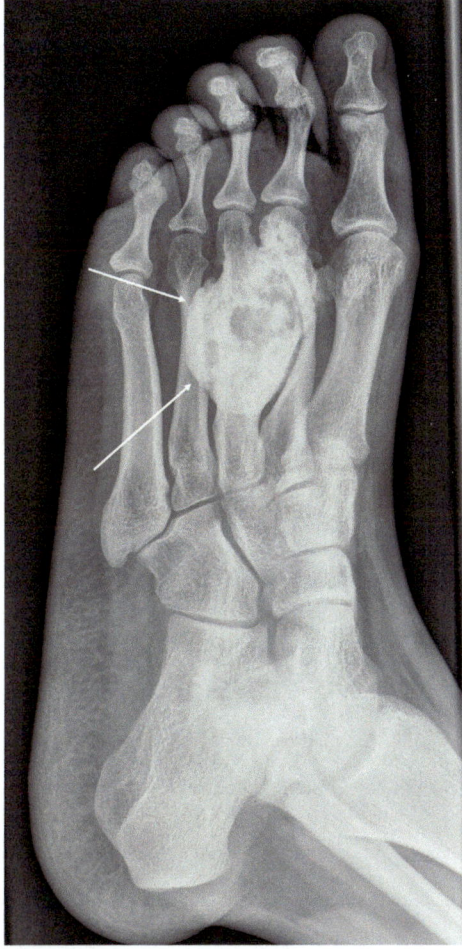

FIGURE 49.5 - OSTEOID MATRIX
Lesion arising from the third metatarsal which has an osteoid matrix characterized by the fluffy, cloud-like appearance

mineralization that appears as punctate arc and ring calcifications (Fig. 49.6). CT is often better than plain film at delineating the type of matrix mineralization.

When evaluating bone tumors

1. Age of patient
2. Tumor location
3. Does it look aggressive?
4. Margins of bone tumor—sharp/sclerotic or indistinct?

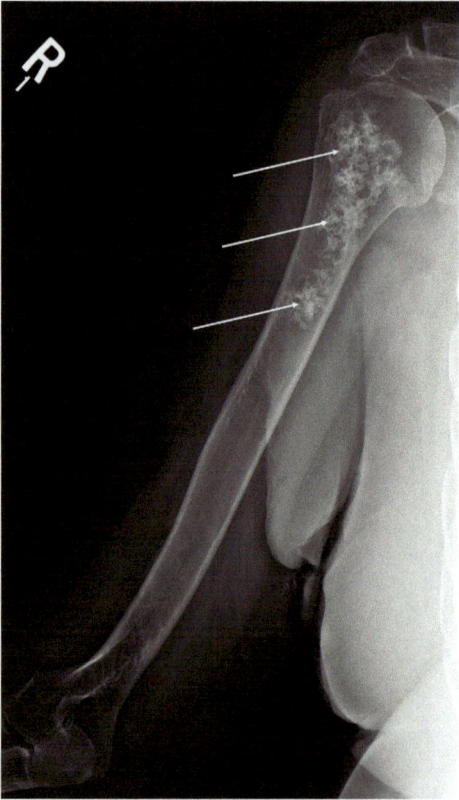

FIGURE 49.6 - CHONDROID MATRIX
Lesion arising in the proximal humerus with chondroid matrix characterized by arc and ring calcifications

5. Periosteal reaction—yes or no? Smooth (nonaggressive) or lamellated (aggressive?)
6. Mineralization: may help to characterize origin of tumor

S: Investigation of a bone tumor begins with radiographs to help differentiate between aggressive and nonaggressive processes.
A: CT and MR are useful for further characterizing malignant bone tumors, evaluating soft tissue extension, and metastatic involvement. They are also imperative for biopsy planning and surgical planning.
F: Radiographs should include at least two views. Cross-sectional imaging is best performed with IV contrast to help in diagnosis and biopsy approach planning.
E: Positive findings of a bone tumor on radiographs warrant a communication to the provider for initiation of tumor workup. The risk of pathological fracture should also be communicated.

Suggested Reading

Miller TT. Bone tumors and tumor-like conditions: analysis with conventional radiography. Radiology. 2008;246(3):662–74.

50 ARTHRITIDES AND INFECTION

Osteoarthritis

Osteophyte formation, asymmetric joint space narrowing, and subchondral sclerosis/cystic change are hallmarks of degenerative or osteoarthritis

The typical radiographic characteristics of osteoarthritis include:

1. *Asymmetric joint space narrowing*—This indicates loss of articular cartilage. For example, the hip migrates superiorly because of the loss of cartilage superiorly along the weight-bearing surface.
2. *Subchondral sclerosis* (*also called eburnation*)—This is caused by trabecular compression and fracture with callus formation.
3. *Osteophyte formation*.

Figure 50.1 is an example of asymmetric joint space narrowing which reflects thinning of the cartilage in the medial aspect of the joint, the area of maximal weight bearing. The body reacts to this change in its weight-bearing surface by increasing the thickness at the margins of the weight-bearing area resulting in subchondral sclerosis and reinforcement of the ligamentous support of the knee through the formation of spurs or osteophytes.

© Springer Nature Switzerland AG 2020
J. Kissane et al. (eds.), *Radiology Fundamentals: Introduction to Imaging & Technology*, https://doi.org/10.1007/978-3-030-22173-7_50

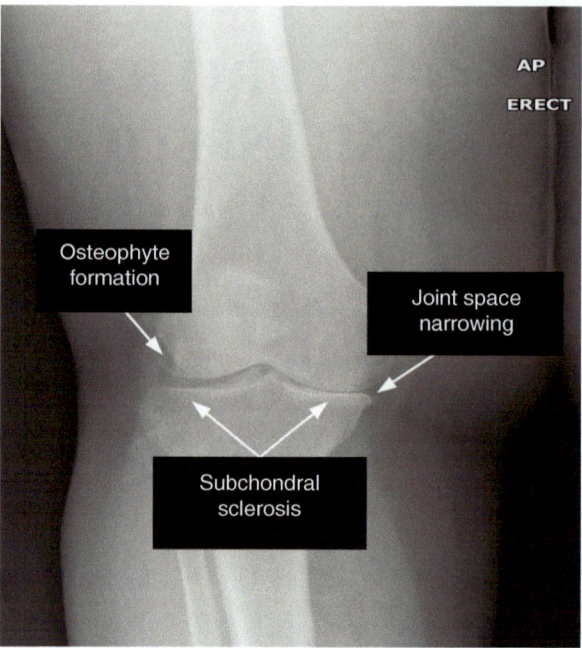

FIGURE 50.1 - OSTEOARTHRITIC KNEE
Right knee displaying osteophyte formation, joint space narrowing, and subchondral sclerosis, consistent with severe osteoarthritis

Rheumatoid Arthritis

Figure 50.2 demonstrates a case of rheumatoid arthritis (RA). In rheumatoid arthritis, there is symmetric joint space narrowing and loss of bone density. These findings help distinguish rheumatoid arthritis from osteoarthritis.

In addition, look for marginal erosions along the edges of articular surfaces in RA. Erosions first occur along the edges of the articular surface because these areas lack articular cartilage and are in direct contact with the inflamed synovial lining of the joint. Articular cartilage offers protection from the inflammation. Therefore, the edges of the articular surface not covered by cartilage are the first areas susceptible to the inflammatory pannus. The locations of these erosions help distinguish rheumatoid arthritis from other arthritides.

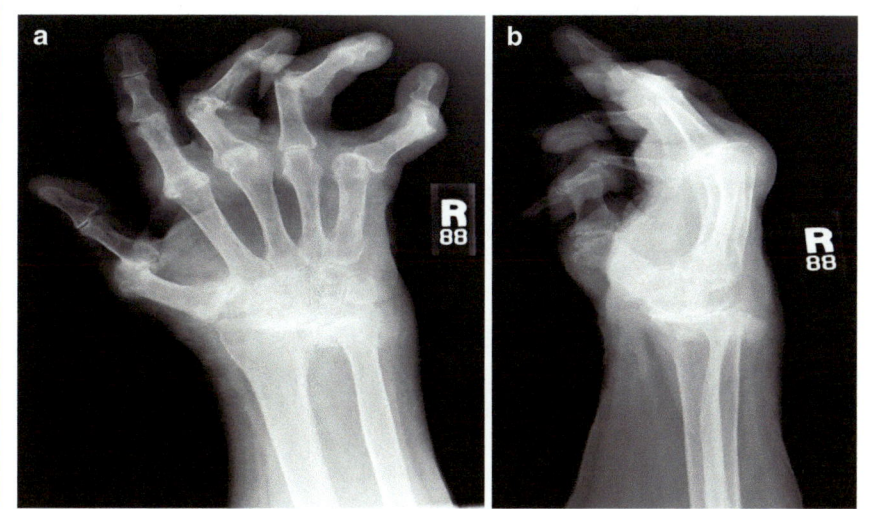

FIGURE 50.2 - SEVERE RHEUMATOID ARTHRITIS DEMONSTRATED IN AP (a) AND LATERAL (b) VIEWS OF THE HAND
Boutonniere deformity of the fifth digit is noted, with hyperflexion at the PIP joint and hyperextension at the DIP joint. There are severe ulnar subluxations of the fingers and carpal bones and marginal erosions. Diffuse joint space narrowing is noted at the carpal joints and the metacarpalphalangeal joints

Differences Between Osteoarthritis and Rheumatoid Arthritis

Note again that in osteoarthritis (OA), there is asymmetric joint space narrowing, subchondral sclerosis, and osteophyte formation. Also note that the main areas of involvement are in the distal interphalangeal joints with relative sparing of the metacarpophalangeal joints and intercarpal joints. Osteophytes formed about the DIP joints are referred to as Heberden's nodes, while those at the PIP joints are referred to as Bouchard's nodes. Osteoarthritis begins peripherally and, as it becomes more severe, progresses to involve the PIP joints. The only exception from the distal to proximal migration of osteoarthritis would be the first (thumb) carpometacarpal joint. This is a common site of osteoarthritis proximally.

On the other hand, in rheumatoid arthritis (RA), there is symmetric joint space narrowing and marginal erosions (which can be quite subtle in the early stages). RA usually involves the intercarpal joints and metacarpophalangeal joints at an early stage (Fig. 50.3). There is ulnar deviation and subluxation in the late stages of RA. You should be able to distinguish osteoarthritis from the rheumatoid-type arthritides in most cases. However, in very advanced disease, degenerative arthritis may be superimposed on preexisting rheumatoid-type arthritis, which may result in a confusing picture with imaging features of both disease processes. Other

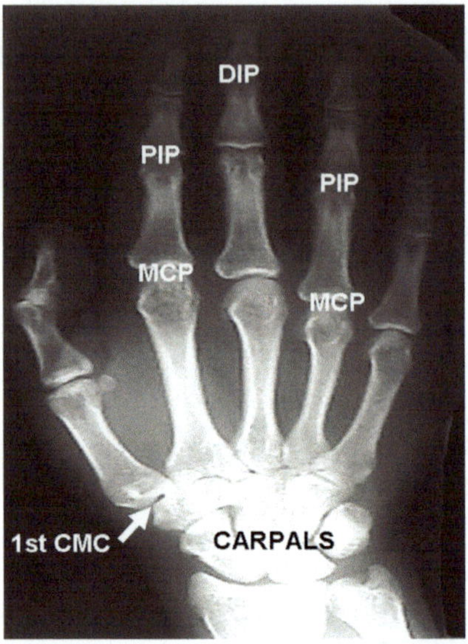

FIGURE 50.3 - ABNORMALITY DISTRIBUTION OF OSTEOARTHRITIS VERSUS RHEUMATOID ARTHRITIS
Osteoarthritis, characterized by joint space narrowing, subchondral sclerosis (also called eburnation), and osteophyte formation, tends to affect the proximal and distal interphalangeal joints as well as the first carpometacarpal joint. Rheumatoid arthritis, characterized by periarticular osteoporosis, marginal erosions, boutonniere deformity, swan neck deformity, subluxations, and dislocations, tends to affect the metacarpophalangeal joints and proximal interphalangeal joints

arthritides, which may look like osteoarthritis, include the arthritis produced by pseudogout (calcium pyrophosphate deposition disease) and hemochromatosis. Other than rheumatoid arthritis, arthritides which produce erosions include psoriatic arthritis, reactive arthritis, and enteropathic arthritis (associated with Crohn's disease and ulcerative colitis).

Gout

Figure 50.4 demonstrates the hand of a patient with gout. You should note the following:

1. *Soft tissue tophi:* Lumpy bumpy pattern of soft tissue swelling that may mineralize in a small percentage of cases.
2. *Juxta-articular erosions:* Erosions occur in the regions of soft tissue tophi. Unlike the marginal erosions of rheumatoid arthritis, gouty erosions are located farther from the joint and have characteristic sharply defined overhanging edges.

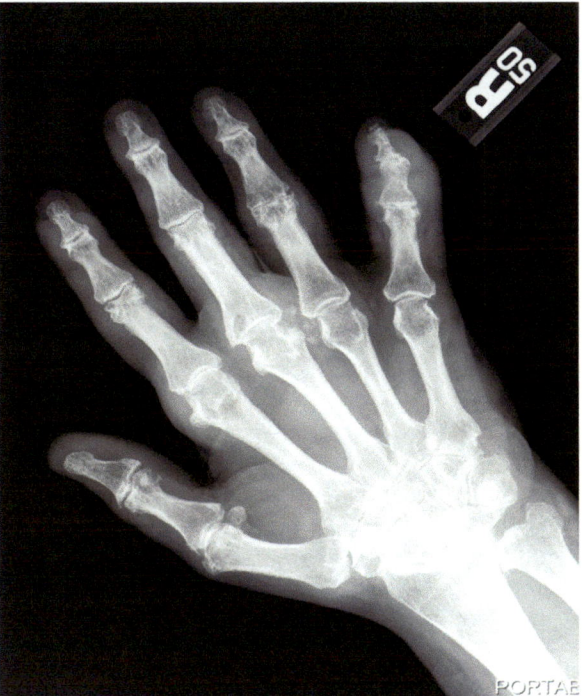

FIGURE 50.4 - GOUT
Nodular soft tissue swelling most impressive in the distal little finger, but also involving the ring, middle, and index fingers. Also note juxta-articular erosions in multiple joints, most conspicuous in the third MCP and fifth PIP. These findings are consistent with tophaceous gout

3. *Joint destruction:* This usually occurs late in the disease and contiguous to the tophus. The joint spaces are characteristically normal in joints that are not destroyed.

In summary, gout is a disease of the soft tissues near the joints, not of the intra-articular portions of the joint itself.

Infection

Bony erosions can also be due to infection of the bone, called osteomyelitis. In adults, osteomyelitis often results from direct extension of soft tissue infection, such as diabetic foot ulcers. Osteomyelitis can also occur hematogenously. Radiographic

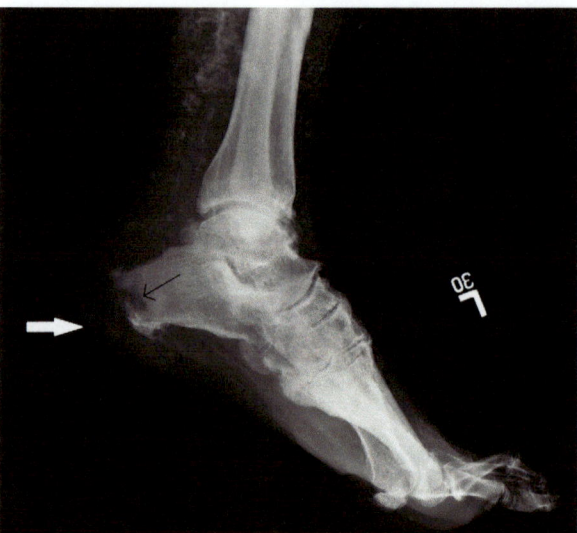

FIGURE 50.5 - OSTEOMYELITIS
Left foot radiograph demonstrating soft tissue ulcer (*white arrow*) of the heel with underlying erosion and osteopenia (*black arrow*) of the calcaneus consistent with osteomyelitis

findings of osteomyelitis include cortical erosions, periostitis, and focal osteopenia (Fig. 50.5). However, findings may take up to 14 days to appear on radiographs. MRI is more sensitive for early imaging evidence of osteomyelitis.

Septic arthritis is an infection of a joint. Radiographic findings of septic arthritis include joint effusion, erosions, and osteopenia. However, similar to osteomyelitis, radiographs may be normal. If suspicion is high, joint aspiration should be performed for further evaluation.

In the setting of suspected infection, soft tissue gas can indicate a potentially fatal infection of the soft-tissue fascia called necrotizing fasciitis. This process can be rapidly progressive, and commonly affected body parts include the extremities, perineum, and trunk. Immunocompromised patients are at an increased risk for necrotizing fasciitis. It is critical to be aware that radiographic findings are often similar to cellulitis and may even be normal until the advanced stages of infection and tissue necrosis. Soft tissue gas is only seen in a minority of cases; therefore, if there is a high clinical suspicion emergent surgical consultation is required.

S: Radiographs may be normal in the setting of septic arthritis. If clinical suspicion is high, joint aspiration should be performed. Radiographs may be normal in the setting of osteomyelitis. If clinical suspicion is high, MRI should be performed.
A: Radiographs are the most appropriate initial exam for suspicion of arthritides and infection. MRI may be helpful to evaluate the extent of infection and any soft tissue or bony abscess that may require surgical or percutaneous intervention.

F: Radiographs may be normal in the early stages of infection (10–14 days in an adult). Radiographic findings of osteomyelitis include focal osteopenia, periosteal reaction, and cortical erosions.

E: Soft tissue gas can indicate a potentially fatal infection known as necrotizing fasciitis. It is critical to remember that no imaging modality can reliably exclude the diagnosis and emergent surgical consultation is required in cases with a high clinical suspicion.

PART VIII
NEURORADIOLOGY

51 CNS ANATOMY

Objectives:
1. Identify the important normal anatomic landmarks on brain CT and MRI.
2. Describe how you would differentiate an enhanced (intravenous contrast) from an unenhanced CT scan of the head.
3. Understand the basic principle of image formation in MRI.

Figures 51.1 and 51.2 demonstrate a normal CT and MRI of the brain. Be sure to become familiar with the labeled structures. An in-depth discussion of the CNS anatomy is beyond the scope of this introductory text.

Note that on CT scans which are performed after administration of intravenous contrast, the circle of Willis, as well as other various cortical vascular structures, are prominently displayed. You should be able to identify the anterior cerebral artery, the middle cerebral artery, the posterior cerebral artery, and the region of the anterior and posterior communicating arteries.

MRI technology uses powerful magnets with magnetic fields several times more powerful than the earth's gravitational field. Hydrogen atoms are normally spinning in a random fashion. When a magnetic field is applied to the atoms, the magnetic poles of the hydrogen atoms are aligned. The magnetic field is then turned off, and the alignment of the hydrogen atoms degrades. With the degradation, a radio-frequency signal is given off which is then recorded and analyzed by the computer. From this information, an image is formed.

© Springer Nature Switzerland AG 2020

J. Kissane et al. (eds.), *Radiology Fundamentals: Introduction to Imaging & Technology*, https://doi.org/10.1007/978-3-030-22173-7_51

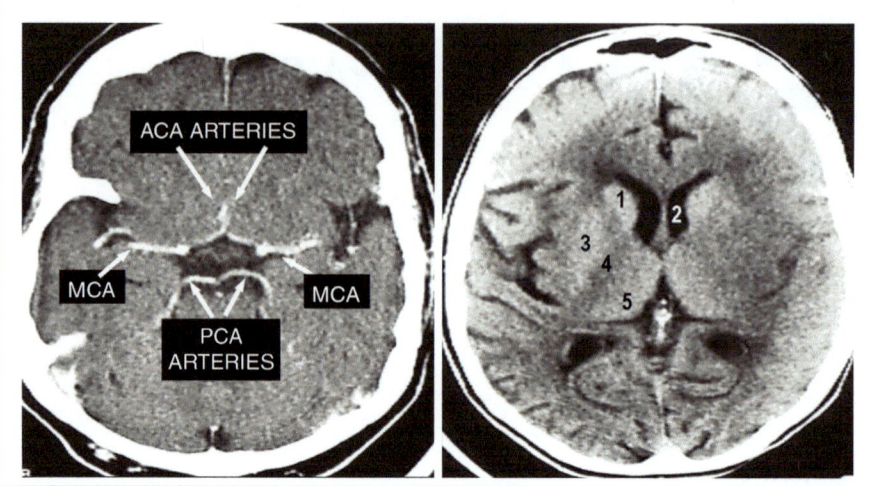

FIGURE 51.1 BASIC CT NEUROANATOMY
The image on the *left* shows the intracerebral circulation (circle of Willis), which is clearly evident post-contrast. On the *right*, a non-contrast image, the following structures have been labeled: (*1*) caudate, (*2*) lateral ventricle frontal horn, (*3*) putamen and globus pallidus, (*4*) internal capsule (extends anteriorly), and (*5*) thalamus

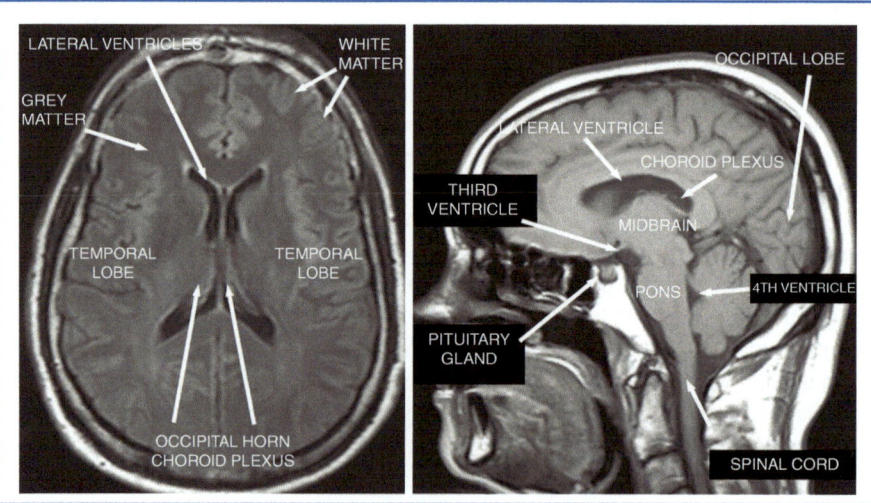

FIGURE 51.2 BASIC MRI NEUROANATOMY

S: Always be mindful of normal anatomic variants and artifacts when interpreting images.

A: For imaging of acute blood and evaluation of bony pathology, CT scan is the method of choice; whereas for brain as well as spinal cord parenchymal pathology MRI is the preferred modality.

F: In CT scans, it is important to look at all three planes of images—axial, coronal, and sagittal. Also remember to look at images in soft tissue as well as bone window settings. In MRI brain, FLAIR and DWI (diffusion) are usually the highest yield sequences. Remember the list of things bright on T1 sequence—methemoglobin, calcium, iron, gadolinium, melanin, and fat.

E: Common artifacts on CT include beam hardening and volume averaging artifacts. Common artifacts on MRI include CSF and arterial pulsation artifacts, susceptibility artifacts at bone-brain and air-brain interface, and motion artifacts.

52 THE CERVICAL SPINE

Plain radiographs of the cervical spine are the initial imaging modality, where the frontal, lateral, and AP views may be supplemented by additional views (like the "open-mouthed" and extension/flexion views). Screening in spine trauma may begin with plain radiographs as traumatic injuries must be ruled out prior to moving the patient for other views and further treatment. Bony evaluation is now more commonly performed with CT which has much higher resolution and can provide multiplanar reformations. MRI is the modality of choice when spinal cord injury or ligamentous or soft tissue injury is suspected. A systematic and thorough review as outlined in the following steps is mandatory.

Systematic Approach to Evaluating the Cervical Spine with CT or Plain Film

(Figs. 52.1 and 52.2)

- Step 1: Count the visualized cervical vertebral bodies. It is mandatory that all seven cervical vertebrae (both the body and posterior elements) as well as the relationship of the inferior aspect of C7 with T1 are visualized.
- Step 2: Check the alignment of the anterior aspects of the vertebral bodies: the anterior vertebral line. There should be a smooth curve that is convex anteriorly as one progresses from superior to inferior in the cervical spine. Loss of this

© Springer Nature Switzerland AG 2020   381
J. Kissane et al. (eds.), *Radiology Fundamentals: Introduction to Imaging & Technology*, https://doi.org/10.1007/978-3-030-22173-7_52

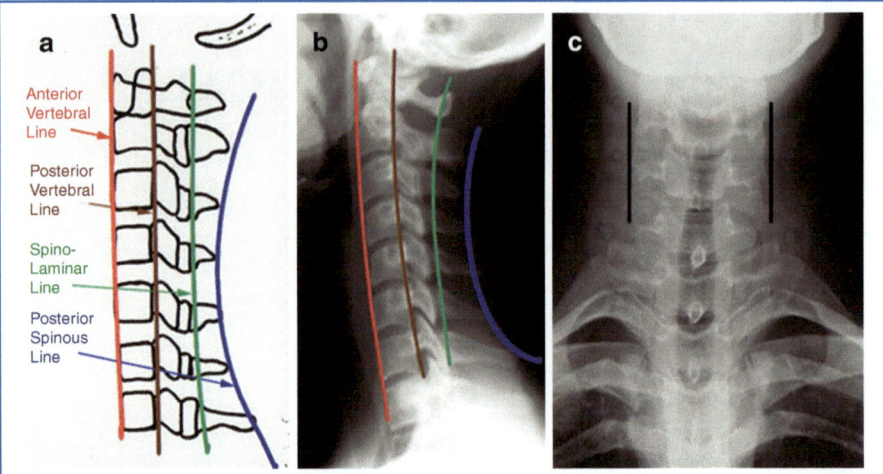

FIGURE 52.1 - CERVICAL SPINE LATERAL AND AP VIEWS
The anatomical landmarks are labeled on the diagram (**a**) and subsequently shown on the lateral radiograph (**b**). Note the undulating, rhythmic appearance of the lateral aspects of the cervical spine, bilaterally (**c**)

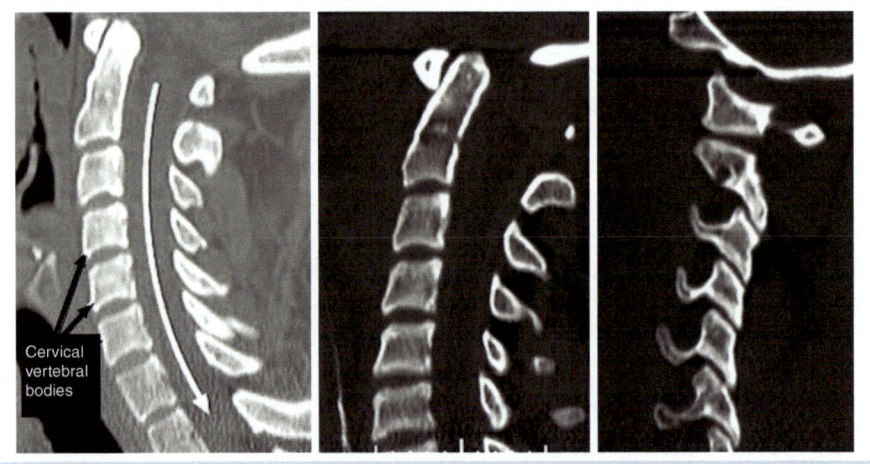

FIGURE 52.2 - CERVICAL SPINE CT SAGITTAL VIEWS
Normal alignment of the vertebrae with maintained body heights and normal facet articulations

curvature may indicate muscle spasm or soft tissue injury if the curvature is straightened or reversed. If the curvature changes abruptly, a fracture is likely.
- Step 3: Check the alignment of the posterior aspects of the vertebral bodies (posterior vertebral line, which represents the anterior aspect of the bony spinal

canal). For obvious reasons, this curvature should parallel the curvature of the anterior aspect of the vertebral bodies. Abnormalities of this curvature have the same significance as those of the anterior vertebral body curvature.

- Step 4: Check the alignment of the spino-laminar line. This is a smooth line drawn along the anterior aspect of the spinous processes (which represents the posterior aspect of the bony spinal canal). Again, any disruption of this smooth curvature should be viewed with suspicion.
- Step 5: Check the distance between the posterior aspect of the anterior arch of C1 and the anterior aspect of the odontoid process. This is the atlantoaxial space (sometimes called the predental space). Any increase in this distance may represent disruption of the transverse ligament that secures the posterior aspect of the dens to the atlas. The upper limit of normal for adults is 2.5 mm. Check the prevertebral soft tissues. As a general rule, think 6 and 2: at C2 they should be maximally 6 mm wide, and at C6 they should be maximally 22 mm wide. An openmouthed odontoid view is helpful to look for fractures of the odontoid process of C1 and the status of the lateral masses of C2 (Fig. 52.3).

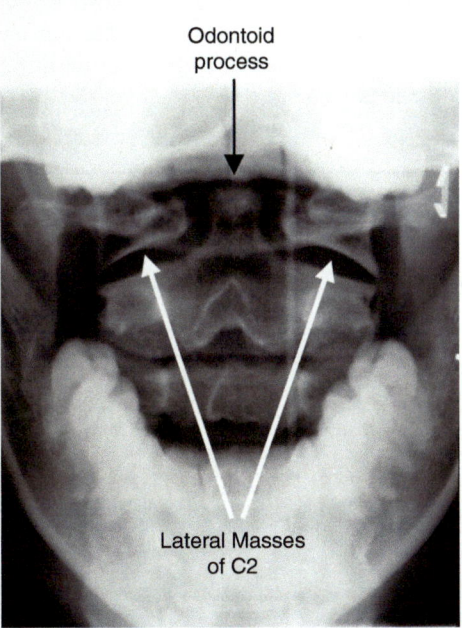

FIGURE 52.3 - OPEN-MOUTHED ODONTOID VIEW
The AP open-mouthed odontoid view provides an unobstructed view of both the odontoid process of C2 and the lateral masses of C1

The approach in evaluating a cervical spine CT is similar to that of a radiograph. However, with multiplanar reformats and better resolution, CT is much more sensitive than plain radiography. With the advent of multidetector CT, bony evaluation of the cervical spine is now done with CT, but the principles outlined above can be applied to any imaging modality.

MRI in the Cervical Spine Evaluation

MRI is very useful for evaluating spinal injuries. It is especially helpful for diagnosing or ruling out spinal cord injuries and acute compression of the spinal cord when clinical examination shows muscle weakness or paralysis. MRI is able to detect subtle changes in the vertebral column that may be an early stage of fracture, infection, or tumor. MRI may be better than CT scanning for evaluating tumors, abscesses, and other masses near the spinal cord (Fig. 52.4).

Evaluation of cervical spine MRI begins with the assessment of alignment, vertebral body heights, and presence abnormal marrow signal. Disc and ligaments are much better seen on MRI as compared to CT. Next, evaluation should include assessment of the cord for compression, canal stenosis, or abnormal signal within the cord. Finally, the pre-/paravertebral soft tissues and muscles are evaluated for hematoma or pathologic masses.

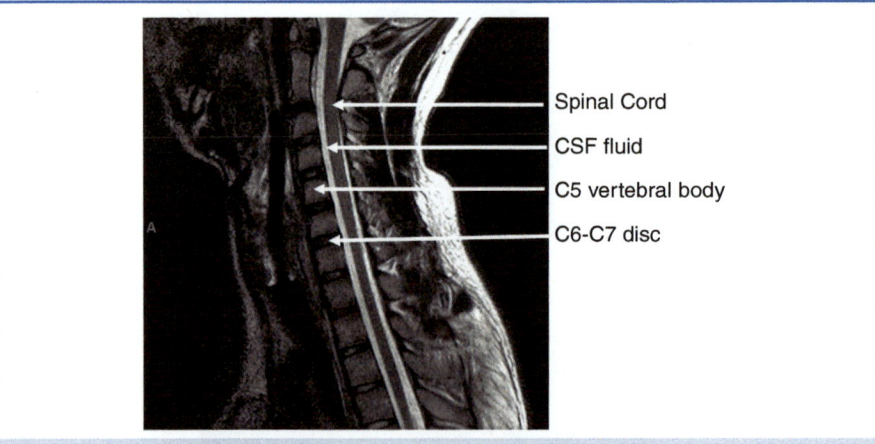

Spinal Cord

CSF fluid

C5 vertebral body

C6-C7 disc

FIGURE 52.4 - SAGITTAL CERVICAL SPINE MRI
T2-weighted MRI of the cervical spine shows normal alignment of the vertebrae with normal bone marrow and spinal cord signal

S: Missing unstable cervical spine fractures or ligamentous injuries may lead to serious injury to a patient like quadriplegia and disastrous medico legal consequences for physicians.

A: Radiographs are very insensitive to acute neck trauma and hence CT cervical scan without contrast is the modality of choice. In significant fractures with or without dislocations of the cervical spine, fractures involving transverse foramina, and skull base fractures, CT angiogram of the neck is strongly recommended to look for arterial dissections. MRI is appropriate after CT if there is suspicion of myelopathy, intervertebral disc injury, or other ligamentous disruption.

F: For avulsion fractures, look for a corresponding donor site on the larger bone. Beware of isolated intervertebral disc, atlanto-axial, and atlanto-occipital widening type distraction injuries where the extent of soft tissue injuries are quite severe, despite an apparently normal radiograph. In patients with extensive spine ossification like ankylosing spondylitis or diffuse idiopathic skeletal hyperostosis (DISH), spine injuries can be disproportionately severe with respect to the degree of trauma.

E: In suspected acute cervical spine injury, the trauma team will often call the radiologist to clear the spine before removing the collar. Any fractures involving the bony spinal canal such as the pedicle, lamina, or articular pillars are highly unstable whereas isolated spinous process fractures are stable configuration fractures and will not result in cord injury.

53 HEAD TRAUMA

Objectives:
1. Understand the role of skull radiographs in head trauma.
2. Describe the appearance of an epidural hematoma on a head CT scan.
3. Describe the appearance of a subdural hematoma on a head CT scan.
4. Describe the appearance of a subarachnoid hemorrhage on a head CT and MRI.
5. Be able to list the findings on CT/MRI in a patient with cerebral contusion.
6. Describe the appearance of diffuse axonal injury on CT/MRI.

Skull Radiograph

With the advent of CT scans, the role of routine skull radiographs in neurologic trauma has become limited. In moderate and severe head trauma, a CT scan is the study of choice. Skull radiographs are only indicated in minor head trauma patients where a CT scan is otherwise not clinically indicated during the initial evaluation.

Skull radiograph may be helpful and can complement other imaging modalities in the following conditions:

1. Depressed fracture is suspected clinically or by the nature of the injury.
2. Penetrating injury by metal or glass is suspected.
3. Radiodense foreign body is suspected.

The basic skull projections used in evaluation of head trauma are the lateral and the fronto-occipital (AP) views (Fig. 53.1).

Epidural Hematoma

Figure 53.2 shows a CT of a patient with a known skull fracture and acute hemorrhage. Blood appears as radiodense (white) material on head CT. The biconvex appearance of the epidural blood is caused by the tight attachment of the dura to the skull. Midline shift is present secondary to the mass effect of the hematoma.

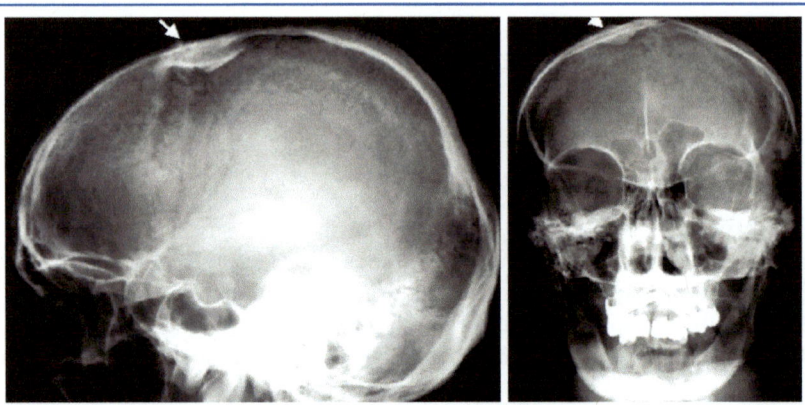

FIGURE 53.1 - SKULL RADIOGRAPH
Lateral and AP views show a depressed fracture of the right parietal bone with displacement of the bone fragment into the skull

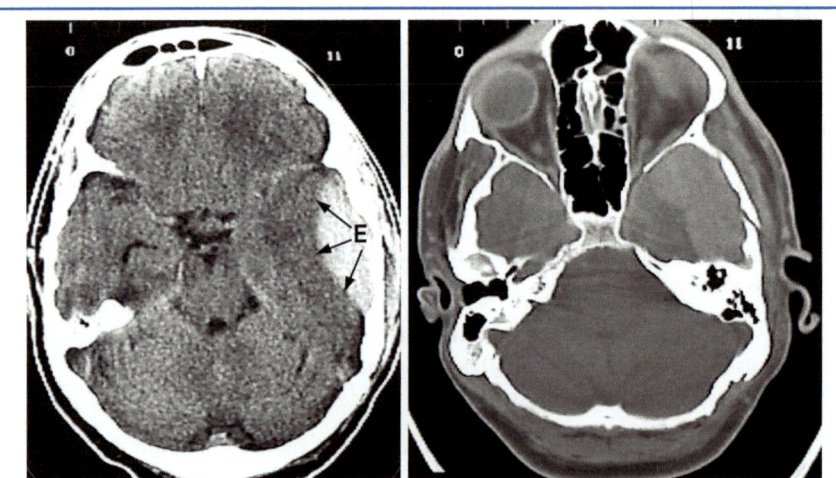

FIGURE 53.2 - EPIDURAL HEMATOMA WITH SKULL FRACTURE
In this trauma victim, there is an epidural hematoma (*E*). It has the typical elliptical shape. There is mass effect, centered on the bleed (*arrows*). The image on the *right* is further evidence of head trauma and the likely cause of the epidural hematoma. Did you notice the left temporal bone fracture?

Subdural Hematoma

Figure 53.3 demonstrates a subdural hematoma which is hemorrhage under the dura. Note that the blood is free to follow the contour of the brain so that it has a flat or concave inner surface.

In the normal evolution of a subdural hematoma, the collection becomes hypodense (more gray) with respect to brain tissue. As more time passes, it becomes isodense (equally dense) with respect to the brain tissue. Diagnosis during this period of isodensity can be difficult. Chronic subdural hematomas that are hypodense with respect to the brain substance are referred to as subdural hygromas.

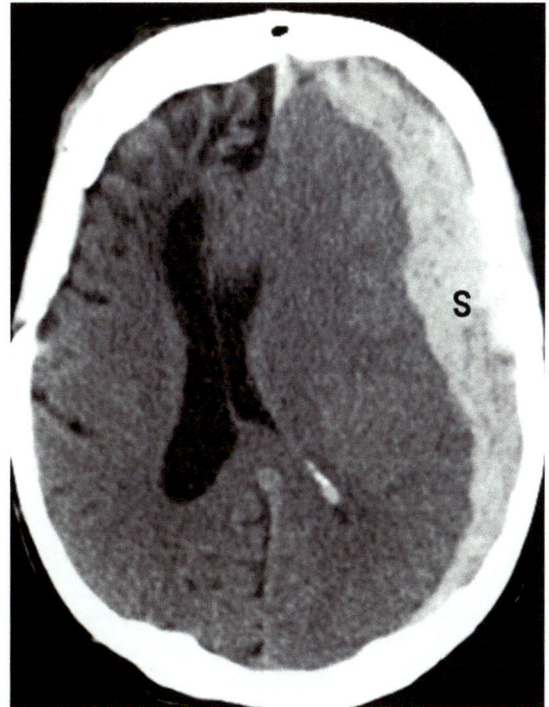

FIGURE 53.3 - SUBDURAL HEMATOMA
In this trauma victim, there is a large left holohemispheric subdural hematoma (*S*). It has a distinctly flat/concave inner surface which allows one to distinguish it from an epidural hematoma

Subarachnoid Hemorrhage

Trauma is the most common cause of subarachnoid hemorrhage (SAH) overall. A large percentage of traumatic brain injuries include of this type of bleeding. On CT scans, SAH appears as a high-attenuating or radiodense (white), amorphous substance that fills the normally dark, CSF-filled subarachnoid spaces around the brain (Fig. 53.4). These findings are most evident in the largest subarachnoid spaces, such as the suprasellar cistern and sylvian fissures. It can also be seen tracking along the sulci, outlining the gray matter. MRI is more sensitive in diagnosing subarachnoid bleed, especially in hyperacute and chronic phases where CT may be completely negative because blood in those states is equal density to brain on CT.

Parenchymal Contusion

Figure 53.5 shows an area of generally decreased attenuation (gray) with an area of lobular increased densities. There is subtle mass effect with contralateral midline shift (to the patient's right). This displacement and low density are caused by edema with the lobular areas representing hemorrhage. This is the radiographic appearance

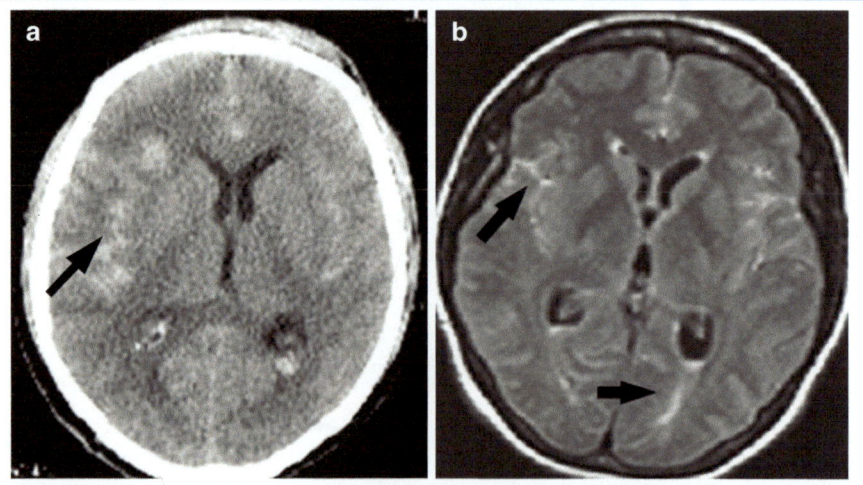

FIGURE 53.4 - CT AND MRI OF SUBARACHNOID HEMORRHAGE
(a) CT shows hyperdensity within the CSF sulci spaces, most prominently along the sylvian fissures (*arrow*), consistent with subarachnoid hemorrhage. (b) MRI on the same patient shows corresponding areas of T2 hyperintensity within the sylvian fissures along with intraventricular hemorrhage

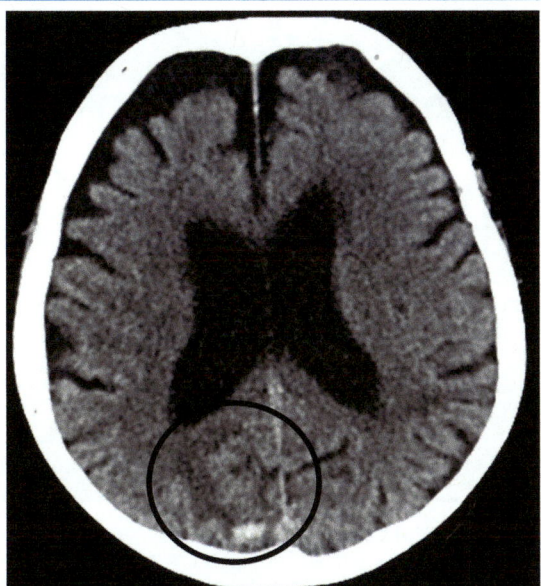

FIGURE 53.5 - PARENCHYMAL CONTUSION
There is blood in the parenchyma with some surrounding edema consistent with a contusion.
Note the subtle mass effect at this level

of a cerebral contusion or, literally, "a bruise of the brain." In all of the above diagnoses, there may be associated findings such as a skull fracture and associated soft tissue swelling external to the skull. These abnormalities may give you a clue as to where to look within the brain for abnormalities, as these findings can sometimes be quite subtle.

Diffuse Axonal Injury

Diffuse axonal injury (DAI) is a frequent result of traumatic deceleration injuries and a frequent cause of a persistent vegetative state. Typically, the process is diffuse and bilateral, involving the lobar white matter at the gray-white matter interface (Fig. 53.6). The corpus callosum frequently is involved, as is the dorsolateral rostral brainstem. On CT, 60–90% of patients with DAI may have a normal CT scan on presentation. Small petechial hemorrhages located at the gray-white matter junction and corpus callosum are characteristic but only occur in about 20%. MRI is the modality of choice for diagnosing DAI. Most common MRI findings are multiple

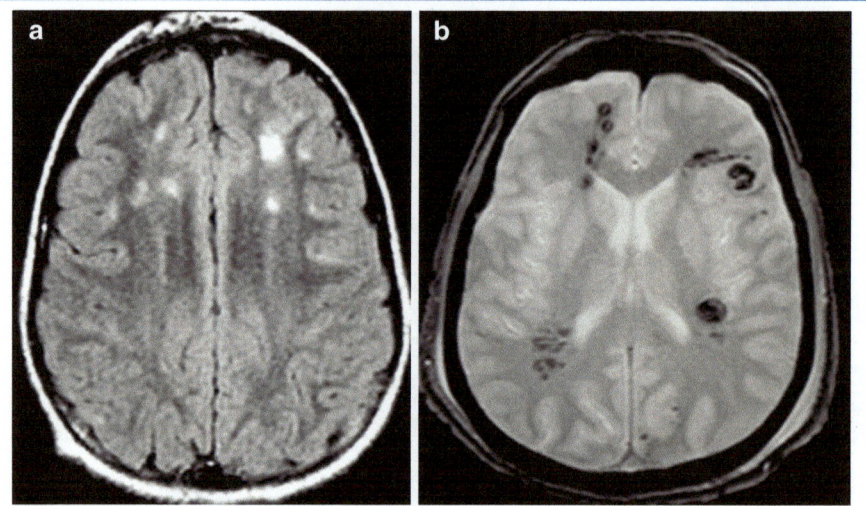

FIGURE 53.6 - HEAD TRAUMA IMAGING
MRI in a young patient with trauma and negative head CT shows multiple areas of T2 hyperintensity at the gray-white matter junction (**a**). The petechial hemorrhages are seen as low signal areas on gradient images (**b**). (Gradient echo is a MRI sequence which is very sensitive to blood products)

focal areas of abnormally bright signal on T2-weighted images in the white matter of the temporal or parietal corticomedullary junction or in the splenium of corpus callosum. Gradient echo sequences are very useful in demonstrating petechial hemorrhages. The paramagnetic properties of blood cause a loss of signal, represented by black areas.

S: In acute head trauma, sometimes it may be necessary to obtain an MRI. Patients should still be carefully screened for ferromagnetic materials/implants. Special attention should be taken to use only MRI compatible materials like oxygen cylinders and other compatible equipment. Also important to remember is the fact that these critical patients are often accompanied by several caregivers, many of whom may not be adequately trained in MRI safety.

A: In acute head injury, noncontrast CT is the modality of choice despite radiation concerns. Radiographs of the skull usually are very low yield and are usually avoided. Skull radiographs are used in infants to screen for skull fractures, especially in the setting of suspected non-accidental injuries. MRI is done after CT if there is suspicion for diffuse axonal injury.

F: Small subdural and epidural hemorrhages may be difficult to differentiate from each other using the usual radiologic criteria. In such cases they are often referred to radiology reports as small extra-axial hematomas, indicating that they are intracranial but lie outside the brain parenchyma.

E: When the patient has a subdural or epidural hematoma, important things the neurosurgeons want to know are the thickness of the hematoma, the amount of midline shift, the degree of mass effect on the midbrain, and presence or absence of uncal and other intracranial herniations.

54 STROKE

Objectives:
1. State the definition of stroke.
2. Understand the role of imaging in stroke.
3. Be able to describe major CT and MRI findings in stroke.

Introduction

Stroke is a clinical syndrome. It is used to refer to a group of clinical syndromes that present with acute mental status change including ischemic infarction, hemorrhage, seizure, tumor, encephalopathy, etc.

Imaging in stroke is used to differentiate:

1. Vascular process from other mimics such as hemorrhage, tumor, vascular malformation, and encephalopathy
2. Hemorrhagic from nonhemorrhagic infarction
3. Arterial from venous infarction
4. Large territory infarct from lacunar-type infarctions

In addition, more advanced CT and MRI techniques can be applied (i.e., CT perfusion, CT angiography, MRI angiography) to guide treatment options and potentially predict outcome.

© Springer Nature Switzerland AG 2020   395
J. Kissane et al. (eds.), *Radiology Fundamentals: Introduction to Imaging
& Technology*, https://doi.org/10.1007/978-3-030-22173-7_54

Imaging Findings in Stroke

When is the optimal time to image "stroke?" The answer generally is "as soon as possible," although this depends on the treatment options available to the patient at the presenting medical care facility. Treatment options include conservative management, intravenous tissue plasminogen activator (t-PA), intra-arterial t-PA, and mechanical thrombolysis. Treatment depends on the timing of onset of symptoms and the clinical status of the patient. The patient's clinical status is assessed using the National Institutes of Health Stroke Scale (NIHSS), a systematic assessment tool that provides a quantitative measure of stroke-related neurologic deficit, based on a 15-item scale measuring the patient's level of consciousness, language, neglect, visual field loss, extraocular movement, motor strength, ataxia, dysarthria, and sensory loss.

Noncontrast CT is usually first obtained (Fig. 54.1). This is a very fast and widely available study. Quite a bit of information can be gained from the basic CT, such as the following: Is there a discernible abnormality? Does it appear to be ischemia or something else, like a mass? Is there bleeding? How much brain tissue is involved? Is there herniation/mass effect that would constitute a neurosurgical emergency?

Ischemia/infarction is not always immediately evident on CT, especially if the patient is imaged very early after the onset of symptoms or if the area of brain involved is small (lacunar infarct).

The early signs of ischemia on CT are:

1. Hypoattenuation (low density) in the affected tissue
2. Loss of gray-white matter differentiation (insular ribbon sign)
3. Sulcal effacement due to brain swelling
4. Hyperdensity in a large vessel (hyperdense MCA sign) or "dot sign" due to acute clot in the diseased vessel

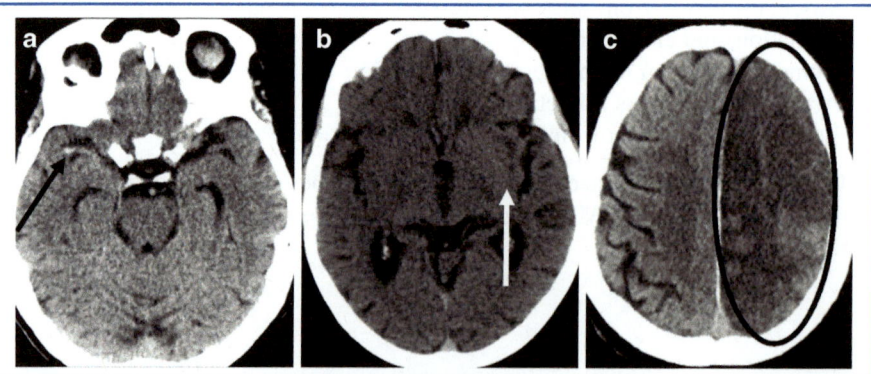

FIGURE 54.1 - CT FINDINGS OF ACUTE ISCHEMIA
The above images represent CT findings of acute ischemia: (**a**) hyperdense MCA, (**b**) loss of gray-white matter differentiation in the insula, and (**c**) sulcal effacement and hyperdensity in the MCA territory

Seeing the distribution of infarcted or ischemic tissue and knowing the arterial supply (Fig. 54.2) to the different parts of the brain, one can infer the vessel(s) affected. The vascular territories of the cerebral arteries described in the figure include ACA = anterior cerebral artery, MCA = middle cerebral artery, and PCA = posterior cerebral artery.

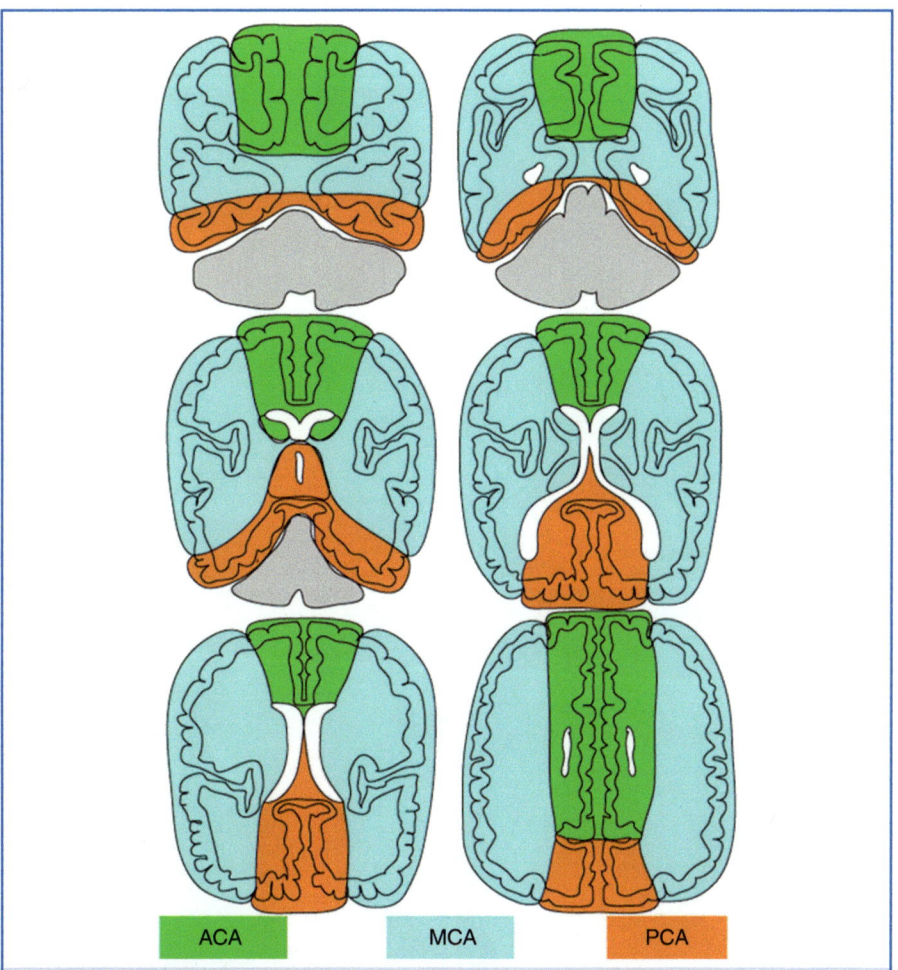

| ACA | MCA | PCA |

FIGURE 54.2 - VASCULAR AREAS OF CEREBRAL ARTERIES
Based on the distribution of infarcted or ischemic tissue, one can infer the vessel that is affected based on the arterial supply to the brain

Although in many instances subtle findings can be seen on CT, sometimes the study can appear essentially normal, especially early on. If this is the case, the patient could clinically still have a "stroke" syndrome and will be treated as such.

MRI is more sensitive for detection of early ischemia and is better at detecting small infarctions, especially in patients with cerebrovascular disease who have chronic small infarcts (Fig. 54.3). Diffusion-weighted imaging can detect ischemia within minutes of the acute event and is generally agreed to be the best indi-

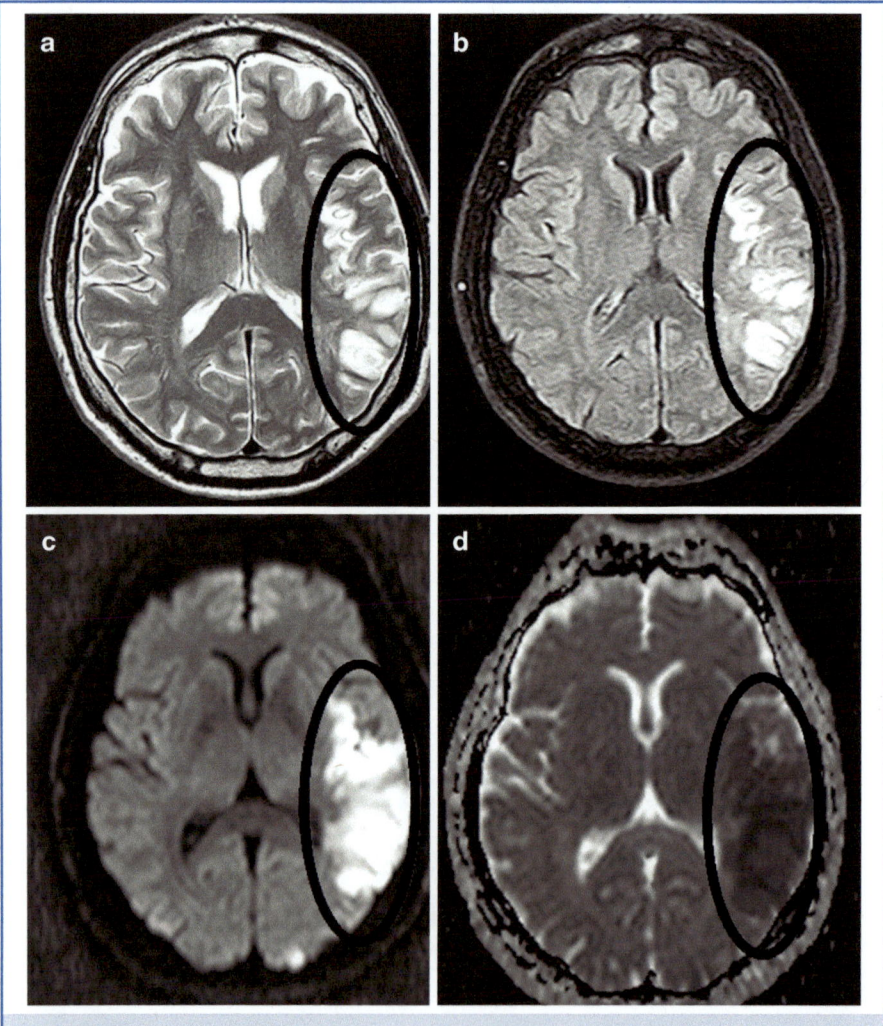

FIGURE 54.3 - ACUTE ISCHEMIA
MRI findings of acute ischemia in the left MCA distribution: (**a**) T2W, (**b**) FLAIR, (**c**) DWI, and (**d**) ADC map

cator of the total infarcted volume. Also, MRI is better at finding other processes which may be causing the symptoms; however, disadvantages of MRI include less availability, higher price, and longer scanning time (a major drawback given the previously discussed treatment window). MRI is not safe for some patients who have metallic foreign bodies or certain devices, most notably older model pacemakers, certain models of artificial valves, cochlear implants, and spinal stimulators.

CT perfusion (CTP) is performed by monitoring the first pass of the contrast bolus through the cerebral circulation (Fig. 54.4). Information can be obtained at four representative levels in the brain or be obtained through a volume of brain tissue. Using this information, color maps of cerebral blood volume (CBV), cerebral blood flow (CBF), mean transit time (MTT), and time to peak (TTP) are generated. This information is used to look for areas of perfusion defect and mismatch, which, in addition to the region of the infarction core, indicate other areas of ischemia and potential infarction, the "penumbra." This may influence further treatment decisions. MRI perfusion operates on basically the same principles, except gadolinium-based contrast is used and perfusion maps are compared with diffusion-weighted images to determine if there is tissue that can potentially be saved. Although the information is similar, CTP is much faster and therefore more commonly used in acute settings, although there is some disagreement among the stroke community as to the added value of perfusion imaging.

CT angiography or venography (CTA or CTV) are noninvasive techniques using thin section techniques and contrast to image the intracranial and extracranial (neck) vasculature. This is useful for identifying sites of occlusion, stenosis, dissection, and/or aneurysm (Fig. 54.5).

Although infarction is more frequently caused by arterial occlusion, venous thrombosis can also lead to ischemia and hemorrhage. Venous infarcts do not follow

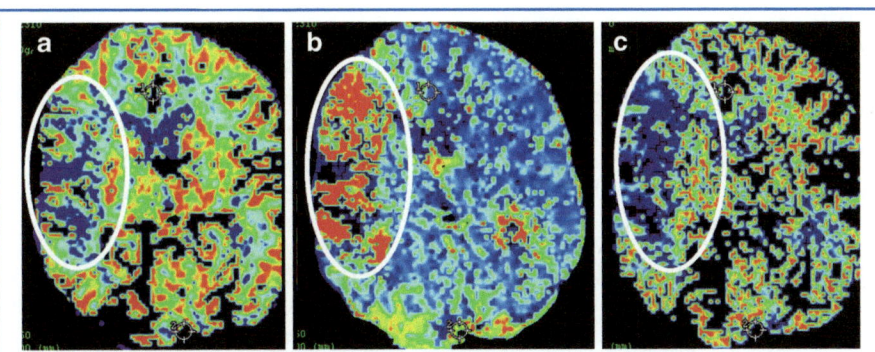

FIGURE 54.4 - CT IMAGES OF AN ACUTE INFARCT
CT perfusion in acute right MCA infarct with all three parameters being abnormal in the affected distribution: (**a**) CBV, (**b**) CBF, and (**c**) MTT

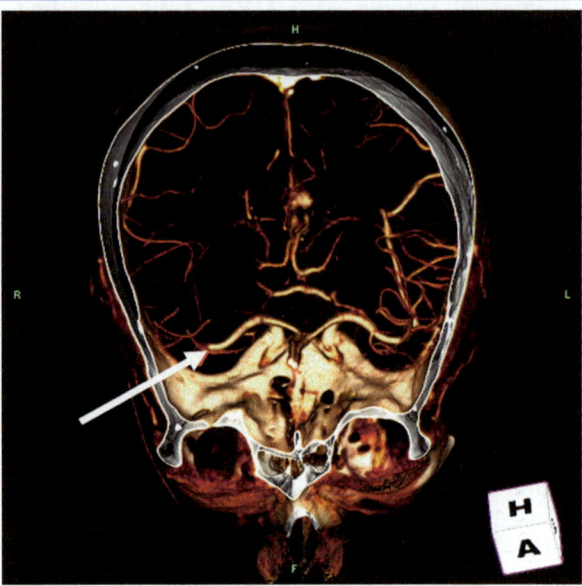

FIGURE 54.5 - OCCLUSION OF MIDDLE CEREBRAL ARTERY
CTA shows acute occlusion of the right MCA (*arrow*)

arterial territories and occur in younger patients with hypercoagulable states or other risk factors. CT venography or MR venography can evaluate the patency of major dural sinuses.

Summary

Options for imaging stroke include CT, CT perfusion, CT angiography, MRI, MR perfusion, and MRI angiography. Not all of these studies are indicated on every patient. CT is faster, more readily available, and, in some ways, easier to interpret. MRI is more expensive, less available, slower, but more sensitive for acute ischemia and useful for finding other causes of patient's symptoms that may not be evident on CT.

S: Acute stroke patients often get iodinated contrast for CT angiogram or catheter angiogram despite an abnormal GFR and risk of renal failure since the benefits often outweigh the risks. This practice may vary and usually depends on prior consensus between the neuroradiologists and the neurologists.

A: CT perfusion carries a high radiation dose, and MR perfusion may be a good alternative. However, this choice is often dictated by comfort level of the clinical stroke team and/or available expertise of the radiologists.

F: Noncontrast CT is the first imaging obtained for suspected stroke patients and the most important task for radiologists is to unequivocally rule out the presence of hemorrhage, so that tPA can be administered to patients often in the CT suite itself, even if acute infarct is not seen, to avoid delay in treatment.

E: In ischemic infarction, neurons are dying by the thousands per minute and "Time is Brain." So, expediting imaging and communication of results to the clinical stroke team is of paramount importance.

55 HEADACHE AND BACK PAIN

Objectives:
1. Understand the role of imaging in the patient with headache and back pain.
2. Be able to describe the major CT findings of subarachnoid hemorrhage.
3. Be able to state other causes of headache.

Introduction

Many disease processes manifest as headache. While headaches are mostly benign and self-limited, imaging is often obtained to exclude acute or life-threatening processes, such as a hemorrhage or mass.

Back pain is one of the most common complaints in health care. It is important to remember that back pain is not a diagnosis but a symptom of a medical condition. Most causes are benign. Imaging is often obtained when there is no response to rest, exercise, and medication to ensure there is no process that needs further intervention.

Intracranial Hemorrhage

Classically, the presentation of "the worst headache of my life" with sudden onset is concerning for subarachnoid hemorrhage (SAH). The most common cause of *nontraumatic* subarachnoid hemorrhage is a ruptured intracerebral aneurysm. Acute blood products are hyperdense (white) on CT, and therefore CT is useful for detection of SAH. CT angiography (CTA) is highly sensitive for the diagnosis of the underlying aneurysm, although catheter angiography remains the gold standard

© Springer Nature Switzerland AG 2020

J. Kissane et al. (eds.), *Radiology Fundamentals: Introduction to Imaging & Technology*, https://doi.org/10.1007/978-3-030-22173-7_55

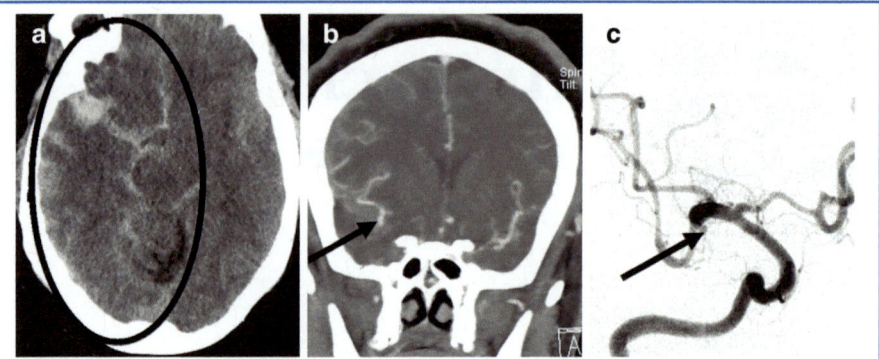

FIGURE 55.1 - SUBARACHNOID HEMORRHAGE
Image (**a**) is a CT which shows predominantly right hemispheric SAH. Image (**b**) is a coronal CTA reformat showing a very small aneurysm of the right M2 segment of the MCA, while the digital subtraction image (*DSA*) shown in image (**c**) shows the same aneurysm

(Fig. 55.1). CSF sampling by lumbar puncture can be done in cases of CT-negative suspected SAH.

There are other types of intracranial hemorrhage which could cause headache though they are frequently associated with trauma. These include subdural and epidural hematomas and hemorrhagic contusions (see Chap. 53, "Head Trauma").

Other Common Causes of Headache on Imaging

Any disease process which alters the intracranial pressure (ICP) or causes hydrocephalus, midline shift, or cerebral edema can cause a headache. This includes brain tumors (primary or metastatic), non-neoplastic masses which can have mass effect or obstruct the ventricles, or idiopathic processes such as pseudotumor cerebri. Infectious processes, including meningitis and encephalitis, can present with headache but often have no or little findings on imaging; rather, the diagnosis is dependent on CSF and serum assay (Fig. 55.2).

Back Pain

Causes of back pain include mechanical problems, injuries, neoplasms, infections, and many other conditions. Intervertebral disc degeneration and herniation, facet arthritis, and muscle spasm are examples of mechanical problems that result in back

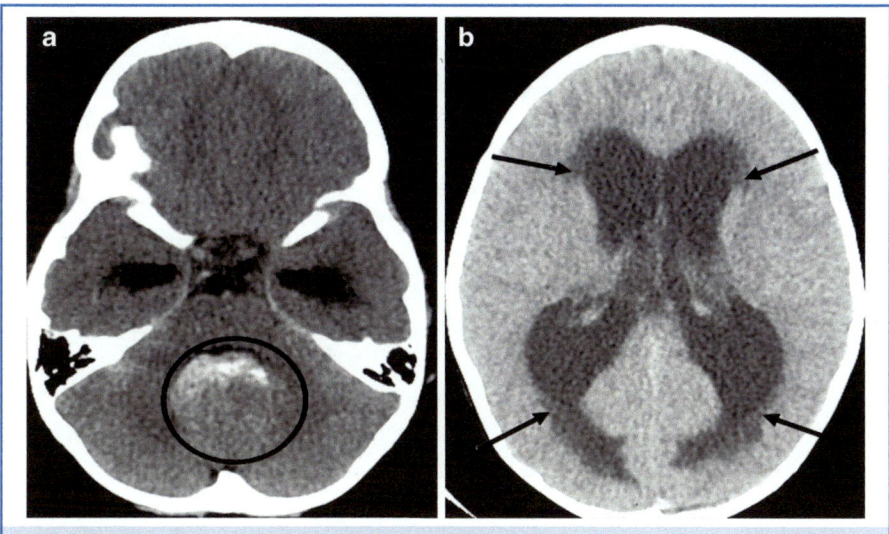

FIGURE 55.2 - HYDROCEPHALUS
CT showing a dense posterior fossa mass (**a**) causing hydrocephalus (**b**)

pain. Injuries to bones, muscles, tendons, and ligaments from sports, trauma such as car accidents, and improper lifting and twisting can result in back pain. Compression fractures in osteoporotic patients may manifest as back pain. Permanent and progressive conditions such are inflammatory and osteoarthritis, scoliosis, and fibromyalgia cause or contribute to back pain. Patients with renal calculi, pancreatitis, pregnancy, and endometriosis may have back pain. Leaking aortic aneurysm and aortic dissection may present as back pain. Osteomyelitis/discitis, primary tumors of the spinal cord or vertebral bodies, and metastatic disease may also cause back pain. And while most causes of back pain are physical, stress, anxiety, depression, and insomnia can present as back pain or exacerbate underlying back pain conditions.

In the absence of underlying conditions such as malignancy or trauma, appropriate treatment may first be exercise, mild medication, physical therapy, and lifestyle modification such as weight loss and management of stress and depression. If these interventions do not help, imaging should be considered. Plain films of the lumbar spine will demonstrate alignment, compression or traumatic fractures, disc space height abnormalities, and changes of arthritis and serve as a road map. CT scan, particularly if other conditions are suspected, will frequently demonstrate other causes such as kidney stones, aortic aneurysm, pelvic mass, etc. MRI is sensitive for the detection of tumors, disc herniation, nerve root impingement, and infections of the bone, discs, and spinal cord (Fig. 55.3).

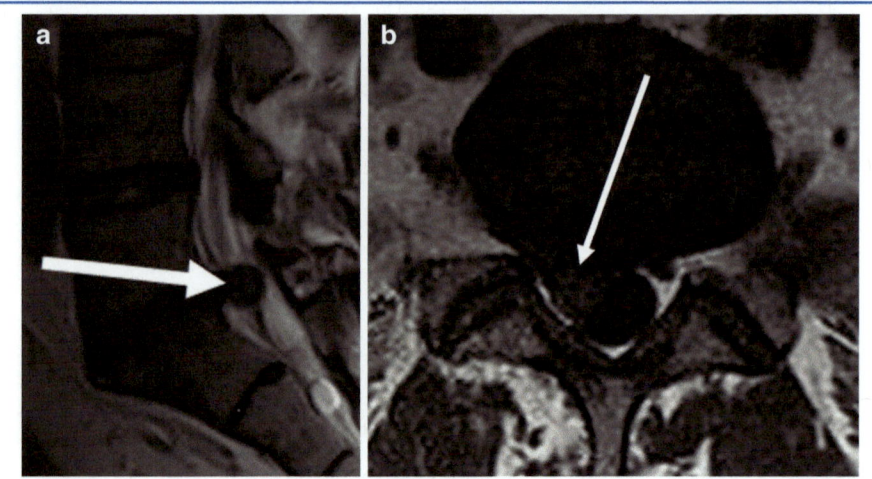

FIGURE 55.3 - LUMBAR DISC HERNIATION
Sagittal (**a**) and axial (**b**) MRI images showing a focal protrusion of the L5–S1 disc (*arrows*) causing moderate mass effect on the thecal sac

Summary

Headache is a very common complaint. Patients with simple headache often have no imaging findings. Moreover, imaging is not needed in the majority of cases of headache. Imaging is used when there is clinical suspicion for a more complicated or acute process, such as hemorrhage, mass, or hydrocephalus. Noncontrast CT is excellent for the initial evaluation of headache to exclude life-threatening processes, with the caveat that some very serious disease processes, especially infectious diseases affecting the central nervous system, can have little or no imaging findings.

Back pain is also very common and imaging is also not always required. Acute situations such as loss of bowel or bladder control or acute muscle weakness should prompt a consideration of imaging with CT and/or MRI. Clinical acumen remains of the utmost importance in the evaluation and treatment of patients presenting with either complaints.

S: Patients with chronic back pain may have spinal cord stimulators, most of which are a contraindication for MRI (although newer MRI compatible versions are being developed). However, most intracranial vascular coils and clips are MRI compatible (each case is individually checked by the MRI technologists).

A: Most cases of headache and backache do not require imaging. In the setting of chronic pain however, if clinical suspicion for pathology is high, evaluation of the brain and spine is best performed with MRI due to the ability of MRI to image detailed anatomy and detect subtle pathology. In the setting of acute trauma however, CT is the preferred modality despite its inability to image detailed anatomy of the brain and spine as it can be used to rapidly detect hemorrhage, bony fractures, and vascular injury.

F: Look at paranasal sinuses carefully in imaging for headaches as sinusitis may be the cause. CT or MRI contrast administration is usually at the radiologists' discretion but should be administered if there is strong suspicion for tumor, intracranial hypotension, and spine surgery within 2 years (to look for abnormal scar tissue). Most degenerative spine imaging does not need contrast administration.

E: Emergent communication with the ER is indicated in subarachnoid hemorrhage. SAH often has associated hydrocephalus due to interference of CSF drainage by the blood. Be careful to evaluate for narrowing of arteries due to vasospasm, which can be lethal.

PART IX
PEDIATRIC RADIOLOGY

56 PEDIATRIC RADIOLOGY PEARLS

Objectives:
1. Recognize the need for greater radiation safety precautions in children.
2. Be familiar with and appreciate common imaging appearances of pediatric chest and abdomen.
3. Identify the differences between pediatric fractures and adult fractures.
4. Recognize the role of radiologic imaging in non-accidental injuries.

While the principles of imaging discussed in this book apply to the pediatric patient, the adage that "children are not small adults" is crucial to the specialty of pediatric radiology. Children have unique safety and appropriateness considerations that influence the modality choice and interpretation of pediatric imaging studies. As a full discussion of pediatric radiology is beyond the scope of this text, this chapter covers a few fundamental topics in pediatric radiology.

Radiation Concerns in Diagnostic Imaging

Radiologists must be careful when using imaging modalities that produce ionizing radiation, such as CT, radiography, and fluoroscopy. Ionizing radiation is known to result in tissue damage and carcinogenesis. The risk of ionizing radiation exposure is directly proportional to the size of the radiation dose and time elapsed after exposure. Growing children are more sensitive to ionizing radiation than adults. Additionally, pediatric patients have a longer life expectancy than adult patients. Therefore a dose of ionizing radiation that may not harm an adult may result in adverse outcome in a child. Pediatric radiologists must be particularly careful when choosing a modality that involves ionizing radiation, balancing the risk to the child against the benefit of the information obtained by the

© Springer Nature Switzerland AG 2020
J. Kissane et al. (eds.), *Radiology Fundamentals: Introduction to Imaging & Technology*, https://doi.org/10.1007/978-3-030-22173-7_56

imaging study. Pediatric radiologists must ask how a radiology test will change a patient's management and if there is a safer modality that will provide the same information without ionizing radiation. If a modality that uses ionizing radiation is deemed appropriate for a child, it is the job of the radiologist, health physicist, and technologist to use an x-ray dose that is appropriate for the size of the child. Further information related to imaging safety in pediatric patients can be found at www.imagegently.org.

Anatomic Considerations in Children

Growing children have unique anatomy which can be confusing to providers not used to looking at pediatric imaging studies. Two common areas of confusion are the thymus and growing bones. When reading a pediatric chest radiograph, it is not uncommon to see the thymus altering the expected contour of the mediastinum. The thymus is a bi-lobed lymphoid organ in the anterior mediastinum that is prominent in young children but becomes small in adults. To the untrained eye, the thymus may be mistaken for a mediastinal mass. To distinguish the thymus from a mass, look for its characteristic sail or wave shape (Fig. 56.1).

The thymus will not exert mass effect on adjacent structure, and you should be able to see normal lung parenchymal markings through the thymus. Growing bone contains cartilage which is not visible on radiographs. When looking at pediatric musculoskeletal radiographs for the first time, it is easy to mistake the cartilage in long bone growth plates as fractures. Smaller bones, such as the carpal and tarsal bones, may not yet be ossified in young children, rendering these bones radiographically invisible. Knowledge of the normal anatomic appearance of growing children is vital to the pediatric radiologist.

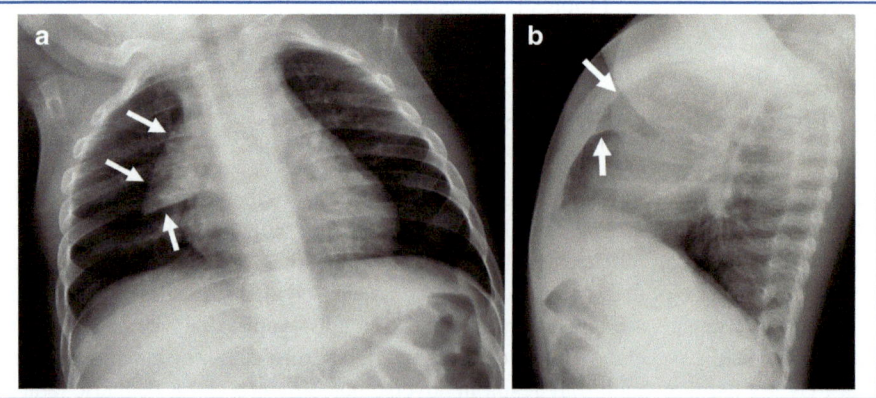

FIGURE 56.1 - PEDIATRIC THYMUS
Characteristic sail sign on AP view (**a**) and anterior location on lateral view (**b**)

Cardiorespiratory Imaging

Children commonly present with cough, fever, or difficulty breathing. When infection or serious cardiorespiratory compromise is considered, it is appropriate to obtain a chest radiograph. Pediatric cardiac problems are relatively rare, but a child with a previously unknown congenital heart defect could present with difficulty breathing. More commonly, children have difficulty breathing due to viral or bacterial lung or airway infections. We will discuss the radiographic appearance of left to right cardiac shunts, viral bronchiolitis, bacterial pneumonia, and stridor.

Congenital heart disease is commonly thought of as being cyanotic or acyanotic. If the cardiac defect results in deoxygenated blood entering the systemic circulation, the patient will present with cyanosis. This is usually evident soon after birth. More commonly, the cardiac defect results in oxygenated blood recirculating back through the pulmonary arteries. These patients are not cyanotic (acyanotic). Ventricular and atrial septal defects are common examples of acyanotic congenital heart disease. In these conditions, oxygenated blood flows from the higher pressure left atrium or ventricle across the septal defect and into the relatively lower pressure right atrium or right ventricle. This results in overcirculation of blood through the pulmonary circulation. Asymptomatic children with a small septal defect will often have an audible murmur on auscultation. A large septal defect may cause the child to have tachypnea or dyspnea. On chest radiography, a symptomatic child may have an enlarged heart, prominent pulmonary vasculature, and interstitial edema as a result of the pulmonary overcirculation (Fig. 56.2).

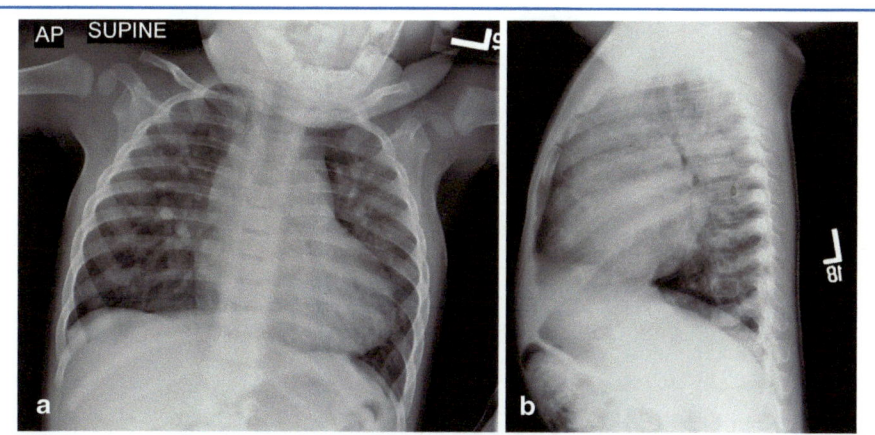

FIGURE 56.2 - ACYANOTIC CONGENITAL HEART DISEASE
AP (**a**) and lateral (**b**) chest radiograph of a 1-year-old with enlarged heart, prominent pulmonary vasculature, and mild interstitial edema in the setting of a large ventricular septal defect

Further evaluation of the septal defect with ultrasonic echocardiography or cardiac MRI will help the pediatric cardiologist and cardiothoracic surgeon plan appropriate treatment.

Children often present with fever and cough. In the acutely ill child, chest radiography is helpful in determining if the source of the patient's symptoms are viral or bacterial, guiding the clinician to the appropriate choice of medical therapy. Infants and preschool children are more predisposed to viral pulmonary infections. The virus infects the airways causing bronchiolitis, an inflammation of the small airways of the lungs. On chest radiography, the inflamed bronchioles and peribronchial interstitial tissues become edematous and more conspicuous, with a symmetric perihilar distribution. Additionally, air trapping may lead to pulmonary hyperinflation. Airway secretions may occlude airways resulting in atelectasis. Pleural fluid is rare (Fig. 56.3).

School age children are still likely to present with viral illness but have an increased incidence of bacterial pneumonia. Bacterial infections cause damage to lung parenchyma resulting in inflammatory exudates filling the infected airspaces. Radiographically, this leads to focal airspace opacification with the adjacent air filled bronchi visible as air bronchograms. Children have underdeveloped collateral air drift pathways, known as the pores of Kohn and canals of Lambert. As a result, pediatric pneumonia infiltrates may have a more round appearance when compared to adult patients (Fig. 56.4).

Pleural effusion is sometimes seen with bacterial pneumonia. Typically, a frontal and lateral chest radiograph is sufficient for the diagnosis of pneumonia. CT is

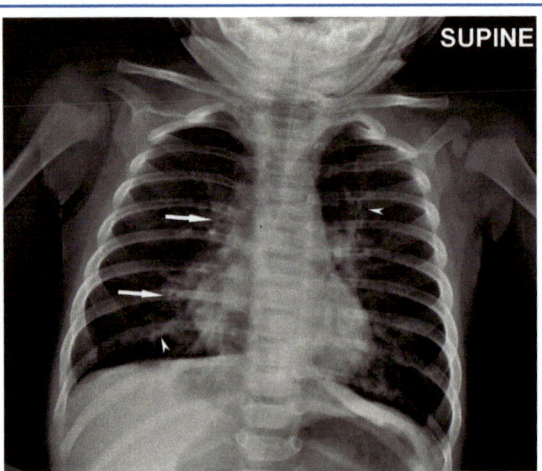

FIGURE 56.3 - VIRAL PULMONARY INFECTION
Peribronchial thickening (*arrows*), hyperinflation, and central non-segmental sites of atelectasis (*arrowheads*)

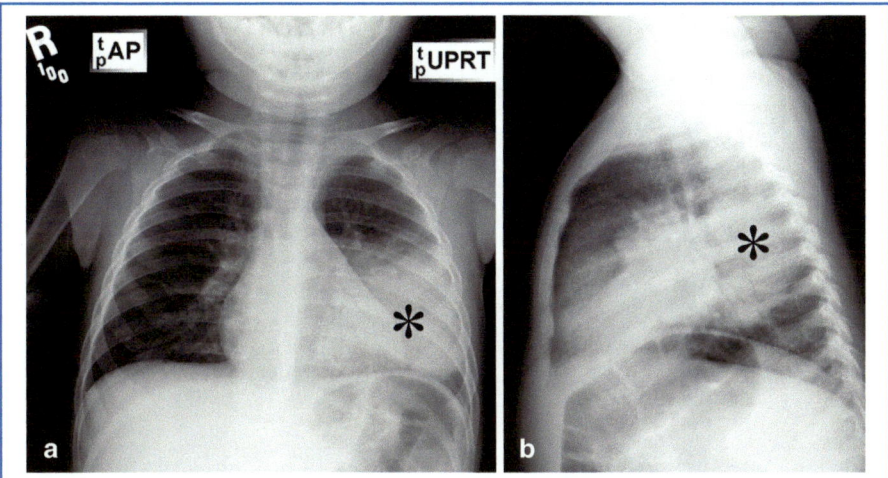

FIGURE 56.4 - BACTERIAL PULMONARY INFECTION
Lobar consolidation (*star*) in the left lung on AP (**a**) and lateral (**b**) chest radiographs

reserved for evaluation of complications such as abscess or empyema, or to look for an anatomic abnormality that predisposes the patient to recurrent pneumonia.

Stridor is a high pitched harsh noisy breath sound that results from obstructed or turbulent airflow through a narrowed airway. Children presenting with stridor require attention to determine the underlying airway disorder. The age of the patient and timing of when the noise occurs in the breathing cycle are clinical clues to the underlying etiology of the stridor. Newborns or younger children with persistent stridor are more likely to have a congenital airway anomaly such as a laryngomalacia, tracheomalacia, vocal cord paralysis, subglottic hemangioma, or a vascular ring. Toddlers who are prone to put objects in their mouth may have an aspirated foreign body. An acute onset of stridor in any child may be related to infection, such as croup, trauma, or aspiration. Inspiratory stridor is indicative of a collapse of the extrathoracic airway. Expiratory stridor suggests an intrathoracic airway obstruction. Biphasic stridor indicates an obstruction between the glottis and subglottis or a fixed obstruction at any level. Armed with this information and the results of a good clinical assessment, the radiologist and clinician can work together to determine the next best imaging step.

The imaging evaluation of stridor should begin with frontal and lateral radiographs of the neck and chest. Attention to the airway can often reveal the etiology of the stridor. Subglottic edema with an air distended hypopharynx is diagnostic of croup (Fig. 56.5).

The lateral neck radiograph will also allow for visualization of the epiglottis. Epiglottitis, although less common than croup, requires emergent care to prevent

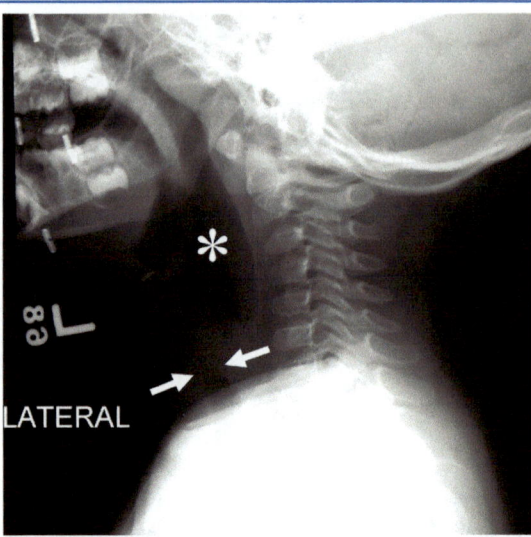

FIGURE 56.5 - CROUP AIR-DISTENDED HYPOPHARYNX (*STAR*) AND SUBGLOTTIC EDEMA (*ARROWS*)

airway compromise. If the neck radiograph reveals a mass in the subglottic trachea, further assessment with direct visualization via flexible laryngoscopy as well as CT or MRI may be performed to look for a subglottic hemangioma. The chest radiograph will allow for visualization of the thoracic trachea. Narrowing or mass effect on the trachea may be due to vascular anomalies of the aortic arch (right aortic arch, vascular ring) or pulmonary artery (pulmonary sling). Such a finding can be further evaluated with upper GI or barium swallow study, with CT or MRI reserved for surgical planning if needed. Aspirated foreign bodies may or may not be visible on radiographs. If a non-visible radiolucent foreign body, such as an aspirated grape, is suspected as the cause of airway obstruction, bilateral decubitus radiographs can be performed to show the lack of collapse on the dependent affected side and appropriate collapse of the lung on the contralateral dependent side.

The decision to pursue imaging beyond neck and chest radiographs in a child with stridor should always be based on the clinical picture and treatment plans. Flexible laryngoscopy is a good way to further evaluate the upper airway. The lower airway and mediastinum are better evaluated with fluoroscopy or cross-sectional imaging with CT or MRI. Airway fluoroscopy is helpful in the assessment of laryngomalacia and tracheomalacia as the diameter of the airways can be visualized dynamically with inspiration and expiration. In addition to the evaluation of possible airway and esophageal vascular compression, an upper GI study will also assess for gastroesophageal reflux. CT and MRI are both very useful in demonstrating peripharyngeal abscess or lesions compressing the airway. Both modalities also demonstrate detailed relationships between soft tissues and vascular anatomy. CT is better in the identification of associated tracheal anomalies such as complete tracheal rings, while MRI characterizes the soft tissue and vascular anomalies without ionizing radiation. The patient's condition may dictate the choice of cross-sectional imaging modality. CT has a much shorter scanning time than MRI. Therefore CT is appropriate if rapid imaging is needed in the acutely ill child or if there is a desire to obviate the need for sedation in a young child undergoing MRI.

Abdominal Imaging

Abdominal pain and vomiting are common complaints in the pediatric clinic. The causes of abdominal pain and vomiting are numerous and diverse. Radiology is helpful in the evaluation of common conditions such as gastroesophageal reflux and urinary tract infections, as well as more acute gastrointestinal problems such as hypertrophic pyloric stenosis (HPS), intussusception, and midgut volvulus.

The proper diagnosis of the vomiting infant or young child often requires imaging to distinguish between benign and life-threatening conditions. Making the correct diagnosis depends on knowing if the vomiting is bilious or non-bilious as well as the patient's age. Gastroesophageal reflux is the most common cause of non-bilious emesis and is readily apparent on an upper GI fluoroscopy study. In infants of 2–8 weeks in age with projectile non-bilious emesis, HPS should be considered. Sonographic evaluation of the pylorus will reveal a thickened, elongated pyloric sphincter resulting in gastric outlet obstruction, confirming the diagnosis (Fig. 56.6).

The infant or young child with bilious emesis raises the emergent concern of malrotation with midgut volvulus. Recall that the midgut is distal to the ampulla of Vater, thus emesis arising proximal to the midgut volvulus will contain bile. The diagnosis of malrotation and midgut volvulus is made with an upper GI study. At the site of the volvulus, typically in the distal second or proximal third portion of the duodenum, a "beak" or corkscrew of twisted bowel will be identified with ingestion of barium (Fig. 56.7).

Midgut volvulus requires emergent surgical intervention to prevent catastrophic bowel loss and potentially death.

Ileocolic intussusception is the most common cause of intestinal obstruction between the ages of 3 months and 4 years. In this condition, part of the intestine invaginates into an adjacent portion of the intestine, similar to a collapsing telescope. While small bowel intussusception is self-limited, ileocolic intussusception requires urgent evaluation and treatment. If left untreated, intussuscepted bowel will become ischemic, leading to a cascade of events from edema to obstruction and eventually peritonitis. The classic presentation of a child with dark bloody "currant jelly" stools is a result of bowel ischemia. Often the presenting symptoms of intermittent abdominal pain in a previously well child are initially mistaken for gastroenteritis. Intussusception should be considered when a child has paroxysms of pain leading the

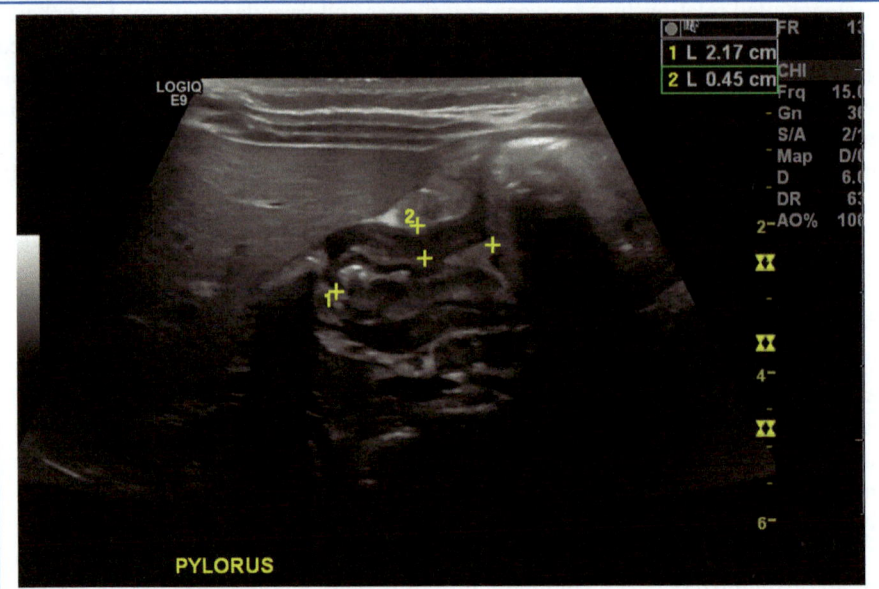

FIGURE 56.6 - HYPERTROPHIC PYLORIC STENOSIS
Ultrasound image demonstrates a hypertrophied pylorus measuring 22 mm in length and 5 mm in thickness

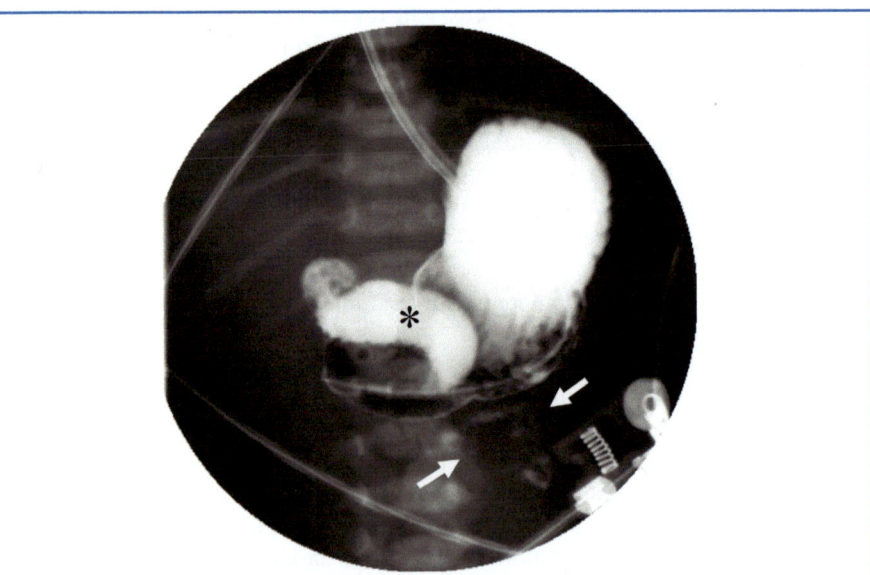

FIGURE 56.7 - MIDGUT VOLVULUS
An upper GI exam shows dilated first and second portions of the duodenum (*star*) with cork-screw appearance of the distal duodenum and midgut (*arrows*)

patient to pull his or her knees to his or her chest. These episodes of pain will result in the child being irritable and inconsolable. However, the child may be playful and content between bouts of pain. Eventually the child becomes weak and tired from the repeated episodes of pain and progression of the intussusception.

The initial radiologic study should be abdominal radiographs followed by abdominal ultrasound when indicated. The abdominal radiographs may be normal or may show a paucity of bowel gas in the right lower quadrant or an area of increased density in the region of intussusception. In some cases, the abdominal radiographs may reveal a small bowel obstruction or sick-looking bowel. On ultrasonography, intussusception appears as a target-like mass, created by the cross-sectional appearance of one bowel loop within another, often in the expected location of the colon in the right abdomen (Fig. 56.8).

Ultrasound may identify a "lead point" and can confirm the presence or lack of blood flow to the affected bowel. Once the diagnosis of ileocolic intussusception is established, pediatric surgical consultation is required before the pediatric radiologist attempts fluoroscopic-guided air enema to reduce or correct the intussusception. Air enema reduction has a high success rate. However the intussusception can recur. So the child usually is observed overnight before discharge. In the 10–15% of ileocolic intussusception that cannot be reduced by air enema, surgical treatment is necessary.

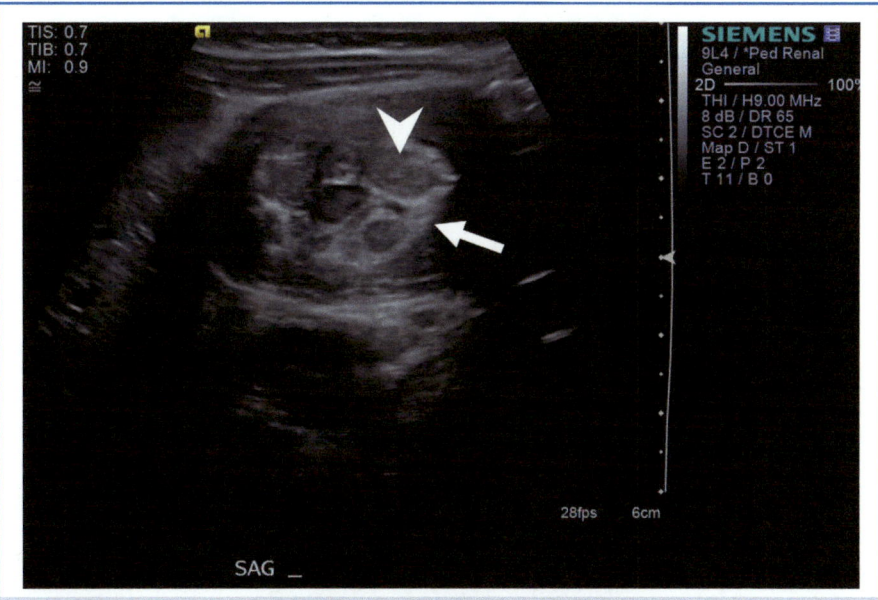

FIGURE 56.8 - INTUSSUSCEPTION
Target appearance of the bowel loops with echogenic mesentery (*arrow*) and small lymph nodes (*arrowhead*)

Young children with urinary tract infections (UTI), specifically pyelonephritis, present with non-specific symptoms including high fevers, decreased appetite, irritability, and vomiting. Older children may have back pain, abdominal pain, high fever, and nausea and vomiting. The initial imaging study of the child with a UTI is ultrasound to assess the size and shape of the kidney and the presence of hydronephrosis or congenital renal anomaly such as renal duplication or malposition. In addition to hydronephrosis, the renal and bladder ultrasound may reveal scarring or evidence of high-grade vesicoureteral reflux (VUR) or obstructive uropathy. Children with a UTI before the age of 24 months, or with an abnormal ultrasound or multiple recurrent UTIs, should also undergo a voiding cystourethrogram (VCUG) fluoroscopic study. The VCUG will look at the anatomy of the urethra in boys and will visualize the presence and extent of VUR in both sexes. The severity of VUR is graded between I and V based on the level of contrast reflux and degree of urinary collecting system dilation (Fig. 56.9).

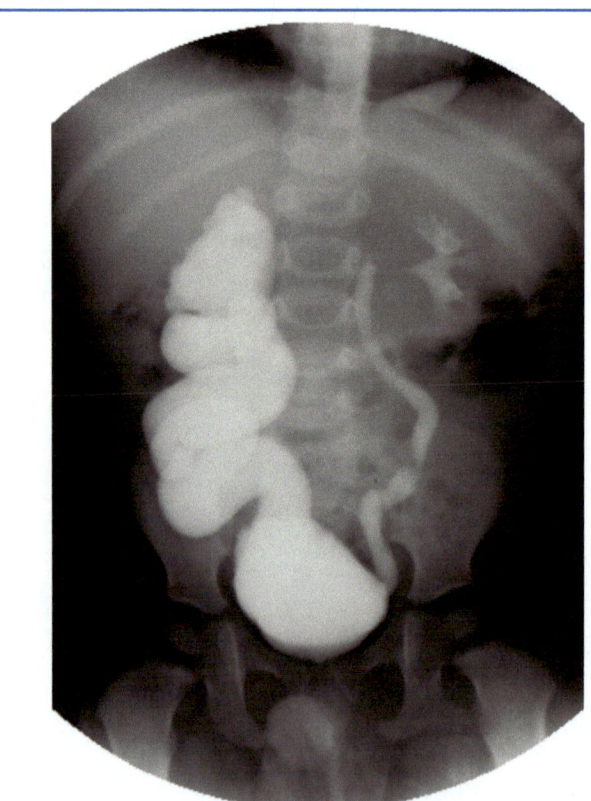

FIGURE 56.9 - VESICOURETERAL REFLUX
Grade V right VUR and grade II left VUR

While most VCUGs are normal, the majority of abnormal VCUGs have lower grade reflux (grade I–III), with a small minority of patients having higher grade IV or V reflux. The results of the imaging evaluation will guide treatment decisions and follow-up. Children with persistent high-grade VUR are candidates for surgical intervention.

Musculoskeletal Trauma

Children are active and adventurous by nature, sometimes resulting in traumatic injury to the musculoskeletal system. The unique anatomy of growing bones results in a musculoskeletal injury pattern and imaging appearance that is different than adult patients. Unfortunately, some children also experience non-accidental trauma. Providers caring for children must always be concerned that the injured child has not been the victim of child abuse. An understanding of pediatric musculoskeletal radiology can help determine if a child has simply had an accident or has been intentionally harmed.

Children's bones differ from those of adults. Pediatric bones contain proportionately more woven than lamellar bone. Strong periosteum is loosely attached to the underlying bone cortex by Sharpey's fibers and can act as a splint in torus and greenstick fractures. Torus fractures are incomplete fractures in which the bone cortex is subtly angulated or buckled (Fig. 56.10).

Greenstick fractures involve the disruption of the cortex on one side of the bone and the bending of the other. Growth plates (physes) at the ends of growing bone predispose children to Salter Harris (SH) fractures. SH fractures involve the physis and adjacent bone with a classification of I–V, with increasing classification number portending a higher risk of complications such as growth arrest. SH I fractures involve the growth plate alone and can be difficult to identify radiographically. Look for soft tissue swelling adjacent to the growth plate and possible displacement of the epiphysis. SH II fractures are the most common and involve both the metaphysis and physis. SH III fractures involve the epiphysis and physis, while SH IV fractures involve the metaphysis, physis, and epiphysis. Both SH III and IV fractures may extend to and disrupt the articular surface of the bone. SH V fractures are physeal crush injuries and, while rare, are subject to development of premature growth plate closure and growth arrest. While most pediatric fractures are imaged with radiographs, MRI and CT are utilized to evaluate subtle or complex injuries.

There are musculoskeletal, visceral, and neurologic manifestations of child abuse. Distinguishing accidental from non-accidental injury can be challenging. The types of accidental trauma for which a child is at risk are closely related to her or his development and what milestones he or she has achieved. Identification of multiple fractures in different stages of healing and/or fractures in which the history does not fit the injury should raise concern for non-accidental trauma. There are a

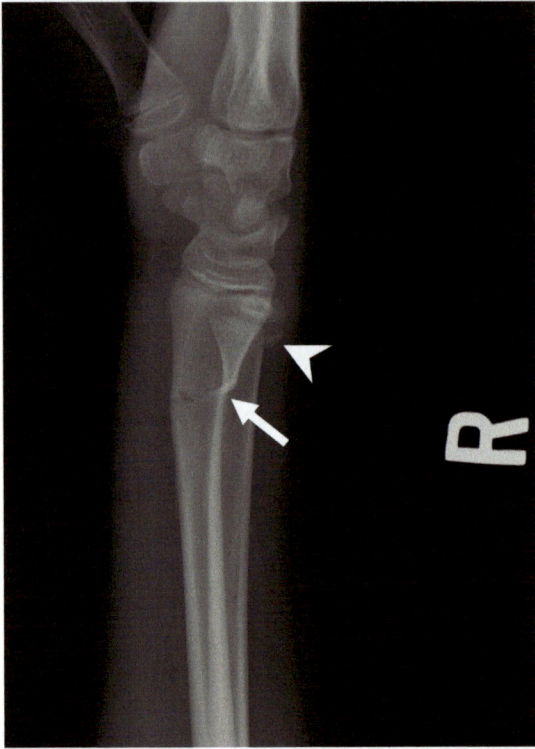

FIGURE 56.10 - BUCKLE FRACTURE
Buckle fracture of the distal radial diaphysis (*arrow*) and salter II fracture of the distal ulna (*arrowhead*)

few fractures with high specificity for abuse, including metaphyseal corner fractures and multiple rib fractures (Fig. 56.11).

These fractures are often readily apparent on radiographs. Visceral non-accidental injuries are relatively uncommon but potentially lethal and include pancreatic injury (with pancreatitis and pseudocyst formation) and duodenal hematoma. Neurologic manifestations include subdural hematoma formation, contusion, and cerebral edema. CT and MRI are the modalities of choice for evaluation of visceral and neurologic trauma.

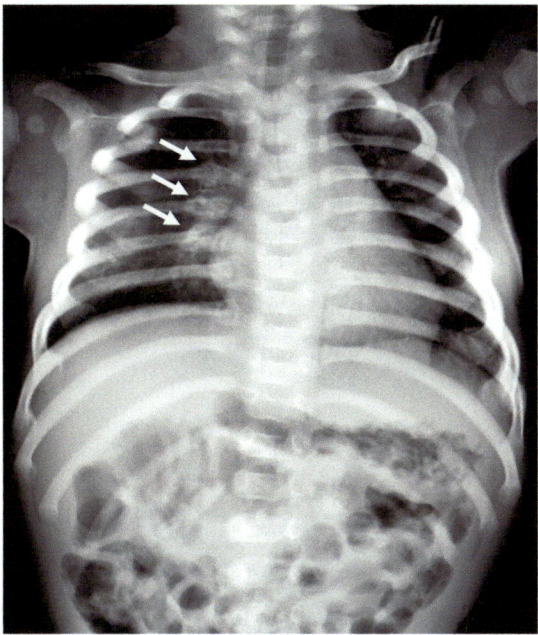

FIGURE 56.11 - MULTIPLE HEALING RIB FRACTURES
Many scattered healing rib fractures (*arrows*)

S: Safe imaging is particularly important in the pediatric age group. This is most important with regards to ionizing radiation as there are increased odds of radiation exposure resulting in a harmful effect as children are actively growing (i.e., highly mitotic, dividing cells) and have a long life expectancy.

A: Along with safety, appropriateness is essential in imaging children. Work with your pediatric radiologist to determine the appropriate imaging for the clinical question while minimizing exposure to ionizing radiation, energy exposure from ultrasound and MRI, and chemical exposure to contrast and sedation.

F: Pediatric radiologists are expert consultants and can help interpret findings that are unique to children such as extremities with growth plates, abdomens with minimal internal adipose (therefore harder to discriminate normal from pathology), and normal from non-accidental trauma.

E: Pediatric radiologists are your best medical "friends" to help identify conditions that need expeditious attention such as CNS bleeding in premature infants, malrotated bowel, and non-accidental trauma.

INDEX

© Springer Nature Switzerland AG 2020
J. Kissane et al. (eds.), *Radiology Fundamentals: Introduction to Imaging
& Technology*, https://doi.org/10.1007/978-3-030-22173-7